MODERN PRACTICE IN

JOHN F. JOHNSTON, D.D.S., M.S.D., F.A.C.D.
University Professor of Dentistry

RALPH W. PHILLIPS, A.B., M.S., D.Sc., F.A.C.D.
Research Professor and Chairman
Department of Dental Materials

ROLAND W. DYKEMA, D.D.S., M.S.D., F.A.C.D.
Professor and Chairman
Department of Fixed and Removable Partial Prosthodontics

INDIANA UNIVERSITY SCHOOL OF DENTISTRY

CROWN AND BRIDGE PROSTHODONTICS

SECOND EDITION

W. B. SAUNDERS COMPANY /
Philadelphia, London

W. B. Saunders Company: West Washington Square,
Philadelphia, Pa. 19105

12 Dyott Street
London, W.C. 1

Reprinted October, 1965, October, 1966, July, 1968, March, 1969 and November, 1969

Modern Practice in Crown and Bridge Prosthodontics

This Book Is Dedicated to Our Wives

LAVONNE JOHNSTON

DOROTHY PHILLIPS

DOROTHY DYKEMA

Without their constant help and understanding, their militant defense of our shortcomings and subtle bolstering of our egos, completion of this project would have been impossible.

PREFACE TO THE SECOND EDITION

In this second edition, *Modern Practice in Crown and Bridge Prostho dontics* has been expanded and portions have been reorganized.

Additional space and increased emphasis have been given to more advanced and diversified techniques that will appeal to the practicing dentist. In the material on ceramics there is much that will be of assistance to the technician.

Despite the introduction of new and advanced information, however, we have retained a conservative approach to clinical operations and have kept firmly in mind the needs of the student. We have also, in this revision, attempted to conform closely to the nomenclature approved by *Current Clinical Dental Terminology*.

During the past five years, it has been the privilege of the authors to attend or to participate in teaching courses in all sections of the country. This provided many opportunities to visit crown and bridge departments and to discuss concepts and techniques, always to our benefit. Especially noteworthy were the contacts with Dr. Donald Smith, Professor Emeritus of Crown and Bridge Dentistry of the University of Southern California, Dr. Ernest Granger, at the University of Pennsylvania, and Dr. Charles Stuart, at the University of Kentucky.

Material was generously made available for our use by the following men: Dr. Miles R. Markley, Dr. R. E. Going, Dr. Frank A. Eich, Dr. R. E. Baker, Dr. P. N. Kondon, Dr. Harry Lundeen, Dr. Bailey Davis, Dr. Fredrick A. Hohlt, Dr. William Gilmore, Dr. Robert E. Willey, and Mr. Russell J. Jones.

We acknowledge with thanks the permission given by Drs. Donald Spees, Lloyd Phillips, John Borkowski, Dwain Love, and Stefan Wittner for use of their preparation outlines; our appreciation goes, too, to others who responded later to our questionnaire.

Willing cooperation was forthcoming from Mr. Richard Scott and his staff in making the illustrations. Drs. Thomas Connell, James Grimes, and Sumiya Hobo gladly provided many new drawings.

Drs. George Mumford and Ray Maesaka have been extremely helpful in the selection and development of material to be used in the area of ceramics and in the chapter on Dentistry for the Young-age Group.

Dean Maynard K. Hine graciously acquiesced in an occasional change of schedules made necessary by pressures connected with this text.

Many manufacturers, listed in the Appendix, have contributed illustrations.

We are deeply grateful to all these people.

The authors appreciate the courtesy of the Virginia State Dental Association, The C. V. Mosby Company, the Tennessee State Dental Association, and the Year Book Medical Publishers, Inc., in giving their consent for the reuse of material previously published in the *Virginia Dental Journal, The Journal of Prosthetic Dentistry,* the *Journal of the Tennessee State Dental Association,* and *Practical Dental Monographs.*

Typing, reading copy, rewriting, research, and editing once again have been done by Lavonne Johnston. Without her keen interest, dedication, and the untold hours devoted to this project, our endeavors would have fallen short of our goal. To her we extend well deserved recognition.

THE AUTHORS

PREFACE TO THE FIRST EDITION

This book is concerned with the construction of crowns to rebuild teeth and fixed partial dentures to replace missing teeth. It has been planned with the particular needs of the undergraduate student in mind. Its purpose is to be comprehensive but not encyclopedic in scope and to present basic knowledge and accepted techniques in a manner which will enable the student or practitioner to assimilate and apply them clinically.

The clinical operations set forth are intentionally conservative so that the student will follow a plan designed to help him avoid difficulties. The experienced clinician will broaden the application of many principles with complete success, at the same time observing the fundamentals.

The authors are firm in their conviction that strict compliance with the procedures advocated for the handling of materials is not only justified but mandatory. There is no doubt that certain of the techniques described here will become obsolete as dental research provides better instrumentation and materials. Likewise, there are other methods of accomplishing the same objectives. However, at the moment, the procedures outlined in this book are proved, fundamentally sound, and simple.

The terminology used does not adhere completely to the recommendations of the Committee on Nomenclature. *Bridge, fixed bridge, fixed partial denture, prosthesis, fixed replacement,* and occasionally *appliance,* are used interchangeably. *Removable prosthesis, removable partial denture,* and *partial denture* are given the same meaning. *Removable bridge* refers only to a prosthesis supported entirely by teeth.

The concept of feeling and enthusiasm for maximal personal effort and concentration in the construction of fixed partial dentures, which the authors have tried to incorporate in this text and hope to pass on to its readers, was first encountered in 1922 in a study club directed by Dr. Frank A. Hamilton. Dr. W. I. McCullough and Mr. Ivan A. Welborn were among the industrious and exacting associates. Dean F. R. Henshaw, Dean G. D. Timmons, Dr. Edgar T. Haynes, and Dr. Glenn J. Pell helped to foster and prolong the activities of the study clubs. Two of the inspiring guest instructors were Dr. Forrest H. Orton and Dr. James Mark Prime.

The published works and direct teachings of Dr. Stanley D. Tylman, Dr. Irving H. Ante, Dr. J. Williams Adams, and Dr. A. O. Klaffenbach, to mention only a few, have for many years been an unfailing guide in both practice and teaching.

In writing this book, our thanks are extended to Dr. Wallace S. Bell for the chapter on orthodontic positioning of abutment teeth; to Dr. Henry M. Swenson and Dean M. K. Hine for the chapter on occlusion factors; to Dr. D. M. Cunningham for his assistance with the chapter on mouth preparation for removable partial dentures; to Dean Gilbert P. Smith, Dr. Kenneth C. Pruden, Dr. Miles R. Markley, Dr. Claude R. Baker, Dr. E. C. Brooks, Dr. L. W. Thom, and Dr. H. D. Grubb for permission to quote from their published articles; to Dr. Frank P. Vedder and Dr. Ernest B. Nuttall for their contributions to the chapters on partial veneer crowns and jacket crowns; to Dr. Basil G. Theofilis for his consent to use portions of his senior thesis in the chapter on jacket crowns, and to Mr. John N. Pettrow for his helpful suggestions on the same chapter; and to Mr. Joseph P. Ficaro for the outline on polishing metal.

The authors gratefully acknowledge the work on illustrations done by Dr. James Grimes, Dr. Ralph Brennan, Mr. Richard Scott, Mrs. Gloria Spray, Mr. Thomas J. Connell, and several other students.

Our appreciation goes to Dean M. K. Hine, Dr. L. Walter Brown, Jr., Dr. Robert P. Dressel, Dr. John D. Adams, and Mrs. Mabel Walker for their willingness to read portions of the manuscript and their counsel and encouragement in overcoming obstacles—many real, some imaginary.

Many manufacturers have willingly supplied photographs, information, and advice. A list will be found in the Appendix.

An attempt has been made to credit all sources from which techniques and ideas have been obtained. It is regretted if any has been omitted.

The authors wish to thank Lavonne Johnston, above all others, for accepting full responsibility for all of the typing, rewriting, and organization of the material, and for editing the manuscript of what it is hoped will be a useful and stimulating text.

THE AUTHORS

CONTENTS

Introduction *1*

1
Preoperative Study *3*

2
Differential Diagnosis and Selection and Planning of Treatment *19*

3
Cutting Instruments *51*

4
Tooth Reduction *59*

5
The Full Veneer Gold Crown *74*

6
The Partial Veneer Crown *94*

7
The Pinledge Retainer *130*

8
The Inlay Retainer *144*

9
The MacBoyle Retainer *151*

10
The Working Cast *155*

11
Individual Dies Constructed from Tube Impressions *197*

12
Wax Patterns 207

13
Spruing, Investing, and Casting 218

14
The Pontic 249

15
Pontic Form 278

16
Soldering 300

17
Glazing and Staining Facings 312

18
Checking and Cementing Crowns and Bridges 320

19
The Veneered Gold Crown 336

20
Porcelains and Porcelain Furnaces 351

21
Esthetic Criteria in a Porcelain Restoration 357

22
The Construction of Bonded Porcelain Veneer Crowns 365

23
The Construction of Bridges with Bonded Porcelain Veneers 385

24
The Porcelain Jacket Crown 398

25
The Construction of Crowns and Bridges with Resin Veneers 430

2
The Resin Jacket Crown 444

27
Bridge Patterns 459

28
Splinting Teeth 480

29
The Construction of Crowns and Bridges in the Preparation of Partially Edentulous Mouths for Clasp-Retained Removable Prostheses *487*

30
Orthodontic Positioning of Abutments and Associated Teeth *505*

31
Crown and Bridge Procedures for the Young-Age Group *519*

32
The Restoration of Mutilated Anterior Teeth *524*

33
Occlusion Factors in Bridge Construction *536*

34
Bridge Failures: Indications and Corrective Measures *551*

35
Complete Oral Rehabilitation *563*

36
Case Histories *567*

Appendix *587*

Index *589*

INTRODUCTION

Dentistry is a clinical art devoted to the betterment of mankind. Among its many ramifications are the relief of pain, the treatment of oral diseases, the maintenance of masticatory efficiency, and the maintenance or restoration of the esthetics of the mouth and face. One of the functions of dental practice, and one that is frequently overlooked, is to combine and coordinate ideas and educational and clinical efforts so that an ever-increasing number of people can avoid wearing complete dentures.

Clinical preventive dentistry may be divided into several phases or specialties. The order in which these can be administered most effectively to achieve retention or stabilization of the dentition is as follows: (1) education of the patient and treatment for the control of caries, (2) operative dentistry, and (3) periodontics (these first three are closely interrelated); (4) the planning and construction of bridges; (5) the designing and insertion of removable partial dentures after the mouth has been adequately prepared; (6) endodontics; (7) surgery; and (8) orthodontics. (Numbers 6, 7, and 8 are adjuncts to expedite 2, 3, 4, and 5.)

If the patient reports to the dentist early in life and is convinced of the dividends to be earned from a policy of preventive therapy, correct mouth hygiene, and prompt repair of the tooth when a carious lesion has penetrated the enamel, there should be little need later for major restorative operations. If a tooth must be lost, it is the duty of the dentist to inform the patient that the space should be filled as soon as possible after surgery. Too often such a suggestion is not made, or if made at all, it is done in a halfhearted manner. The significance of keeping the arch intact is not stressed, nor are the sequelae from lack of replacement discussed and presented emphatically.[1] Since the loss of one tooth can effect changes in positions and contact relationships of all teeth remaining in the mouth, the desirability of replacing the missing tooth, and of *recommending such*

1

services at the same time that the removal of the tooth is advised, becomes obvious. "Replacing a tooth can be more important than saving the tooth."[2]

The following quotations succinctly summarize the popularity and momentous potentialities of the fixed partial denture prosthesis:

". . . In my own experience the fixed bridge, where indicated and properly installed, has been found the most successful, not only from the standpoint of health and natural function, but from the standpoint of appearance and lasting qualities. The fixed bridge is the easiest to care for, comes nearer to satisfying the patient's pride and peace of mind, and seems more nearly a part of his natural masticatory mechanism than any removable appliance."[3]

"Patients do appreciate the effort to provide the same service to all, regardless of cost. They respond by offering to do their part. There is no doubt that improvement in the dentist's aptitude and skill and in his ability to construct restorations of the highest specifications will result in a better type of practice. People in a community learn quickly who is a good dentist and who is a poor one."[3]

REFERENCES

1. Brown, L. W., Jr.: Dentistry's zone of silence. J.A.D.A., *55*:843, Dec. 1957.
2. Adams, J. W.: Personal communication.
3. Grubb, H. D.: Partial dentures with precision attachments. J.A.D.A., *42*:154, Feb. 1951.

1

PREOPERATIVE STUDY

In order that subsequent discussions may be understood and methods and meanings may be grasped readily, terminology must be clarified.[1]

DEFINITIONS OF TERMS

Crown and bridge prosthodontics is the science and art of the complete restoration of a single tooth, or the replacement of one or more teeth by a nonremovable partial denture.

A **crown** is a restoration that reproduces the entire surface anatomy of the clinical crown of a tooth (Fig. 1). It may be a metal casting, a metal casting with a veneer of tooth-colored porcelain or resin, or a so-called jacket crown constructed of porcelain or resin. The prepared tooth stump may be sound, or it may be partially rebuilt by a cast metal core or a cast core and post, cemented to the remaining tooth structure, or by amalgam. Occasionally the tooth stump may be restored with resin or zinc phosphate cement.

A **bridge** is a nonremovable prosthesis, or fixed partial denture, rigidly attached to one or more abutment teeth, replacing one or more lost or missing teeth (Fig. 2).

A **removable bridge** is a prosthesis, or removable partial denture, entirely supported under occlusal force by natural teeth and maintained in position by clasps or other attachments. It replaces one or more, usually more, missing teeth and should be bilateral in its retention (Fig. 3).

A **partial denture** is a removable prosthesis replacing one or more missing teeth, which receives its major support under occlusal force from

3

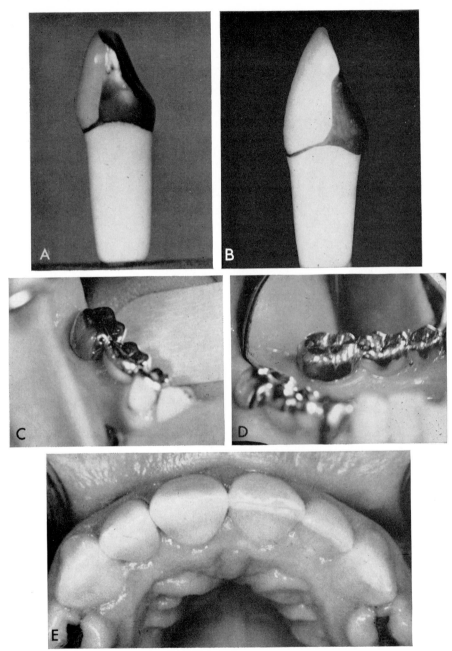

FIGURE 1.   *A,* A crown with a veneer of tooth-colored resin.

B, A crown with a bonded porcelain veneer.

C, D, Full veneer gold crown retainers on second molar abutments (buccal and lingual views).

E, Porcelain jacket crowns on right central and lateral incisors.

the structures underlying its base.[2] It is maintained in position by clasps and rests or intracoronal attachments (Fig. 4).

A bridge may be divided into four component parts:

The **abutment** is the natural tooth (usually two or more) or a root which supports the prosthesis and to which it is attached.

The **retainer** is the restoration rebuilding the prepared abutment tooth, by which the bridge is attached to the abutment and to which the pontic is connected.

The **pontic** is the substitute for the lost tooth, esthetically and functionally; usually, although not necessarily, it occupies the space formerly filled by the natural tooth (Fig. 5).

The **joint,** or **connector,** is the part of a dental bridge that unites the retainer with the pontic or which joins the individual units of the bridge. It may be rigid, e.g., the solder joint, or nonrigid, as are the subocclusal and dovetail occlusal rests.

REQUIREMENTS OF BRIDGE CONSTRUCTION

There are two kinds of requirements in bridge construction. The first is a concept of certain intangibles that may be defined as an appreciation of (1) forces developed by the oral mechanism and by the resistance of the tooth and its supporting structures to them, (2) modifications of normal tooth form that are designed to reduce forces or increase resistance to them, and (3) establishing and maintaining normal tissue tone.

The second requirement exacts a superior level of technical proficiency and concern in (1) the removal of caries from the abutment or from any associated tooth, the loss of which might affect the design or life of the bridge; (2) the sterilization or cleansing of the tooth surface; (3) the protection of the pulp during preparation of the tooth and construction of the bridge; (4) the restoration of the tooth surface in such a way that it will function normally and comfortably and not abuse the supporting structures; (5) the restoration of multiple areas of occlusion; and (6) a comprehensive and applicable knowledge of tooth form.[3]

The construction of crowns and bridges, especially bridges, where and when they are needed, must be considered an accessory to preventive dentistry. Discernment and dexterity are more of a requisite here than in any other segment of this profession. Anatomy, ceramics, the chemistry of resins, colorimetry, dental materials, metallurgy, periodontics, phonetics, physics, radiology, and tooth form—all of these must be aptly applied for successful diagnosis and practice in the field of crown and bridge prosthodontics. Adams[4] has stated that the preparation of an upper cuspid for a partial veneer crown is the most significant test of a dentist's clinical skill. While this opinion may not be accepted universally, undeniably the construction of a complicated bridge is a challenge.

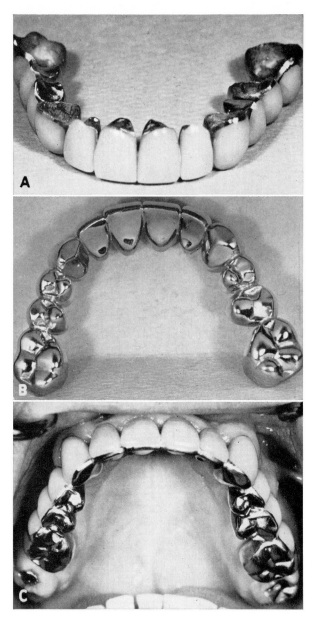

FIGURE 2. See facing page for legend.

The beginning student may feel that he is confronted with, and confounded by, a bewildering jumble of facts, many with exceptions attached, and with a multitude of technical procedures, each of which is subdivided into numbered steps for its execution. Although much of this must be memorized to provide a doctrinal background so that initial laboratory and clinical operations may be done with some understanding and dispatch, perception and application soon become automatic. Many of the items discussed later in the text under examination can be observed and accom-

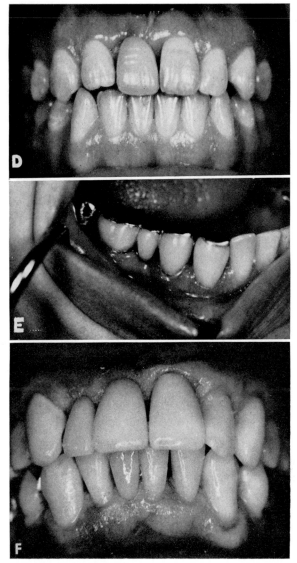

FIGURE 2. Six views of five bridges.

A, A twelve-unit maxillary bridge with veneered gold crown retainers on the right first molar, right cuspid, left cuspid, left second bicuspid, and left first molar. All units are veneered with resin except the incisors, on which Steele's facings were used.

B, The twelve-unit bridge, or fixed partial denture, from the occlusal. Notice the size and position of the solder joints, the form of the embrasures, and the spillways crossing the marginal ridges.

C, The twelve-unit bridge cemented to the abutments.

D, A three-unit bridge replacing the maxillary right central incisor. It is retained by pinledges on the left central and right lateral incisor abutments.

E, A three-unit bridge replacing a mandibular right second bicuspid. The retainers are veneered gold crowns on the first bicuspid and first molar. There is a separate veneered gold crown on the cuspid and a single-unit full veneer gold crown on the second molar.

F, A maxillary four-unit bridge with bonded porcelain veneer crown retainers on the right cuspid and left central. The right lateral and central incisor pontics are bonded porcelain veneers. The occluding three-unit mandibular bridge has pinledge retainers on the right lateral and left central incisors. The pontic has a Steele's facing with porcelain incisal. The abutments were realigned orthodontically.

7

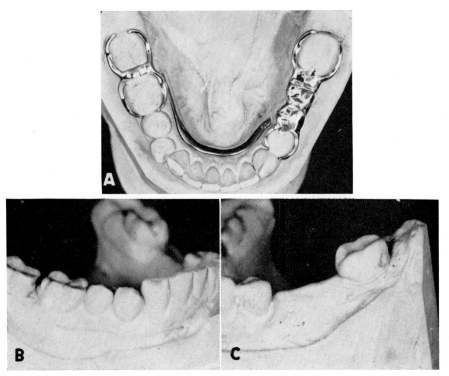

FIGURE 3.   A removable bridge.
A, Occlusal view, bridge in place.
B, Groove cut above contact areas of approximating inlays to make room for clasp to cross occlusion.
C, Guiding planes on molar and bicuspid. Rest seat in molar.

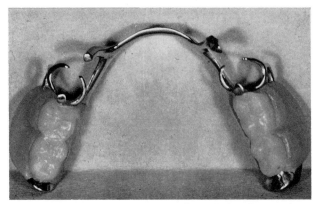

FIGURE 4. A partial denture. This is a bilateral distal extension (Class I) removable partial denture with two Roach-Akers clasps and two secondary retainers.

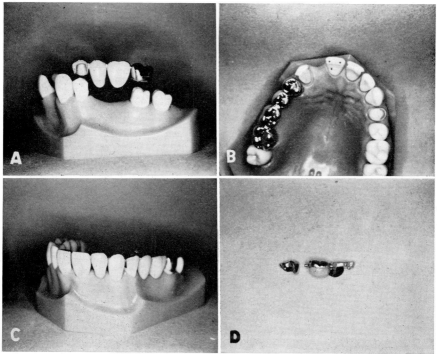

FIGURE 5. *A,* A four-unit bridge, or fixed partial denture, suspended above a model and displaying its component parts. The retainers are a partial veneer crown above the first bicuspid abutment and a full veneer gold crown above the second molar abutment. The pontics replace the second bicuspid and first molar. The joints, or connectors, are solder.

B, An occlusal view of the four-unit bridge, showing the reduction from normal tooth form in the dimensions of the pontics. Two other abutments can be seen. The upper right cuspid is prepared for a partial veneer, or three-quarter, crown; the right central will receive a pinledge. The left central incisor preparation is for a partial veneer crown; the left first bicuspid will be restored with a veneered gold crown.

C, The bridge (*A*) seated, with the pontics in contact with the ridge tissue, but without pressure against it. A labial view of the upper right anterior bridge replacing the lateral incisor. Retainers and abutments are discussed under *B.*

D, The subocclusal rest, one type of nonrigid connector.

plished simultaneously with the steps in procedure. Each has a special purpose; the order in which these are noted is not indicative of their relative influence.

BENEFITS DERIVED FROM
INSTALLATION OF A BRIDGE

If a bridge is built soon after the loss of a tooth, the patient should benefit in many ways. The bridge should contribute to mastication; it should augment the ability of the patient to enunciate; it should restore and preserve contacts between the abutments and the approximating teeth, and

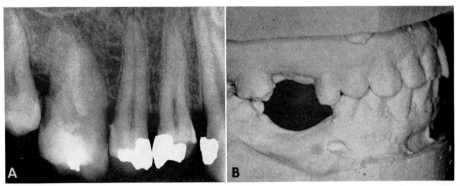

FIGURE 6. *A,* Radiograph of maxillary right posterior showing first molar extruded so that alveolar process contained only conical apical half of root. Extension of crown beyond occlusal plane was so great that correction was not advisable. Second molar tipped mesially into distal surface cervical concavity of first molar. Extraction advised.

B, Diagnostic casts showing relation of maxillary and mandibular edentulous spaces.

also all others in the arch; and it should maintain the positions of the opposing teeth and the normal tone of the supporting structure.

When a space is unfilled for a long time, there will be some shifting of positions of the teeth approximating the edentulous area and possibly extrusion of the opposing teeth (Figs. 6 and 7).[5] Even here a bridge should substantially aid mastication, help reinstate contacts of appropriate strength, size, and location, and improve the health of the alveolus and periodontium and prevent further injury to them. Any bridge at all times should create the illusion of natural teeth.

INDICATIONS FOR BRIDGES

A bridge is indicated whenever there are properly distributed and healthy teeth to serve as the abutments, provided that these teeth have suitable crown-root ratios and that after radiographic, diagnostic cast, and oral examinations seem capable of sustaining the additional load. These criteria may be defined as follows:

Proper distribution ordinarily means the presence of an abutment tooth (or teeth) at each end of the edentulous space, and an intermediate abutment (pier) when in the posterior the over-all length of the prosthesis will include the area of more than five teeth.

A tooth is considered *healthy* if the supporting bony structure is not being dissipated by alveolar atrophy (Fig. 8); if the soft tissue and periodontal membrane are in normal condition; and if the pulp is vital and responds typically to accepted stimuli, or, when the tooth is pulpless, if the root canals are adequately filled and the apical alveolus is not resorbed. A tooth may be carious and be restored to health by treatment. Gingivitis and other irregular conditions must be eliminated or controlled.

Crown-root ratio or periodontal support may be determined and evaluated by the application of a rule hereinafter designated as "Ante's law,"[6] which states that "in fixed bridgework the combined pericemental area of the abutment teeth should be equal to or greater in pericemental area than the tooth or teeth to be replaced." While there may be some deviation from this rule, the pericemental area of the abutments often being as much as 15 or 20 per cent less than an equal amount, it should be computed when planning a bridge. The accepted and desired crown-root ratio is 1:1½ in linear measurement.[7] (See Fig. 8B.) Here, also, a less favorable proportion frequently can be acceptable when there is an absence of mobility and the patient has a healthy mouth and supporting tissue and an occlusion that at that time is nondestructive.

Radiographic examination will disclose the crown-root ratio, the presence of periodontal pockets, the quality and thickness of the periodontal

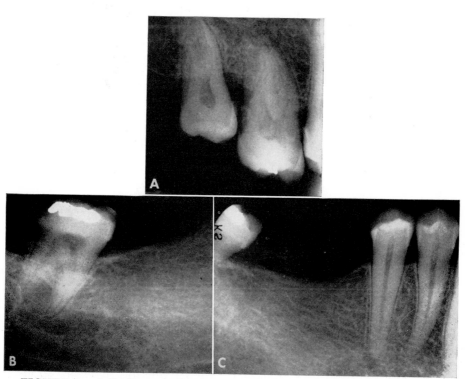

FIGURE 7. *A,* Radiograph showing maxillary second molar. Crown-root ratio, root form, and space length all point to fixed partial dentures. (See *B* in Fig. 6.)

B, Mandibular molar (see *B* in Fig. 6) has poor root form, although crown-root ratio is 1:1½. Crown form and length and space length contraindicate fixed prosthesis.

C, Bicuspids have 1:2½ crown-root ratio, and splinted would give good support for a bridge. Since the left quadrant is intact, situation calls for occluding fixed prostheses.

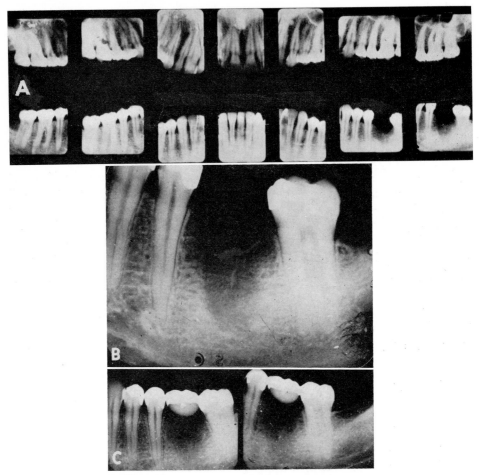

FIGURE 8.   Radiographs.

A, A full mouth radiograph showing healthy, alveolar structure.

B, A detail of the radiograph shown in *A,* illustrating acceptable alveolar bone, good crown-root ratio, and normal periodontal membrane.

C, The same area shown in *B* two years after placement of the three-unit fixed partial denture, or bridge. The abutment teeth are healthy. Ante's law and crown-root ratio are demonstrated satisfactorily. The pontic has a cast gold occlusal and a Sanitarypontic facing; the connectors are a distal solder joint and an anterior subocclusal rest.

membrane, rarefied apical areas, root contour, depth of caries, and height of the alveolus.

Examination of diagnostic casts (Fig. 9) will help ascertain the long-axis relationship of the proposed abutment teeth, mesial and distal space width, relationship of the opposing teeth to the abutments and to the spaces, tipping, adverse forces, the amount of tooth reduction necessary to arrive at retentive preparations and compatible paths of insertion, and sometimes the association of the gingival line to the cementoenamel junction.

Oral examination will reveal tissue tone, evidences of premature contact, extent of caries, depth of the gingival crevice, minute details of tooth

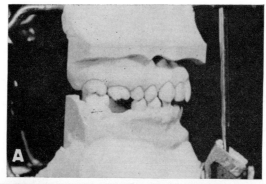

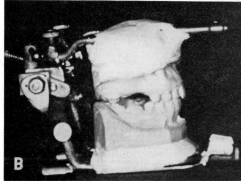
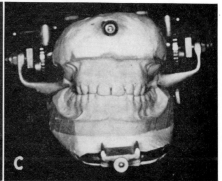

FIGURE 9. Diagnostic casts.

A, Lower first molar missing; second bicuspid rotated; upper molar extruded but can be reduced; plus vertical overlap. Bridge indicated.

B, C, Note position of upper right third molar and length of space. Bridge contra-indicated.

form, and in lateral and protrusive excursions it will show relationships in occlusion that may not be discernible from articulated casts.

The designated abutment teeth may be deemed capable of sustaining the anticipated load if the considered opinion of the operator would suggest success after reviewing distribution, health, crown-root ratio, radiographic and oral examinations, and his previous experience. However, there may be intangible or external factors, such as eating or smoking habits, that could motivate against construction.

CONTRAINDICATIONS TO BRIDGES

A bridge is contraindicated (1) when the space to be filled is of such length that the additional load generated from the occlusion of the pontics will impair the health of the tissues around the teeth that may be designated as abutments; (2) when the space length will require, for rigidity, a beam of such dimensions that embrasures will be greatly reduced in area and the underlying tissue overprotected; (3) when a previous prosthesis has shown

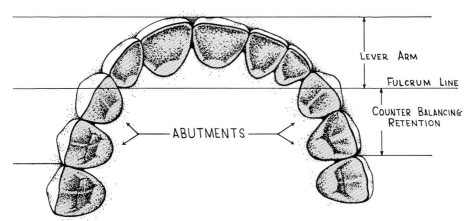

FIGURE 10.   Lever arm and extended retention. A drawing of a clinical nine-unit anterior bridge illustrating the fulcrum line running through the tips of the cuspid abutments; the length of the lever arm from the fulcrum line to the most anterior point on any pontic; and the distal extension of retention onto the first bicuspids, included as abutments. If one of the central incisors had remained to serve as a pier, counterbalancing retention, derived from the first bicuspids, would have been unnecessary.

that the associated mucous membrane reacts unfavorably to such an environment; (4) when, in the anterior, there has been such a loss of alveolar process that the pontics in the fixed prosthesis would be excessively long and unsightly or when a contoured partial denture base would be needed to restore face form; (5) when the fixed prosthesis would occlude with natural teeth or with a fixed prosthesis only on one end for half or less of its length; and (6) when there may be some question as to the ability of the remaining supporting structure around the abutment teeth to accept any additional load without bilateral bracing.

A bridge must be built so that it will restore arch form and occlusion. If the form of the prosthesis is an arc of a circle, a lever arm will be projected unless the span is segmented by a pier. The point of greatest leverage on the bridge must be supported by an abutment, or the areas of retention must be extended in each direction away from the space far enough to counteract the lever arm and establish counterbalancing retention (Figs. 10 and 11).[8]

The shape and length of the root of the abutment must meet certain specifications. A long root, with flattened, parallel sides, is vital for a good abutment. When the root is round or conical, the stability of the tooth will be lessened, and when this is coupled with a lack of length, the terminus of a fixed prosthesis should not be attached to a single tooth.

When the proposed abutments have exposed root areas that are sensitive and that cannot be covered by the retainers, the construction of a bridge often is contraindicated, because the added stress may aggravate the sensitivity. If improvement can be effected, usually it is obtained by a removable bridge with bilateral bracing.

If the height or quantity of the alveolar process and periodontal membrane around the tooth to be used as an abutment is being reduced by some adverse force, the bridge should not be made unless such activity can be restrained both before and after construction.

Mouth hygiene cannot be maintained unless a bridge receives painstaking attention. If a mouth shows habitual lack of care and the patient does not respond to counsel for improvement, then the effort, time, and

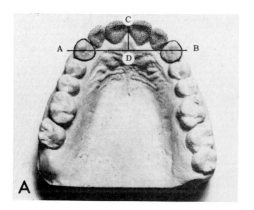

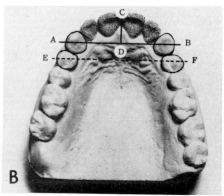

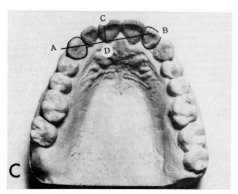

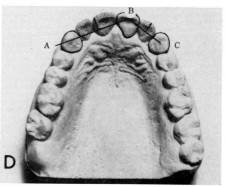

FIGURE 11. *A,* Line AB represents the fulcrum line around which the bridge tends to rotate or tip when force is applied to the incisal edges of the pontics of a bridge replacing all four maxillary incisors. Line CD is the lever arm. The longer the lever arm, the greater is the resultant force that tends to tip the bridge. This force often causes gradual anterior drifting and tipping of the cuspid abutments, together with periodontal breakdown, and tends to offset the retentive qualities of the abutment preparations.

B, The use of the first bicuspids as abutments in addition to the cuspids will offset the effect of the lever arm by providing retention and support, which is located to the distal of the line of rotation.

C, Allowing a lateral incisor to remain when constructing an extensive anterior bridge effectively shortens the lever arm. However, in most cases the adjacent cuspid still will be needed for adequate support and retention and to compensate for the lever arm.

D, The use of an intermediate abutment in the form of a central incisor creates two fulcrum lines, AB and BC, and considerably shorter lever arms. When one lever arm is subjected to force, the opposite terminal abutment tends to compensate for the leverage produced. Seldom will both lever arms be in function at the same time.

expense attending the construction and cementation of a bridge may be wasted. If it is impossible for a person to observe strict oral hygiene because of a physical handicap, a fixed prosthesis is contraindicated.

When the supporting bone has receded or the occlusion may be destructive, a removable bridge, designed to have bilateral retention and bracing, should take precedence over a unilateral fixed bridge.

Adolescent Mouths

Bridges may be contraindicated in the mouths of adolescents when the teeth are not yet in occlusion or when the pulps are excessively large, prohibiting retentive preparations. When a bridge is constructed under the latter circumstance, it may possibly be considered as temporary, to be remade when the patient is more mature and the pulps have decreased in size. The teeth then must be reprepared for a new bridge. At times it is wiser to build a space maintainer designed to hold the abutments and opposing teeth in position. This should be mandatory if the teeth have not made contact with the opposing arch.

Aged Mouths

Bridges are contraindicated in the mouths of elderly patients when there is a noticeable lack of resiliency in the periodontal membrane and when, through abrasion, the increased size of the occluding surfaces has intensified the forces to be absorbed by the thin or dense periodontal membrane and rigid alveolar process. The several exceptions here will be prompted by the length and location of the space; the general mouth condition; the radiographic evidence concerning the periodontal membrane and the alveolar process; and the general physical condition of the patient, his desire for a more complete chewing apparatus, and his reaction to other types of prostheses.

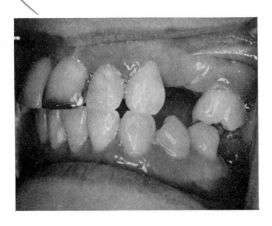

FIGURE 12. Maxillary bicuspids missing, space closed. Mandibular first bicuspid in center of opposing space. Cuspid abutment has end-to-end relationship with occluding cuspid. Molar abutment occludes only on mesial half. Lower first bicuspid must be recontoured to permit correct shaping of upper pontic. Incisal edge of cuspid abutment must have additional thickness of metal in incisal of retainer. Molar retainer must have circumferential retention to support molar.

Abnormal Occlusion

A bridge is contraindicated where the occlusion is abnormal and closure produces forces that will react adversely on the supporting structures (Fig. 12).[9] Such a relationship may preclude construction of pontics that have acceptable form or it may rotate one or more of the abutments to such an extent that the stability of the retainers will be uncertain. If these faults cannot be adjusted or eliminated by inlays, crowns, or equilibration,[10] there should be few deviations from this rule.

The use of a rotated tooth in bridge construction may be debatable. Quite likely it will be awkward to prepare. Retentive form, occlusion, and esthetics must be cleverly contrived. However, when the operator puts forth the effort to overcome the objectionable features, many such teeth will serve well as abutments.

$$* \quad * \quad * \quad * \quad * \quad *$$

The demands placed upon all the materials and fabricated restorations and prostheses used and placed in the oral cavity are heroic. Occlusal forces are in the magnitude of thousands of pounds per square inch. Temperature changes induced by foods and liquids are instantaneous and may be as much as 65° C. The pH alters swiftly from alkalinity to acidity. The oral environment is warm and moist and conducive to corrosion. The soft tissues and the dental pulp are easily traumatized and irritated, calling for constant vigilance.

Because of these and many other exacting conditions that must be met by materials and techniques, the oral environment and the problems it causes continue to intrigue the scientist, and research is proceeding at an accelerated rate. It is conceivable that very soon the criteria favorable to all oral operations will become more inclusive.

When it is designed correctly and constructed competently (Fig. 13), a fixed partial prosthesis begets a happy patient. There is a growing acceptance of bridge construction by the public and the profession. Advances in

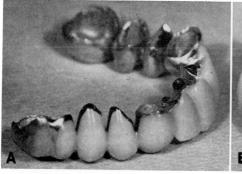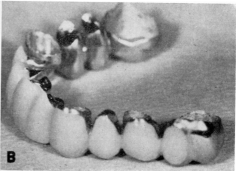

FIGURE 13. Correct design.
Lateral views of the twelve-unit bridge shown earlier. Note the minimal ridge covering areas on the pontics, the embrasure form, and size and location of the joints.

armamentarium, resulting in indirect techniques and more freedom for the patient, have contributed to this acceptance. Participation in this movement is a rewarding experience for all concerned.

REFERENCES

1. Boucher, C. O., ed.: Current Clinical Dental Terminology. St. Louis, The C. V. Mosby Company, 1963.
2. Applegate, O. C.: Essentials of Removable Partial Denture Prosthesis. 2nd ed. Philadelphia, W. B. Saunders Company, 1959, p. 5.
3. Grubb, H. D.: Fixed bridgework. J. Pros. Den., *3*:121, Jan. 1953.
4. Adams, J. W.: Lecture, Postgraduate course, Indiana Univ. School Den., April 1954.
5. Brown, L. W., Jr.: Dentistry's zone of silence. J.A.D.A., *55*:843, Dec. 1957.
6. Ante, I. H.: The fundamental principles of abutments. Michigan State D. Soc. Bul., *8*:14, July 1926.
7. Smith, G. P.: Objectives of a fixed partial denture. J. Pros. Den., *11*:463, May–June 1961.
8. Dykema, R. W.: Fixed partial prosthodontics. J. Tennessee D. A., *42*:309, Oct. 1962.
9. Simpson, R. L.: Failures in crown and bridge prosthodontics. J.A.D.A., *47*:154, Aug. 1953.
10. Nuttall, E. B.: Diagnosis and correction of occlusal disharmonies in preparation for fixed restorations. J.A.D.A., *44*:399, April 1952.

Klaffenbach, A. O.: Biomechanical restoration and maintenance of the permanent first molar space. J.A.D.A., *45*:633, Dec. 1952.

Shooshan, E. D.: Adequate operative dentistry and its significance in maintaining oral health. J. Pros. Den., *6*:710, Sept. 1956.

Tylman, S. D.: To what degree can the partially edentulous patient be rehabilitated biologically and mechanically by means of crowns and fixed bridges? J. Ontario D. A., *30*:255, 314, Aug. and Oct. 1953.

Yurkstas, A. A.: The effect of missing teeth on masticatory performance and efficiency J. Pros. Den., *4*:120, Jan. 1954.

Yurkstas, A. A., Fridley, H. H., and Manly, R. S.: A functional evaluation of fixed and removable bridgework. J. Pros. Den., *1*:570, Sept. 1951.

2

DIFFERENTIAL DIAGNOSIS AND SELECTION AND PLANNING OF TREATMENT

Diagnosis consists of the recognition of an abnormality and a thorough investigation of the severity of a condition and the reason why it has occurred. Treatment, or correction, must be based on a case study that ignores no phase of the over-all situation and follows the most promising course to its culmination.

There are five steps in diagnosis and selection of treatment:

(1) a comprehensive study of existing conditions;

(2) an evaluation of the potential of the remaining teeth and their supporting structures, as related to (a) the load to which the abutments will be subjected and their abilities to sustain this load, and (b) the relative retentive and esthetic qualities of retainer preparations on the abutments;

(3) a discriminating assessment of the relationship of one arch to the other, with the optimal load-bearing ability of the bridge structure;

(4) an eventual selection of a method of restoration that gives consideration to the esthetic requirements imposed by the patient as well as his caries index, oral hygiene, and anticipated cooperation;[1] and

(5) a plan of treatment that will accomplish this satisfactorily.

The existing vertical dimension and maxillo-mandibular relationship are accepted and maintained in the majority of cases, and in the construction of either a fixed or a removable prosthesis the most conservative approach is always attempted. The authors define "conservative" to mean *conservation of tooth structure and the surface enamel* unless the caries index, the need for maximal retention, the presumable susceptibility to caries, or the most effective position of a clasp requires that a tooth be crowned.

THE IMPORTANCE AND METHODS OF TREATMENT PLANNING

Rules must be established as a starting point for the selection and planning of treatment, but it must be remembered that the ideal case is seldom found. While this chapter and others will refer to many instances of minor divergence from suggested procedures, there can be no change in the basic principles of selection, planning, construction, and maintenance.

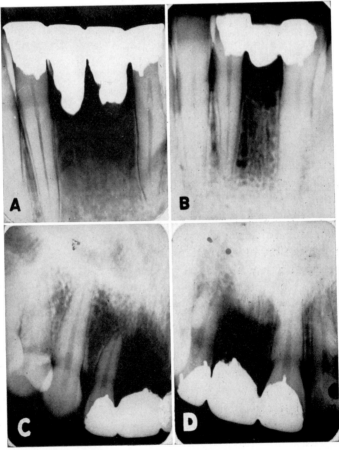

FIGURE 14. Radiographs.

A, Mandibular lateral incisors with high alveolar process and good crown-root ratio.

B, Support is reduced on central incisor abutment, but because of short span is still acceptable without splinting.

C, D, Maxillary lateral incisor with almost 1:1 ratio, but because of spacing, short span, and crown-root ratio of central, it was considered safe. Bridge has been worn for 18 years with no apparent change.

Step-by-step treatment planning is imperative in order that teeth may be preserved, time saved, costs kept to a minimum, and the most satisfactory (or most practical) type of restoration inserted. A "most satisfactory or practical" restoration means one that will produce the maximum in chewing efficiency for the longest period of time, with the least tendency toward a destructive influence on the abutments, the opposing teeth, and their supporting structures.

Dr. Howard Raper[2] expresses his concept of a dental restoration in this

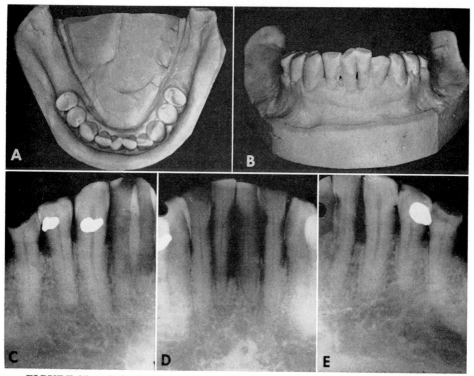

FIGURE 15.   *A,* Occlusal view of mandibular cast. Second bicuspids severely abraded.
B, Labial view. Central incisors extruded. Cuspids and bicuspids abraded by occluding porcelain denture teeth.
C, Left bicuspids and cuspid have good supporting alveolus and good crown-root ratio.
D, Central incisors mobile; right lateral poor; left lateral two-thirds denuded on mesial.
E, Right bicuspids and cuspid have acceptable bony support. It was recommended that all incisors be extracted, and that a treatment bite rim with anterior teeth be worn to increase posterior vertical dimension and to permit mandible to reposition.

Two treatment plans might be considered: (1) A ten-unit bridge would splint all remaining teeth and could be contoured for retention and support of a Class I removable partial denture. (2) If the lower anterior ridge receded grossly, the bicuspids and cuspid on each side could be splinted and contoured to retain and support a Class I, Mod. I, partial denture.

With either plan of treatment, vertical dimension of the second bicuspids must be increased. The second plan could be successful because of occlusion with maxillary complete denture.

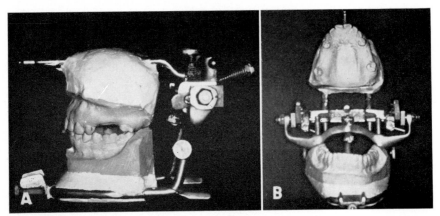

FIGURE 16. Diagnostic casts.
A, Long maxillary posterior space; distal abutment tipped mesially.
B, Distal abutments are third molars; one is tipped buccally; spaces are long. Removable bridge indicated and constructed.

way: "It is a mechanical repair, a treatment for a local disease, and a prophylactic against a systemic disease."

In order that a restoration or prosthesis can be made to coincide with Dr. Raper's definition, all phases of the construction must be considered in advance. He has implied that there must be properly placed contact areas with adequate strength; correct contour of proximal, buccal, and lingual surfaces; harmonious occlusal carving; marginal fit with no overextension or other discrepancies; and protection of the cusps to prevent fracture of the buccal or lingual walls.

These things cannot be accomplished without diagnosis and formulation of a plan of treatment that will fix in the mind of the operator all the existing limitations and all the modifications that may be inaugurated to overcome them.[3, 4, 5] These steps entail examination of radiographs (Figs. 14 and 15), diagnostic casts (Fig. 16), and the mouth (Fig. 17); consultation with the patient; exploration of the carious or otherwise dubious abutment and associated teeth; an understanding of the periodontal factors; consideration of the feasibility of orthodontic positioning of abutment or opposing teeth; and arrangement of appointments so that prepared teeth will be left unrestored for minimal periods only.[6] Likewise, the time surrendered by the patient must fit into the schedule of the dentist, yet discommode the patient's normal routine as little as possible.

Radiographic Examination

Radiographs should reveal the status quo in all sections of the mandible or maxilla and many times in the temporomandibular joint. Edentulous spaces should be examined for residual roots and rarefied areas. The radio-

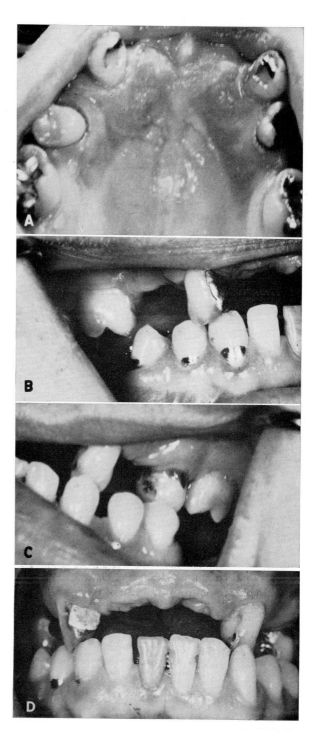

FIGURE 17. Examination of the mouth.

A, B, C, Six teeth that must be explored and evaluated before making decision regarding treatment plan. Position of cuspid and caries index suggested orthodontic repositioning of cuspid abutment and veneered gold crowns as retainers.

D, Labial view showing upper left cuspid locked to lingual of mandibular teeth.

graphs should be scrutinized to appraise the amount and quality of the supporting structure. The root areas within the alveolar process should be measured and compared in length to the portion of the tooth extending beyond the crest of the alveolus. The thickness of the periodontal membrane should be observed for evidence signifying abnormal pressure not in line with the long axis of the tooth. Apical rarefaction should be noted. The continuity of the cortical layer should be inspected for alveolar atrophy.

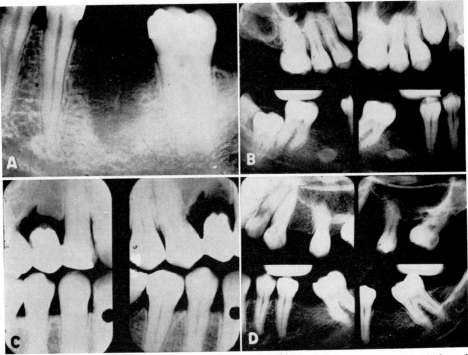

FIGURE 18.   *A*, Root length, crown-root ratio, edentulous area, and periodontal membrane of uniform thickness show bicuspid and molar to be good risks for abutments.

B, C, Radiograph shows retained maxillary cuspid and mandibular third molar and root fragment (?) in alveolus of mandibular space. Cuspid and molar were removed; sockets were allowed to heal. The lower second bicuspid has a conical root and a large crown; however, the crown-root ratio is good and the space is short. Bridges were built.

D, Radiograph shows good alveolar bone and crown-root ratio around upper second bicuspid and cuspid and lower second molar and bicuspid. Upper molar was considered unfavorable for abutment, because of tipping and pocket. It was retained until extraction was necessary.

FIGURE 19.   *A*, Articulated casts (right side), mandibular molar having been extracted for a long time, and second molar unsupported mesially. Maxillary first molar extruded in an arc, with distal cusps extending into space.

B, Radiograph of mandibular second molar. Crown-root ratio 1½:1. Root fused. Apical thickening of periodontal membrane. Second bicuspid shows evidence of abnormal occlusion.

C, Maxillary first molar restored in distal half, making it possible to recontour occluding surface, without probability of sensitivity or shock.

D, Mandibular bicuspids have all requisites for abutments.

E, Articulated casts (left side).

Legend continued on facing page.

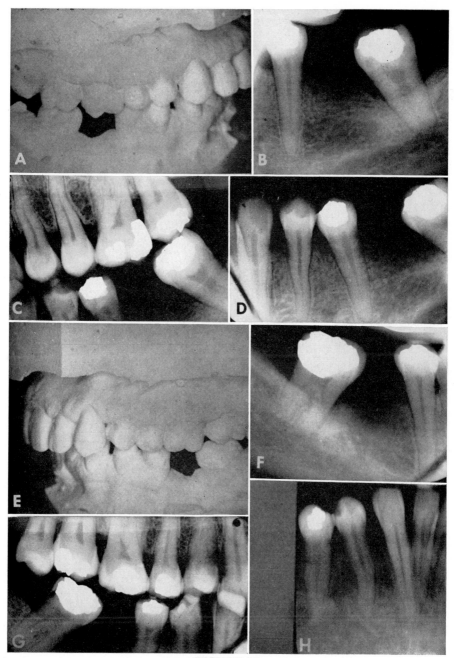

FIGURE 19.

F, Radiograph of left mandibular second molar and second bicuspid. Crown-root ratio about the same as on right side but roots are not fused, making situation better for bridge support.

G, Extruded maxillary third molar should be extracted and distal of first molar shortened to coincide with occlusal plane.

H, Left mandibular bicuspids. Second bicuspid effective abutment.

Despite bone loss around lower second molars and their acquired mesial inclinations, fixed partial dentures are indicated. Including the first bicuspids for anterior support might be considered; however, the length of the bicuspid clinical crowns is not suitable for splinting, and there is no other reason for reducing the height of the gingiva.

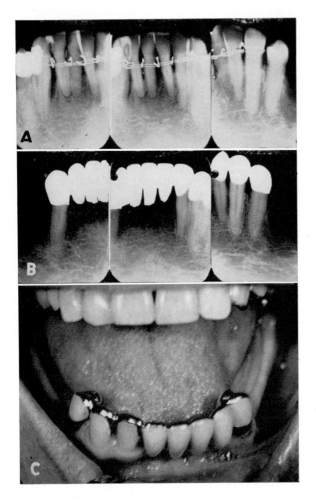

FIGURE 20. Nonacceptable radiographic situation.

A, Radiographically, situation is not acceptable. Did not respond to periodontal treatment. Incisors and one cuspid removed.

B, Radiograph of bridge constructed with four abutments.

C, Bridge shown in *B*. The three splinted abutments will stabilize the single bicuspid on the left side of the arch. It has good bony support and will receive bilateral bracing from removable partial denture.

In addition, the long-axis relationship of the proposed abutment teeth should be calculated.

An acceptable situation radiographically would be one in which (1) the root length within the alveolar process is greater than the combined lengths of crown and root outside it (Fig. 18), (2) the alveolar process in the edentulous area is well filled (although there can be exceptions to this following recent extraction), (3) the periodontal membrane appears to be of uniform thickness and not undergoing undue lateral stress, and (4) the long-axis relationship of the abutment teeth is within 25 to 30 degrees of being parallel. Construction of the bridge still may be termed acceptable, even if the alveolus has receded beyond the prescribed ratio, provided examination shows that splinting can be done (Fig. 19).

A situation would be termed nonacceptable (1) if the radiographs disclose manifestations contrary to the above, (2) when there is apical resorption, (3) when there is pocketing that would not respond to treatment (Fig. 20), (4) when there is an involvement of the bifurcation, (5) when there is an apical area to be treated by a root-end resection that would adversely alter the crown-root ratio; and (6) when the supporting alveolus around roots that are excessively curved and that have received pressure along their sides when force was exerted in the direction of the long axis already shows evidence of a reaction. If it is thought that a bridge will stabilize the proposed abutment (Fig. 21), the end result might be favorable.

Diagnostic Casts

Diagnostic casts (often referred to as "study casts") are positive reproductions of the maxillary arch and hard palate and of the mandibular arch, mounted in accurate relationship on an articulator capable of lateral and protrusive movements similar to those which commonly take place in the mouth. *Casts of the arches cannot be termed "diagnostic casts" until they have been so mounted and so related.*

Construction of Diagnostic Casts. A perforated commercial alginate tray should be used. For the maxilla it should extend apically beyond the gingival line and distally to the terminal molars or the tuberosities, and it should clear the buccal and labial surfaces by not less than 3.0 mm. It usually is necessary to increase the height of the palatal area to adapt and support the impression material.

After the tray has been checked in the mouth, the patient is asked to rinse. Alginate, sufficiently precise for diagnostic casts, is used for the impression because of its simple and convenient technique and working qualities. Mixing should follow the manufacturer's directions as to relative quantities and spatulation time.

A bit of alginate is placed to the distals of the terminal teeth and also rubbed on the occlusals, using the finger as an instrument. This precludes voids and bubbles. The tray is filled and, with the patient in an upright position, is placed in the mouth. A saliva ejector will help to keep the patient comfortable unless an excess of alginate has been inadvertently forced back into the throat. Gelation time will be approximately four minutes. As a rule, downward pressure on the tray handle will remove the impression, although occasionally it will be necessary to use finger pressure in the area of the tuberosity.

After the impression has been washed, stone is mixed, using 22 to 25 ml. of water and 100 gm. of stone.* (See Fig. 22.) It is spatulated until it will mound without slumping and is vibrated into the impression in small increments, starting at the posterior on one side and pulling the stone around the arch. Bulk is added until the impression is overfilled. Stone is then mounded on a glass slab and the inverted impression is pushed into the stone, which is adapted to the borders of the impression with a spatula. The stone should set for a minimum of 1 hour.

---

* Vel-Mix, Kerr Mfg. Company, Detroit, Mich.

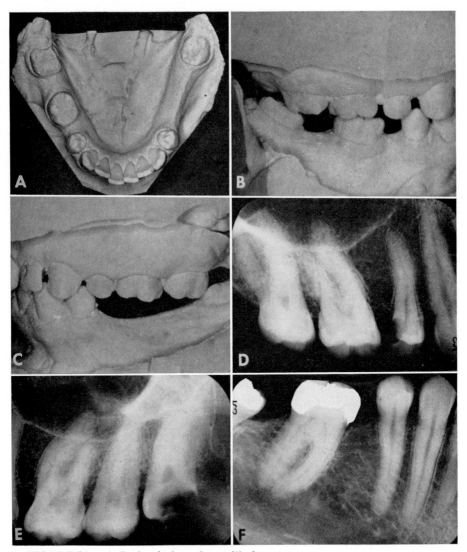

FIGURE 21.   *A,* Occlusal view of mandibular cast.

B, Right lateral view of articulated diagnostic casts. Mandibular third molar occludes only on mesial half.

C, Left lateral view of diagnostic casts. Maxillary second molar slips below lower occlusal plane.

D, E, Radiographs of maxillary molars. Carious left third was extracted.

F, G, Radiographs of right mandibular molars. Third inclined mesially. All force against this tooth absorbed by flat mesial surface of root. No evidence of adverse reaction.

H, I, Radiographs of left mandibular molar and bicuspid. Indications are that lower right posteriors could support any type and extent of load. Treatment plan suggested included a bridge from right first molar to first bicuspid and a Class III, Mod. I, partial denture. The third molar and right first molar were to have crowns with supporting circumferential ledges with the clasps rebuilding the teeth to contour. The left bicuspid would be treated the same way on the lingual but with a retentive clasp arm on the buccal.

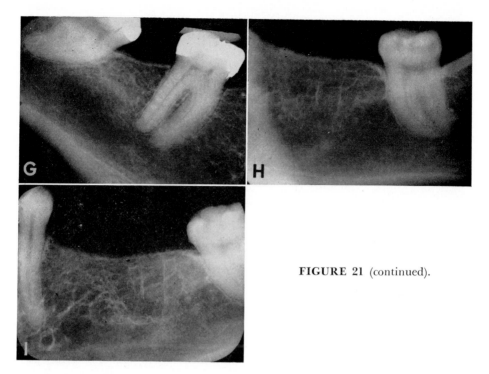

FIGURE 21 (continued).

The lower impression tray should extend distally to the terminal teeth or over the retromolar pad. It should go no more than 3.0 or 4.0 mm. below the lingual gingival line, it should not deform the muco-buccal fold posteriorly, and it should not depress either frenum. Again using the finger as an instrument, impression material should be placed distally to the terminal teeth and along the labial surfaces and cervically to the anteriors. An impression tray should always be held in position by the operator until setting has occurred.

The lower impression is poured in the same way as the upper, but in order to make final trimming less arduous, any stone that rises above the lingual borders of the impression should be removed with a spatula (Fig. 23). The casts should be trimmed symmetrically and short enough in the posterior so there will be no interference in occluding them.

Registration. A face-bow registration is a requisite. A bite fork is covered with three thicknesses of pink baseplate wax and the patient is asked to close so that the upper teeth indent the wax 2.0 mm. The bow is positioned on the face, adjusted to center on the condyle regions, locked (Fig. 24), and transferred to the articulator. The upper cast is mounted.

The patient should be assisted or guided in practicing closing the mandible. A wax registration is then made without allowing the teeth to touch if the objective is to appraise the occlusion. A Kerr Bite Frame and Kerr's Bite Registration Paste* are excellent for this purpose if the existing

---

* Kerr Mfg. Company, Detroit, Mich.

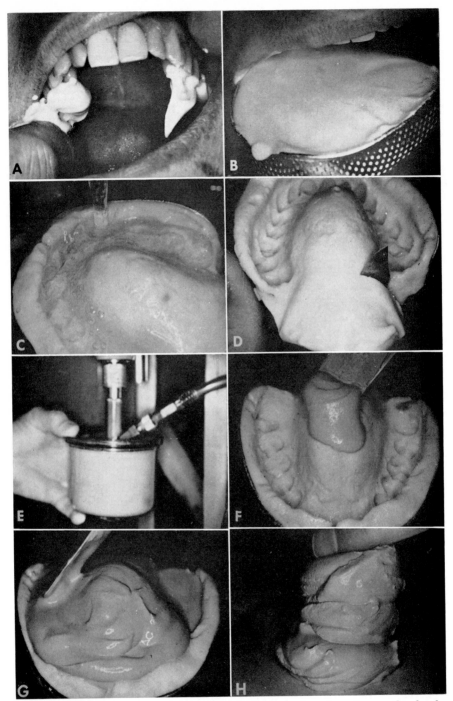

FIGURE 22.　*A,* Alginate placed to distal of terminal teeth and on occlusals of posteriors.

　B, Tray filled.

　C, D, Washing and trimming impression.

　E, Mixing stone in vacuum.

　F, First increment of stone. It flows under vibration. Thin film will enter teeth without forming bubbles.

　G, Impression filled.

　H, Mound of stone onto which inverted and filled impression will be placed.

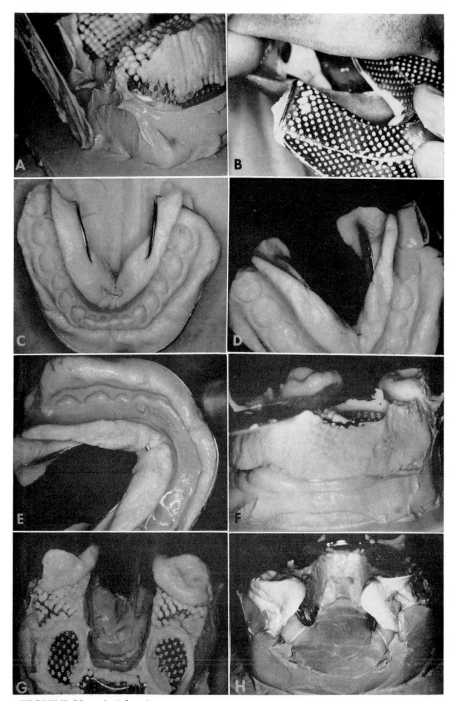

FIGURE 23. *A,* Adapting stone to borders of impression.

B, Placing lower tray in mouth with rotating motion. Tray displaces one corner of mouth while fingers of other hand open and widen orifice. No alginate should be left on lower lip.

C, Lower impression.

D, Stone is added at one end and, using vibration, is pulled in thin layer around to opposite end.

E, Occlusals filled. There should be no bubbles in cusp tips.

F, Inverted impression placed on mound of stone.

G, Adapting stone to lingual border and removing excess.

H, No excess stone around lingual border.

31

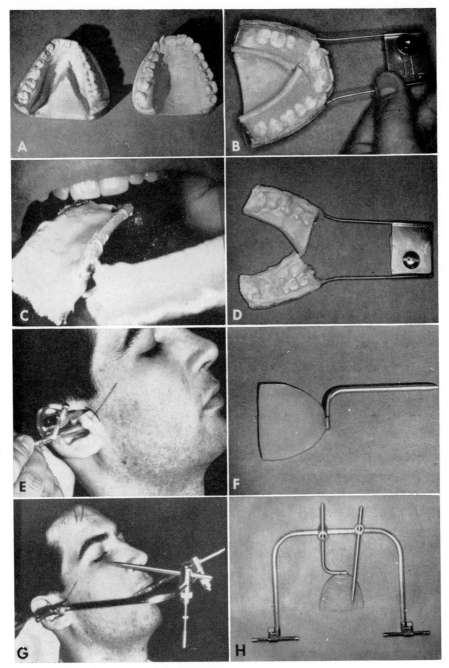

FIGURE 24. *A,* Poured and trimmed casts.
B, Fitting Kerr Bite Frame.
C, Placing Bite Frame, with paste, in mouth.
D, Registration.
E, Arbitrary point for positioning face-bow.
F, Bite fork covered with wax.
G, Face-bow adjusted to patient.
H, Face-bow locked and removed from patient.

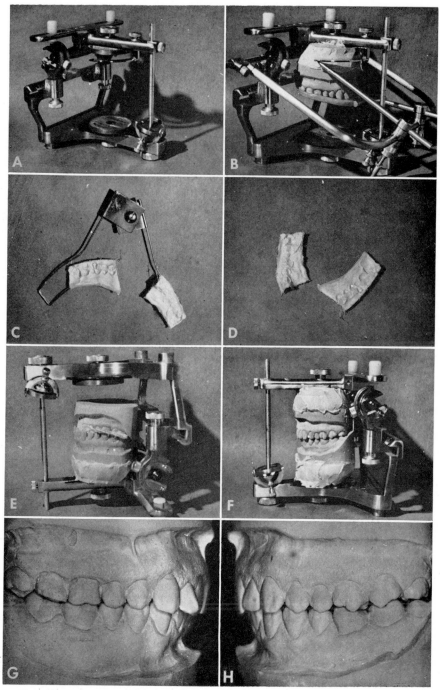

FIGURE 25. *A*, Articulator.
B, Upper cast mounted to face-bow setting.
C, D, Registration for relating lower cast.
E, Articulator reversed. Lower cast related to upper with Bite Frame registration.
F, Both casts mounted.
G, H, Right and left occlusion.

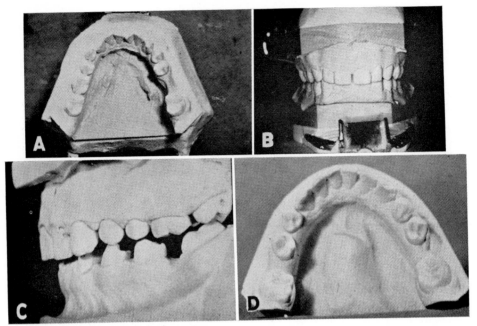

FIGURE 26. Diagnostic casts.

A, Mandibular first molar space; normal mesio-distal width; abrasion on occluding surfaces; square teeth; path of insertion satisfactory on two abutments.

B, Diagnostic casts articulated correctly.

C, D, Teeth have drifted following extraction of first molars, creating handicaps of reduced space, rotated abutments, slightly extruded upper first molars, and the problems of re-establishing occlusal plane and occlusion.

centric occlusion is being accepted. The lower cast is mounted and the preliminary diagnostic casts are now ready for examination and study (Fig. 25).

Prior to taking impressions, the occlusion should have been checked closely and equilibrated. After mounting, if other occlusion factors must be corrected, this should be done both on the casts and in the mouth. The extent of changes will determine the necessity for making and occluding new casts.

Value of Diagnostic Casts

Diagnostic casts are essential in the planning of a bridge (Fig. 26). They enable the operator (1) to evaluate the forces that will act against the bridge; (2) to decide whether any grinding or rebuilding of teeth will be obligatory so that a suitable or improved opposing occlusal plane can be formed; (3) by use of the surveyor, to locate the path of insertion and outline the reduction necessary to make the abutment preparations parallel and to arrive at a design for maximal esthetics; (4) to visualize the directions in which force will be applied to the finished restoration and to plan reduction in the size or changes in the form of the opposing cusps, if such actions are warranted; (5) to select, contour, and position the facings and to use them as guides in preparing the abutments; and (6) to resolve the plan of procedure for the entire mouth.

"Plan of procedure" refers to a determination of the sequence of restorations. For instance, in order to develop the occlusal plane of the bridge more competently, it might be logical to restore opposing teeth first. Again, sometimes there is a likelihood that a bridge will function more effectively and with less chance for trauma if its construction is delayed until occlusal balance is achieved by grinding, by placing a crown or some other restoration on the opposite side, or by a combination of both.

Mouth Examination and Consultation with the Patient

Mouth examination provides an opportunity for studying tissue conditions, the quality of the surface tooth structure, the movements of the teeth

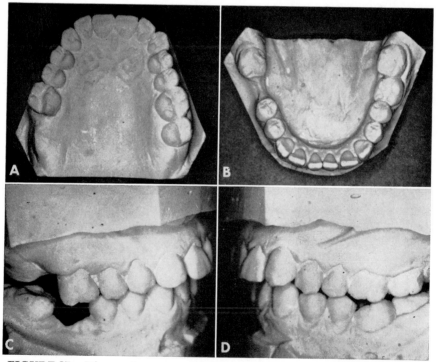

FIGURE 27.   Diagnostic casts.

A, B, Upper and lower casts, occlusal view.

C, Right lateral view. Lower bridge will occlude only on anterior half, placing an added load on the bicuspid abutment and retainer. Two crowns should be considered; also the possible need for splinting the upper molar and second bicuspid to prevent distal movement of the molar.

D, Left lateral view. Upper first molar must be recontoured, making distal half shorter and mesial longer. Lower second molar, now in first molar position, must be built into occlusion, which will necessitate reshaping the distal half of the second bicuspid.

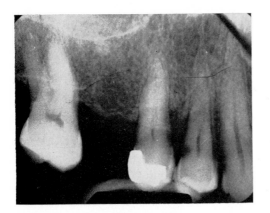

FIGURE 28. Radiograph showing receded alveolar support around molar and bicuspids. Long-axis relationship good. Using three abutments would distribute load and probably would extend service of first bicuspid.

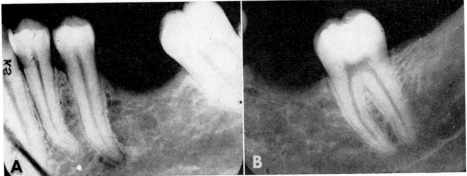

FIGURE 29. *A,* Radiographs showing good alveolar support, crown-root ratio, and root form.

B, The molar has a mesial tip, but it can be prepared without obvious risk. Bridge indicated.

under pressure or the excessive mobility of teeth by finger manipulation, and the oral hygiene and tolerance of mouth tissues to previous restorations. Mouth mirrors, explorers, dental floss or tape, water, and air are used for this type of examination.

Consultation with the patient should be conversational, rather than limited to direct questions and answers, because such an approach will often expose the patient's misgivings and hopes. Of course, in order to gain specific information, conversation must be augmented by some questioning. It is advisable to tell the patient frankly the anticipated nature of the operation, the extent of preparations to be made on the teeth, the need for anesthesia, the type of discomfort, fatigue, and inconvenience that may be experienced, and the amount of time to be spent. Absolute cooperation, respect, and trust from the patient must prevail from the beginning. These intangible but vital requisites make the technical work more facile and pleasant for both the patient and dentist.

The initial consultation is not the time for a discussion of fees. This should take place after all phases of the examination have been completed and findings coordinated, and the patient has been told what method and type of treatment will give him the most comfort and the longest period of useful, nondestructive service. "The size of the patient's purse should not alter the dental truth. He has the right to be well-advised and to be given time to consider that advice. Then, and only then, should the fee be quoted and the method of payment, sequence of operations, and appointments arranged."[7]

Exploration of Abutments and Associated Teeth

Exploration of abutments and associated teeth differs from *examination* in that it encompasses the removal of caries or old and doubtful restorations in order to ascertain the proportion of the remaining tooth substance and the probability of pulp exposure. Usually radiographs and oral examination will contribute ample information, but if there is any suspicion regarding the residuum of tooth structure, an exhaustive exploration of the abutment tooth must be made before planning continues. If any other

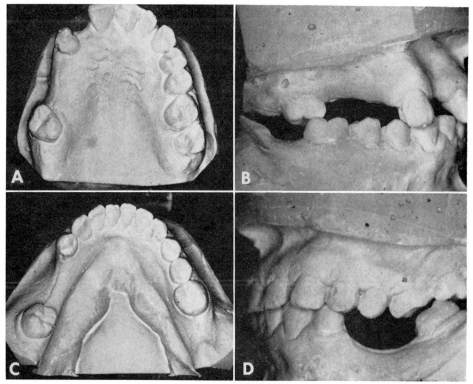

FIGURE 30. *A, B,* Diagnostic casts viewed from occlusal and right. Lateral incisor, first and second bicuspids, and first molar lost. Posterior space long for a bridge unless construction is sturdy. Occlusion on molar not completely favorable to cantilevering lateral incisor pontic. Long-axis relationship of three abutments good.

C, D, Lower left space long for fixed prosthesis unless two abutments are used anteriorly.

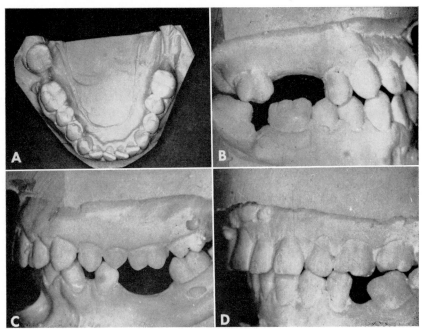

FIGURE 31. *A,* Occlusal view of diagnostic cast. Third molar has moved mesially. Both second molars missing.

B, Lateral view of occluded diagnostic casts. Bicuspid and molar lost. Principal force of occlusion will be on pontics. To prepare opposing arch prior to building upper bridge, lower first molar and third molar should be connected by a small pontic, with both joints and molar soldered. First molar must be recontoured to occlusal plane. Maxillary bridge will be more comfortable and will serve longer if it has continuous occlusion. Also, mastication will be improved.

C, D, Maxillary first molars have extruded in an arc and must be "leveled" before occluding prostheses are built.

tooth, the loss of which might affect the proposed prosthesis, has a carious lesion or a dubious restoration, it, too, should be explored before the treatment plan is formulated.

Consideration of Periodontal Factors

The occlusion should be equilibrated, a prophylaxis given, and any required surgical treatment, such as a gingivectomy or reduction of the ridge, instituted before abutment preparations are planned. The gingiva, the periodontal membrane, and the alveolar process should be brought to the highest level of health attainable before abutments are prepared. Although one of the purposes in placing a bridge is to promote the well-being of the oral structure, an optimal state must be established beforehand. When this is apparent to the patient, he will comply with suggestions regarding his part in maintaining oral hygiene.

There should be no more recession than would be normal for the age of the patient, but variation is expectable, inasmuch as this is governed to some extent by occlusal wear. If the alveolar process has receded without undue irregularity and if this recession has not resulted in pocketing or the bifurcation has not been implicated, the tooth may be used as a single or a splinted abutment. If the bony support is weak, all facets of the case should be scanned before such a tooth is used as an abutment, applying Ante's law in estimating the support.

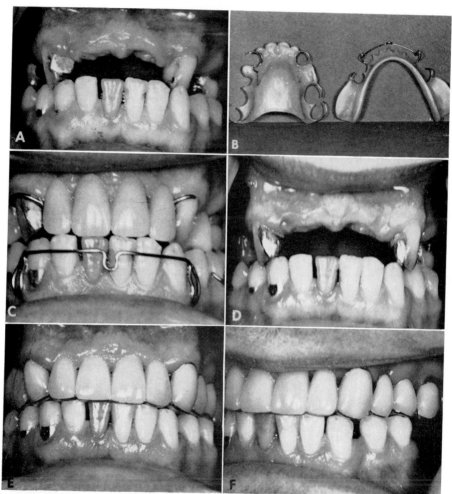

FIGURE 32. *A,* Labial view showing maxillary left cuspid locked to lingual of mandibular teeth.

B, Working retainers that were used to improve tooth position. The upper left cuspid clasp is free of acrylic resin over most of its length so that it can be activated to cause labial movement of the tooth. The labial wire on the lower will be used to move the incisors lingually and together.

C, Appliances in the mouth. The mandibular posterior supplied teeth are set high to increase the vertical dimension so that the left cuspid will be free to move into proper position.

D, Left cuspid has moved to position. Teeth have temporary amalgam restorations.

E, F, Bridge cemented.

Both on the diagnostic casts and in the mouth, the *form,* the *distribution,* and the *position* of the opposing teeth must be heeded, and the plan of construction and the esthetic concept deferred to these factors (Fig. 30). The form or length of an opposing tooth can be altered a little by grinding and to a major degree by the construction of a crown or an inlay, or by splinting two teeth (Fig. 31). Distribution may be revamped by extraction or multiple abutments.

When mandibular bicuspids occlude buccally to opposing teeth, a greater amount of metal may be displayed unless drastic changes are made in the preparations. Not infrequently, also, when an abutment is unopposed, with no teeth posterior to it, the treatment plan must include a greater number of supporting teeth at the anterior end of the prosthesis to offset the increased leverage on the anterior abutment.

Orthodontic Positioning of Abutment or Opposing Teeth

Distribution and position of abutment teeth can often be improved by orthodontics. Minor and uncomplicated treatment can be done by general

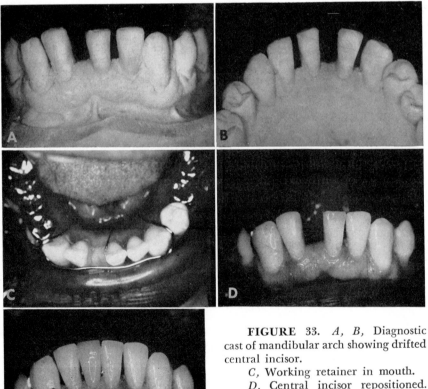

FIGURE 33. *A, B,* Diagnostic cast of mandibular arch showing drifted central incisor.

C, Working retainer in mouth.

D, Central incisor repositioned. Tooth was tipped instead of being moved bodily. While this result is less desirable, it is workable.

E, Bridge cemented.

practitioners, thus decreasing the difficulties in preparation and construction and adding materially to the life of the restoration (Fig. 32). This phase of the restorative procedure deserves more attention than it normally receives (Fig. 33). (See Chapter 30.)

Planning Appointments

Arranging appointments is an individual office matter. In this respect, however, in every office it should be emphasized that preparations on vital teeth should be completed in one visit and it must be remembered always that *abutment teeth should be left unrestored for the shortest possible period of time to prevent movement, sensitivity, and annoyance to the patient.*

THE FOUNDATION

The ideal clinical crown for an abutment is one of average length or longer, of square form, and of more than average bulk. Nevertheless, short teeth may be used when the preparations are altered to develop resistance to displacement. Frail teeth may be employed also, provided that the spaces to be filled are correspondingly narrow and the opposing forces are relative. Taper or ovoid teeth may be prepared as abutments if the pulps have receded enough to allow safe and sufficient reduction of tooth structure. This will have occurred in most instances.

The length of the root segment supported by the alveolar process should be 1½ times that of the crown of the abutment and the root should not be conical. The apical segment of the root should not be curved to create an area that will crush or bruise the periodontal membrane under masticating force. The previous load or types and strength of forces should be assessed and if the reaction is adjudged favorable, roots of this type may be accepted for the support of fixed prostheses.

The abutment teeth should have a near-parallel relationship with each other and a normal long-axis relationship to the opposing teeth, although there may be many digressions from this requirement.[8] Teeth that are tipped mesially or distally can be used as abutments without apprehension if the inclination is not so great as to interfere with preparation. Teeth which are tipped buccally or lingually are less qualified abutments because, when such teeth are used, rotation or torque can damage supporting structure or cause retainers to become loose.

A tooth free of caries is likely to have a pulp less prone to future pathologic reactions; also, it permits the most nearly perfect type of preparation since minimal coronal reduction is possible. Still, teeth that have caries involving areas not usually included in the preparations may be used as

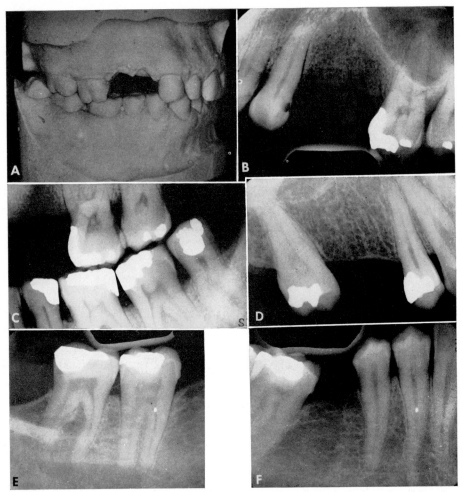

FIGURE 34. *A,* Diagnostic casts showing contour of gingival tissue resulting from unsupported removable prosthesis. Partial denture must not be worn, because tissue should be allowed to recontour prior to the construction of a bridge. Mandibular third molar should be extracted to protect distal of second molar from pocketing, even though it has abraded and is integrated with incisal guidance.

B, C, Radiographs of arches shown in *A.* Periodontal treatment needed before and after bridge is constructed.

D, A molar inclined mesially, but this is an excellent situation for a bridge.

E, F, Second molar and second bicuspid are good abutments. Plus contact on mesial of bicuspid retainer should move first bicuspid into contact with cuspid. Bridge cemented following this treatment and necessary equilibration.

abutments provided that the caries is removed, the pulp is protected against thermal shock, and the tooth is restored to "prepared form"* by a gold casting or amalgam. In a few circumstances, if the carious area does not approach the margin of the preparation and if the retainer will be sup-

---

* "Prepared form" is the shape of the reduced tooth when it is completed to receive the specific type of retainer or restoration which is planned. It must provide maximal retention and resistance to caries and fracture, and encourage biologic acceptance of the treatment as a whole.

ported by tooth structure, cement or resin may be used instead of metal. When caries is extensive and little dentin remains in the crown area, extraordinary care must be used during the preparation to conserve tooth structure.

If the tooth is pulpless, it may be rebuilt with a crown and used as an abutment if there is no apical rarefaction or root resorption and if the root canal can be enlarged to receive a post for the support of a cast or amalgam core. This post must be of a length equal to or greater than that of the crown or retainer. Because the remaining coronal structure of a pulpless tooth is brittle, it is seldom capable of supporting the restoration without one or more posts being extended into the root area.[9]

Splinting

An abutment tooth usually is required at each end of the space to be restored, but if the construction of a bridge were to create a lever arm of some length, additional terminal abutment teeth, splinted, would be in order. (Other exceptions are discussed in Chapter 27, Bridge Patterns.)

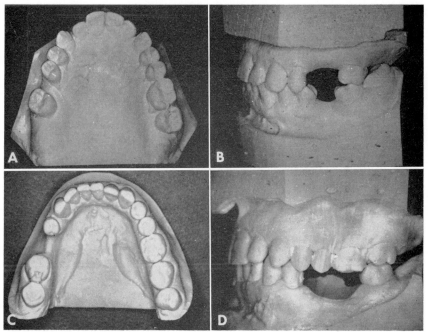

FIGURE 35. *A,* Maxillary diagnostic cast. First molar missing, with second molar moved mesially. Space less than bicuspid width. A bridge may be needed to support molar or second bicuspid and to aid mastication. Hygiene frequently difficult in such cases.

B, Mandibular third molar should be extracted and spaces restored with bridges.

C, Bridge indicated, but space between bicuspid and cuspid should be kept the same. Food packing will be no problem unless bicuspid retainer is overcontoured on mesial.

D, Maxillary first molar must be recontoured. Bicuspid abutment must be carefully evaluated. Many of these bridges fail unless cuspid is also included.

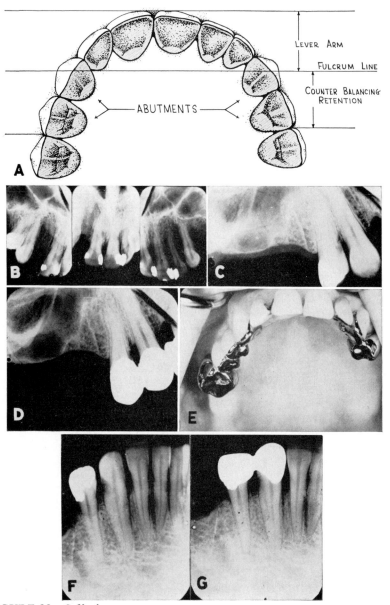

FIGURE 36.   Splinting.

A, Cuspid and bicuspid retainers splinted to form "multiple abutments."

B, C, Good alveolar process and crown-root ratio on cuspid and first bicuspid. Lateral incisor space.

D, Splinted cuspid and bicuspid abutments; cantilever lateral incisor pontic.

E, The three-unit bridge.

F, Reduced support around first bicuspid; too weak for partial denture abutment.

G, Splinted first bicuspid and cuspid; now a strong abutment.

The term *splinting* denotes the rigid joining of two or more approximating teeth (Fig. 36). In bridge construction splinted abutments are called *multiple abutments*. This practice is employed when the supporting structure is weak around one or more of the terminal abutment teeth, or when the space is long or curved or embraces the corner of the mouth in such a way that extra abutments are needed to offset the destructive rotating force generated from the tip of the lever arm. This situation occurs in the maxillary arch, particularly when replacing a cuspid, a cuspid and a lateral, or a cuspid and a first bicuspid.

A lever arm is seen in every upper anterior bridge, but the line of force directed against maxillary anterior fixed restorations comes from the lingual, as a rule, and therefore the lever arm is not such a serious factor. Shorter ones are found in the anterior segment of the mandibular arch and occur frequently with the construction of bridges supplying the bicuspids. Here punctilious planning is essential in the design of the pontics and in the retentive characteristics incorporated in the abutment preparations.

Splinting is a procedure demanding ingenuity, scrupulous attention to details in the preparation of the teeth, modification of the form of abutment castings, and precision in the placement and dimension of solder joints. Unless kept to appropriate size, the joints diminish embrasure space and cause stagnation of underlying soft tissue owing to lack of stimulation from the massage of food particles. (See Chapter 28, Splinting Teeth.)

THE PATH OF INSERTION

The path of insertion is that line or direction in which the prosthesis may be seated simultaneously on all the abutments without causing lateral force or torsion on any one of them. Any semblance of an undercut or a convergence must be avoided or eliminated if the bridge is to be seated. The presence of any undercut may be disclosed by taking an impression, pouring a plaster cast, and checking it with the surveyor.

Several circumstances control or influence the path of insertion. The most important are the long-axis relationship of the abutment teeth and the long-axis relationship of the abutment teeth with those adjacent. Malaligned teeth approximating abutments sometimes interfere with the proposed path of insertion, making it necessary to change the path slightly or to alter the form of the offending approximating tooth by grinding or by placement of a restoration.

The logical path of insertion can be confirmed on the diagnostic cast with the analyzing rod of the surveyor checking the long-axis relationship of the crowns (Fig. 37). It should assume a direction most compatible with the long axes of all the involved crowns, and one that will necessitate minimal cutting on all the surfaces to be included in the preparations.

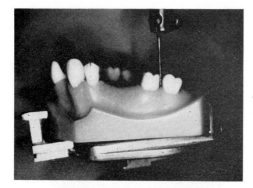

FIGURE 37. Path of insertion marked on bicuspid abutment. Distal of molar prepared to same angle.

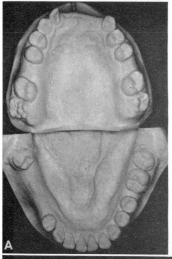

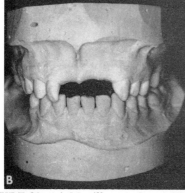

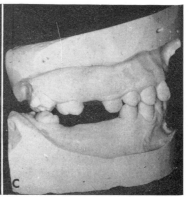

FIGURE 38. *A*, Maxillary and mandibular casts. All edentulous areas in upper arch can be filled with bridges. The cuspids and the lateral incisor will give good support for a six-unit prosthesis; however, if there is doubt, the left bicuspid should be included. The third molars are of questionable value but need not be condemned unless hygiene or periodontal considerations dictate removal. Lower right space is very long, and inclination of molar abutment must be considered. Space on left may be used for clasping.

B, Vertical overlap favorable for bridge construction.

C, Upper bicuspid abutment must be shortened and lower molar "leveled" and recontoured for clasping. Space is too long and abutments are too short for a bridge to be successful.

When more than two teeth are to be used as abutments, one, not necessarily a terminal abutment, serves as the norm and the others are prepared parallel to it.

With this survey marked on the teeth and with radiographic information of root direction and periodontal membrane condition in mind, a calculation should be made concerning the amount of cutting indicated on the other abutment teeth in order that this designated direction may be used as the path of insertion. If esthetic considerations are to be emphasized and exaggerated cutting avoided, generally some departure from the most retentive preparation will be compulsory on one or more abutments whose long-axis directions are not parallel to the guiding tooth.

Except for the young patient, selection of a path of insertion on tipped teeth is a simple matter since pulp recession ordinarily will assure safety in the reduction of the crown. Many times this is obvious to the experienced operator during the oral examination, after the size and location of the pulp horns have been verified by radiographs. Nevertheless, with few exceptions, cuts for parallelism should be traced on the diagnostic cast by a surveyor.

SPACE LENGTHS

The length of the space has a definitive bearing on the type of construction. The ideal space is that of only one missing tooth, unless the third molar is involved. Before the acceptance of this tooth as an abutment, it should be judged as to fitness in regard to long-axis relationship, crown-root ratio, relationship of the crown to the surrounding soft tissue, shape of the root (conical or curved), and type of occlusion.

The wisdom of constructing a bridge supplying three approximating missing posterior teeth may be debatable in the majority of instances, especially in the mandibular arch (Fig. 38). To avoid a springing reaction in the center of the span, the bridge must be bulky and solder joints large; thus the embrasure areas will be reduced in size, with a resultant lack of stimulating massage of food on the underlying tissue. Also, it is hard to satisfy Ante's law under such conditions. In the maxillary arch, however, many bridges, constructed from cuspid to second molar, have provided long periods of clinical service. It has not been proved that any type of removable bridge would have served to better advantage.

ABUTMENTS IN ABNORMAL POSITIONS

Abutment teeth, even in short spaces, must be examined critically for rotation, tipping, and recession. If the rotated tooth has erupted in that position, the supporting structure probably has not been seriously impaired, but if the rotation has occurred because of the loss of an approximating tooth or the extrusion of an opposing tooth, the rotated abutment may be much less desirable. Sometimes the crown form must be changed considerably when constructing a retainer for a rotated tooth. On the other hand, if the abnormal position of a rotated tooth is mechanically and esthetically satisfactory and if retention can be secured by restoring the tooth as it is, minimal change in form should be contemplated.

The rotation of an abutment can either reduce or increase the normal space length. The problem of constructing a pontic of abnormal size should be recognized in advance, as a slight decrease or increase in the mesio-distal width of the abutment teeth can be embodied in the construction of the retainers so that the pontic may be more nearly normal in size.

Tipping mesially or distally usually will reduce space lengths; consequently, there must be some alteration in crown form when the retainer is carved, and also a more careful analysis of the occlusion, connectors, and embrasures when constructing the pontic. Inordinate tipping can preclude the use of the tooth as an abutment. The force of occlusion, the degree to which the tooth may be stabilized, the capacity of the supporting structure, and pocketing must be considered, as well as the willingness of the patient to accept the actual and ensuing state of affairs.

When an abutment is inclined buccally or lingually, the space length is not perceptibly affected, but the position of the connector will be altered. The resistance to forces directed against a bridge supported by one or more such teeth will be less substantial than when the abutments are in normal position. The ability of the supporting structure to withstand these abnormal forces should be reviewed. When a tooth is tipped to the buccal or the lingual, the path of insertion on all of the teeth to be used may be a compromise. The solution can be aided appreciably by surveying the diagnostic casts.

PREPARATION OF OPPOSING ARCH

To facilitate making a bridge, it is often mandatory to change slightly the length and occlusal form of opposing teeth. Retainers may then be constructed to direct the forces as desired, pontics may be placed in more normal positions with better form, and the teeth may occlude with minimal interference.

Occasionally a tooth will have extruded into a space to such a degree that reduction of length and alteration in shape become impossible. The interfering tooth must be removed in such an instance, even if this should entail building another bridge.

If one of the opposing teeth has been lost, resulting in enough drifting or tipping to nullify the continuity of the opposing occlusal plane, those teeth which remain should be restored with crowns, inlays, or a splint, prior to construction of the bridge. If restorations already in place are effectual in terms of margins and preservation of the teeth, but are lacking in occlusal or embrasure form, they should be reshaped.

* * * * * *

The student should realize that all these complex factors cannot be readily defined or positioned in order of their significance. Relative importance will change with individual mouths. In fact, each succeeding case presents new problems and new difficulties to the novice. These principles will be applied to the examples cited throughout the text so that in planning a bridge the student or dentist will learn to make use of such diagnostic aids automatically. Gregory's[10] observation that "after years of practice, each new case is a variation of one previously handled" should become a slogan in the profession.

Rules of procedure included here, if followed diligently, will result in gratification for patient and dentist alike. Experience will modify thinking and technique and will broaden judgment, but to avert chaos for the beginner, one method should be mastered before versatility is attempted. It is to be hoped that the contents of this chapter and those that follow will equip the student with a firm foundation for progress.

REFERENCES

1. Dykema, R. W.: Fixed partial prosthodontics. J. Tennessee D. A., *42*:309, Oct. 1962.
2. Raper, H.: Personal communication.
3. Smith, G. P.: Factors affecting the choice of partial prosthesis—fixed or removable. D. Clin. North America, March 1959, pp. 3–12.
4. Lakermance, J., and Laudenbach, P.: Indications and contraindications for fixed prostheses. Rev. Stomat., *63*:46, Jan.–Feb. 1962.
5. Tylman, S. D.: Fixed partial denture prosthodontics. Internat. D. J., *10*:58, March 1961.
6. Contino, R. M., and Stallard, H.: Instruments essential for obtaining data needed in making a functional diagnosis of the human mouth. J. Pros. Den., 7:66, Jan. 1957.
7. Adams, J. W.: Lecture, Postgraduate course, Indiana Univ. School Den., April 1958.
8. Schweitzer, J. M.: Oral Rehabilitation. St. Louis, The C. V. Mosby Company, 1951.
9. Markley, M. R.: Pin reinforcement and retention of amalgam foundations and restorations. J.A.D.A., *56*:675, May 1958.
10. Gregory, G. T.: Personal communication.

Abramson, I.: Role of endodontics in crown and bridge prosthesis. J. Maryland D. A., *1*:28, No. 1, 1958.
Ante, I. H.: The fundamental principles of fixed and removable bridge prosthesis. Dominion D. J., *42*:109, 1930.
Bastian, C. C.: Consideration of some of the clinical problems of crown and bridgework. W. Virginia D. J., *17*:120, Jan. 1943.

Coelho, D. H.: Ultimate goal in fixed bridge procedures. J. Pros. Den., *4:*667, Sept. 1954.

Ewing, J. E.: Surgical crown and bridge prosthodontics. J. Pros. Den., *4:*523, July 1954.

Granger, E. R.: Occlusion in temporomandibular joint pain. J.A.D.A., *56:*659, May 1958.

Grubb, H. D.: Fixed bridgework. J. Pros. Den., *3:*121, Jan. 1953.

Landa, J. S.: An analysis of current practices in mouth rehabilitation. J. Pros. Den., *5:*527, July 1955.

Miller, S. C.: Periodontics and restorative dentistry. J.A.D.A., *47:*282, Sept. 1953.

Nuttall, E. B.: Diagnosis and correction of occlusal disharmonies in preparation for fixed restorations. J.A.D.A., *44:*399, April 1952.

Nuttall, E. B.: Development of basic prosthodontic principles of crown and bridge. Pennsylvania D. J., *21:*6, May 1954.

Pruden, W. H., II: Today's approach to fixed partial denture prosthesis. J. New Jersey D. Soc., *32:*11, Sept. 1960.

Shooshan, E. D.: Adequate operative dentistry and its significance in maintaining oral health. J. Pros. Den., *6:*710, Sept. 1956.

Tylman, S. D.: To what degree can the partially edentulous patient be rehabilitated biologically and mechanically by means of crowns and fixed bridges? J. Ontario D. A., *30:*255, 314, Aug. and Oct. 1953.

Tylman, S. D.: Discussion of the biologic factors involved in the fixed partial denture. J. Canad. D. A., *23:*67, Feb. 1957.

3

CUTTING INSTRUMENTS

Sound enamel and dentin must be cut away to produce retentive form for individual crowns and retainers. Attachment to teeth must be achieved without increasing dimensions and adding further to the load that abutments must withstand. The one basic method that has been universally accepted makes use of rotating cutting or abrading instruments, such as carbide or carbon steel burs, diamond or carborundum stones and disks, and impregnated paper disks.

Faster dental engines, frictionlesss handpieces, and superior cutting tools, recently developed, enable the dentist greatly to reduce operating time and discomfort to the patient. This statement does not imply that teeth may be cut painlessly without the use of local anesthetics. It does mean that there will be less pressure required and less vibration with these mechanical advances.

In any grinding operation on teeth, involving stones or accelerated speeds, consideration for the pulp cannot be over-emphasized. The dentin and the pulp are subjected to a series of insults, such as caries, instrumentation, placement of restorative materials, and thermal and traumatic shock. One of the most active irritants is the heat generated by the high-speed cutting tools used in modern cavity preparation. If the heat is not controlled and dissipated, severe pulpal reaction may occur.* Lubrication and cooling are essential.[1] Air is NOT an adequate coolant.[2, 3]

Cocoa butter, as it becomes diluted with saliva, serves very well with a carborundum stone or disk to increase the speed of the operation and keep the tooth at a permissible temperature. Better than cocoa butter is lukewarm water, in either a stream or a spray. Water must be used with a

---

* Every precaution must be exercised to minimize irritation.

diamond stone, not only as a coolant but also as a cleanser to keep the surface of the stone free of debris so that it may work with maximal efficiency. It is thought by many that overly rapid cutting can bring about changes within the pulp which will cause the tooth to be sensitive after restorative operations are completed. Davila Alonso et al.[4] maintain that little permanent change will occur in the pulp unless it is directly traumatized. It is agreed that lubrication and coolants contribute a great deal to the comfort of the patient during and possibly following the operation.

Certain precautions must be taken during the preparation of a tooth. A disk that is being used to cut through and remove a portion of a mesial or distal surface must be guided and steadied so that it will not bind and as a result jump out of control, cutting or abrading the gingiva, tongue, cheek, lip, or another tooth. Instruments must be handled on the buccal and lingual surfaces so that gingival tissue will not be injured or abraded to a point that prevents healing and return to original form. There must be no contact of the cutting instrument with an approximating tooth not included in the treatment plan. Mobile tissue may be retracted and protected by the fingers, mirrors, or tongue blades. Sometimes an assistant must help.

There are many series of carbide and steel burs and dozens of designs and sizes of stones, both diamond and carborundum. The steel burs manufactured in this country have a uniform system of numbering, although corresponding numbers listed by different companies will vary in size. Carborundum stones have less similarity as to numbers and sizes than burs. The evolution of the tungsten carbide bur and the diamond stone has been so rapid and opportunistic that even at the present time the numbers and sizes shown in the various catalogues frequently have little relation. Therefore, the numbers and types of only a few companies will predominate in this text, but the reader should realize that suitable carbide burs and diamond stones can be obtained from other sources.

In addition to diamond and carborundum stones and metal burs, paper disks, impregnated with grits of several kinds and finenesses, will be needed for a number of the steps in the preparations to be described later. One brand of disk, utilizing a snap-on mandrel,* is illustrated (Fig. 39), but other disks are equally efficient. With few exceptions, stones, burs, and disks are made for both the straight and the contra-angle handpiece.

Beginning students should proceed cautiously when first operating in the oral cavity. Increased rotational speeds are recommended only when the operator has become highly trained, with an exceptionally accurate concept of what the finished preparation should be, and with the ability or willingness to concentrate and avoid overreduction of teeth. (See Chapter 4.)

Baker[5] has said: "The crown and bridge field, because of its very na-

---

* E. C. Moore Company, Dearborn, Mich.

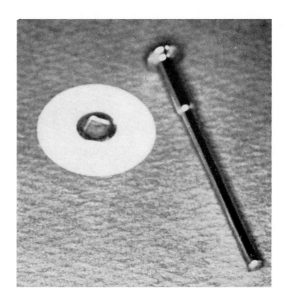

FIGURE 39. Moore's disk and mandrel.

ture, inspires a major interest in the technicalities necessary to its application. Because of this inspiration, we must be alert that technicalities in themselves do not form the basis for suggested treatment.

"Technological advancement is most desirable and of great aid to the dentist, increasing the success of most of his endeavors; yet while it serves the *convenience* of the procedure, it can in no way alter the fundamental requirement."

Concepts of fundamental requirements have changed somewhat since the advent of accelerated speeds in tooth reduction. However, retention and stability of restorations and prostheses will not be lessened even if some contours in prepared form are altered slightly to facilitate the use of new instruments and techniques. Comprehension and acceptance of such changes or advances are inevitable.

Many handpieces and contrivances have been designed to power rotating cutting instruments and each lends itself to a given technique. When skill has been acquired, the choice of such equipment should be a personal matter. The instruments to be used for each abutment preparation, for shaping facings, and for polishing metal will be named and illustrated in the sections devoted to such operations.

REFERENCES

1. Peyton, F. A.: Effectiveness of water coolants with rotary cutting instruments. J.A.D.A., 56:664, May 1958.
2. Weiss, M. B., Massler, M., and Spence, J. M.: Operative effects on adult dental pulp. D. Progress, 4:10, 1963.
3. Stanley, H., and Swerdlow, H.: Biological effects of various cutting methods in cavity

preparations: the part pressure plays in pulpal response. J.A.D.A., *61:*450, Oct. 1960.
4. Davila Alonso, H. M., VanHuysen, G., and Johnston, J. F.: Changes in pulp and periodontal tissues of teeth subjected to crown prosthesis. J. Pros. Den., *10:*350, March–April 1960.
5. Baker, C. R.: Personal communication.

Leff, A.: New concepts in the preparation of teeth for full coverage. J. Pros. Den., *5:*392, May 1955.
Miller, I. F.: Fixed dental prosthesis. J. Pros. Den., *8:*483, May 1958.
Pruden, K. C.: Abutments and attachments in fixed partial dentures. J. Pros. Den., *7:*502, July 1957.
Smith, G. P.: The marginal fit of the full cast shoulderless crown. J. Pros. Den., *7:*231, March 1957.

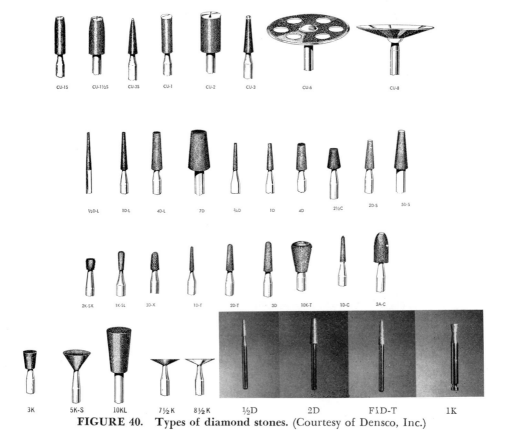

FIGURE 40.   Types of diamond stones. (Courtesy of Densco, Inc.)

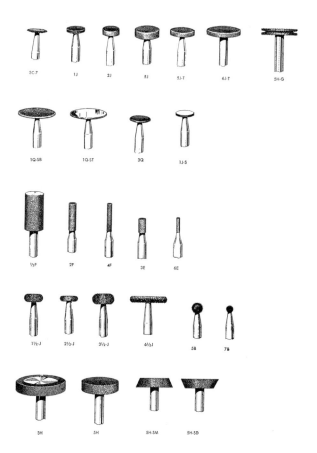

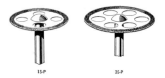

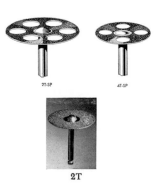

FIGURE 41. Types of diamond disks. (Courtesy of Densco, Inc.)

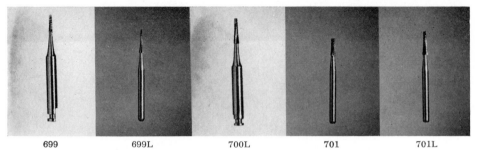

699   699L   700L   701   701L

FIGURE 42. Densco carbide burs. (Courtesy of Densco, Inc.)

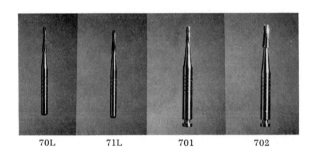

70L   71L   701   702

FIGURE 43. Premier "Ela" carbide burs. (Courtesy of Premier Dental Products Co.)

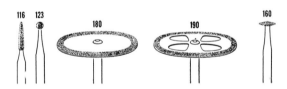

116   123   180   190   160

FIGURE 44. S. S. White diamond stones. (Courtesy of The S. S. White Dental Manufacturing Co.)

170 170L 700 701

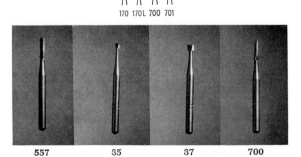

557   35   37   700

FIGURE 45. S. S. White carbide burs. (Courtesy of The S. S. White Dental Manufacturing Co.)

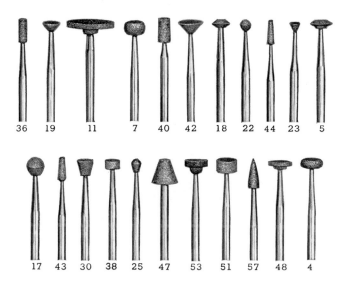

FIGURE 46.   S. S. White "carborundum" stones. (Courtesy of The S. S. White Dental Manufacturing Co.)

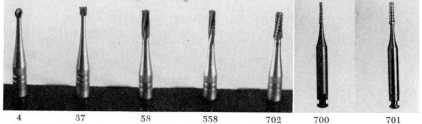

FIGURE 47.   R & R steel burs. (Courtesy of The Ransom & Randolph Co.)

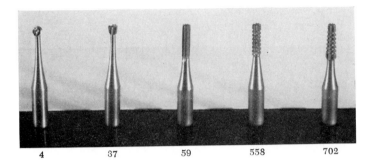

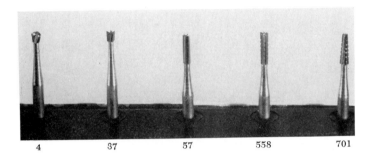

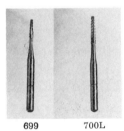

FIGURE 48. **R & R carbide burs.** (Courtesy of The Ransom & Randolph Co.)
Top row: Right angle handpiece. Center and bottom rows: Friction grip.

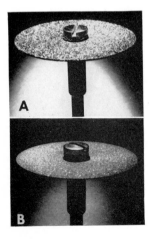

FIGURE 49. *A,* Carborundum separating disk.
B, Steel separating disk. Used when proximal cuts must
be very thin and extension labially held to minimum.

4

TOOTH REDUCTION

Section I. PRINCIPLES AND STANDARD TECHNIQUES

The extracoronal reduction of teeth in the forming of preparations to receive cast retainers may be divided into basic steps. Each will have variations, depending on the position of the tooth in the mouth, its length, contour, angle of eruption, rotation, and the kind or type of retainer to be employed. However, regardless of variation or tooth, the fundamental approach, procedures, and accomplishments are the same.

STEPS IN TOOTH REDUCTION

These steps may be classified as follows:
(1) proximal slices;
(2) shortening the occlusal surface or
(3) incisal edge;
(4) preparing convex lingual, labial, or buccal surfaces and concave lingual surfaces;
(5) rounding corners and completing the cervical finishing line;
(6) making shoulders to include labial or buccal and proximal, or all axial surfaces; and
(7) cutting grooves, ledges, or pinholes, or a combination of these.
The order in which these are discussed may vary from the sequence of application.

59

The Proximal Slice

The object of the proximal slice is to parallel or adjust the mesial or distal surfaces (or both) to the path of insertion for retention; to eliminate the bulge on the surface, which would prohibit making and seating a casting adapted to the cervix of the tooth; to create space for a thickness of metal in the casting that will be sufficient for strength and restoration of tooth form; to afford access for rounding corners or cutting grooves or retentive boxes; and to extend the proximal cervical margins into areas immune to caries (Figs. 50 and 51).

With the possible exception of the inlay, all abutment preparations can include proximal slices. A disk usually is associated with this step, and proximal reduction begins at the incisal edge or occlusal surface, ending at or just under the gingival crest or cementoenamel junction. Basically, it will be parallel to the path of insertion, may follow the plane of the surface being reduced, and can have many relationships with the long axis of the tooth.

Most frequently it will be made with the cutting instrument or disk used in the straight handpiece. Occasionally the cervical margin of a prox-

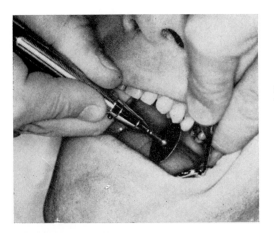

FIGURE 50.   Disk is in position to make proximal slice. Second and third (hidden) fingers of right hand, resting on incisors, support handpiece. Thumb and first finger hold and control handpiece and second finger supports it. Lip and cheek are retracted by first and second fingers of left hand and by mirror held between thumb and first two fingers. Lower lip and tongue protected by mirror.

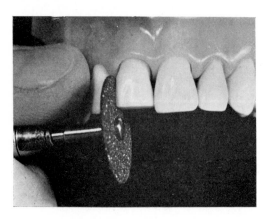

FIGURE 51.

imal cut will be completed using a taper fissure bur or fine taper stone in a contra-angle handpiece. Proximal surfaces may be reduced very rapidly and satisfactorily at accelerated speeds by using a small taper stone or a carbide bur in the contra-angle handpiece. For partial coverage on anteriors, a lingual approach is required. The danger of possibly overtapering the preparation and loss of retention remains the same.

Reducing Occlusal Surfaces

Occlusal reduction opens a space for an irregular and strong metal plate, which will connect and stabilize the circumferential segments of the retainer and protect the tooth against caries, irritation, or fracture. At the same time provision will be made for natural wear or future equilibration and for recontoured occlusal surfaces which re-establish occlusion or decrease leverage or stress on the supporting structure (Fig. 52).

Occlusal reduction can be very simple when the tooth to be prepared has been abraded so that the surface is relatively flat, and it may be complicated when the tooth has sharp cusps, prominent ridges, and deep grooves and sulci. All occlusal surfaces should be prepared to reproduce roughly the contour of the uncut surface. If the tooth is flat or abraded, a small wheel stone with a square edge will answer the purpose. If the occlusal surface is unworn, the groove pattern may be cut out with a taper fissure bur to the depth desired in the finished preparation. Stones with V-shaped cutting edges, or inverted cone or cylindrical stones, are indicated for the reduction of cusp tips and ridge planes.

Areas of contact in centric occlusion and in masticatory excursions must be observed carefully to be certain that minimal clearance has been obtained. On teeth tipped so that one or more cusps or a marginal ridge may be out of occlusion, cutting should be done only in those areas which have remained in contact or, in any position, are within 1.0 mm. of the opposing teeth.

FIGURE 52. Handpiece with water spray attachment. Position of handpiece will be rotated so that occlusal surface may be reduced to conform to contour of cusp planes.

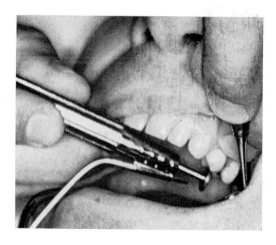

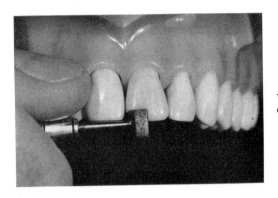

FIGURE 53. Position of stone when reducing incisal edge. Approach can be from lingual, labial, or proximal.

Reducing Incisal Edges

An incisal edge is shortened to forestall fracture of the labial enamel, to procure space for connecting and strengthening metal that later may be adjusted for equilibrium, and to provide the bulk of material or materials needed to restore the tooth to esthetic and functional form (Fig. 53).

Incisal edges may be shortened with any of a variety of wheel stones. Ideally, this cut should be at right angles to the line of force from the opposing teeth. Reduction of an upper incisal edge resembles that done on the lingual planes of buccal cusps of maxillary bicuspids and molars, while the shortening of the incisal edge on a lower anterior tooth can be compared with the same cutting operation on the buccal surface of buccal cusps of mandibular bicuspids and molars.

Preparing Convex Lingual, Labial, or Buccal Surfaces and Concave Lingual Surfaces

Reduction of the lingual surface of either a maxillary anterior or posterior tooth gives room for the metal that will absorb and dissipate forces of occlusion and connect the retentive proximal sections of the retainer (Fig. 54). It also permits the rebuilt tooth to be normal, reduced, or recontoured in size and form, and makes possible an external encircling band of metal that will increase retention, strengthen and prevent splitting of the tooth, and add substance for later abrasion and adjustment. The lingual surface of a mandibular tooth is reduced so that retention may be increased, caries inhibited, and the tooth size either maintained or reduced.

The preparation of convex lingual and labial or buccal surfaces may be done with wheel stones rotating in line with the long axis of the tooth, or with cylindrical stones cutting at right angles to the long axis. When the tooth is in normal position and is aligned with other abutment teeth, the contours of lingual and buccal reduction should be the same as, or should slightly accentuate, those of the untouched surfaces. On lingual surfaces a cylindrical stone, held parallel to and rotating at right angles to the long axis, may be preferred if it is used so that no cervical undercut will be formed and so that the occlusal half of the surface will be prepared to conform to the natural lingual contour.

Labial and buccal surfaces are cut down so that the tooth may be contained within metal to increase retention, hinder the progress of caries, decrease the chances of breaking, and supply space for veneers that will be pleasing in appearance.

Whereas the buccal surface may be prepared in the same way as the lingual, the labial surface often is prepared more easily and better with a wheel stone, either round or square, cutting parallel to the long axis. In this manner, one-half of the surface can be reduced so that depth may be gauged and the curves of the preparation defined; then the other half can be prepared with the first half serving as an example. The gross reduction of a labial surface may be done with a wheel stone, with imperfections being smoothed out with a cylindrical stone moving laterally and cutting at right angles to the long axis.

Concave lingual surfaces are prepared for the same reasons as convex lingual surfaces. Although any type of wheel stone or a cylindrical stone may be used on convex surfaces, the choice on the concave surface is restricted to a small wheel stone with a round edge, or a round stone, if the preparation is to be smooth and have a uniform depth.

Before any cutting is done on a concave lingual surface, the occlusion should be checked so that points of contact and excursion paths may be mentally diagrammed. It will be beneficial if these areas are cut to a

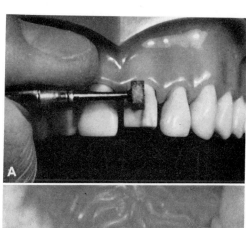

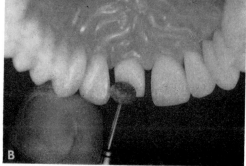

FIGURE 54. *A,* Reducing labial one-half at a time, using same stone which cut incisal.

B, Round-edge stone for lingual.

greater depth than the parts of the surface that are not in occlusion. Once again it is recommended that, like the labial surface, the concave lingual be prepared one-half at a time so that uniform reduction and contour may be more readily produced. In a tooth with deep pits or grooves in the cervical third, either a fissure or a round bur should be used for assurance that no caries has penetrated beyond the enamel fold.

Forming the Cervical Margin

The phases of reduction discussed previously will leave the tooth angular at the line angles, the occlusal margin, and along the labio-incisal, and extremely uneven at the cervical margin. Corners must be rounded in order that the measurements of the casting will be equalized and the cervical finishing line may be adjusted to the configuration of the gingival crest. (See Fig. 55.) The cervical margin must be given form, rather than an indefinite feather edge, so that patterns may be carved with exactness and castings finished precisely.

This is a critical aspect of the preparation. One of the primary points of axial reduction, requiring great care and concentration, is to produce a prepared form that will make the cervical margin of the preparation the largest diameter of the clinical crown, without the tooth being too tapered for maximal retention.

The axial line angles may be rounded and reduced with sandpaper disks or with stones having either flat or angled cutting surfaces presenting away from or toward the shank. Sandpaper disks may be used with the straight handpiece, while stones should be used with the contra-angle.

Rounding the corners and establishing the finishing line on the proximals should be completed with a taper stone in the contra-angle handpiece, one small enough in diameter to enter the space between the prepared tooth and the approximating tooth, and long enough to reach the cervical of the preparation and still extend occlusally beyond the tooth.

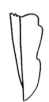 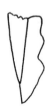 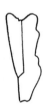 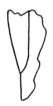 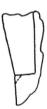

FIGURE 55. Types of finishing lines or cervical margins. Left to right: The feather edge—to be avoided since it is indefinite and makes difficult exactness in carving patterns or finishing castings; the chisel edge—satisfactory and produced very often in lingual and proximal reduction; the bevel—used where shallow caries has made it necessary to cut deeper; the chamfer—the ideal finishing line to be developed when routine preparation does not produce a chisel edge; the shoulder—for areas to be veneered and for jacket crowns. (The shoulder can be beveled. Circumferential shoulders require excessive cutting of tooth structure.)

The cervical finishing line on the buccal and lingual surfaces may be formed with a cylindrical stone having a round tip or by one of the so-called self-limiting diamonds or carbides.

Forming Shoulders

A shoulder preparation facilitates neither the fitting and seating of a casting and sealing the tooth nor the taking of an impression and polishing a seated restoration. The only aim of such extensive reduction should be to guarantee correct depth in the covering of porcelain or resin when constructing veneered and jacket crowns. Here, the tooth structure incisally or occlusally to the shoulder must be reduced an extra amount pulpally, usually about two-thirds of the width of the shoulder. When cutting a shoulder, angling the handpiece to cause an undercut at the cervical must be avoided at all costs (Figs. 56 and 57).

Before a preparation is started, it is well to consider the material that will be used in the restoration, to note its requirements for strength and esthetics, to study the radiograph for pulp size, and to calculate the width that will be needed in the shoulder and determine whether it can be secured under the existing conditions.

Shoulders may be formed with many types of stones or burs. On anterior teeth they may be cut with a straight handpiece, using crosscut or small fissure burs or cylindrical stones. Wheel stones, impregnated only on the flat edge and with smooth surfaces rotating against the tooth, may be used also. When tooth surfaces are reduced from incisal to cervical with wheel stones, the resultant cervical chamfer should be squared with any of the instruments mentioned. Shoulders must almost always be smoothed with hand instruments.

Posterior shoulders can be cut in the same way but the contra-angle handpiece will be more convenient, although a little more difficult to control.

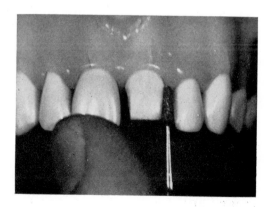

FIGURE 56. Rounding corners prior to taking tube impression and cutting shoulder.

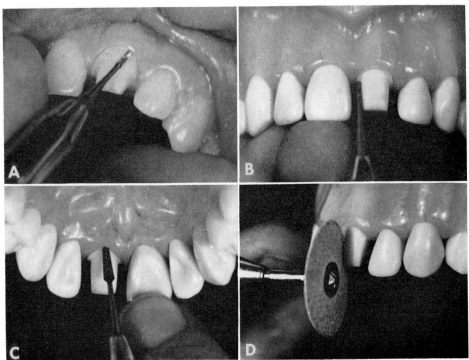

FIGURE 57.   Cutting shoulder and smoothing preparation.

Making Grooves

Grooves are used in preparations to increase resistance to displacement lingually, buccally, incisally, or occlusally; to add to the bulk of metal in the casting in such a way that it will have form to give it rigidity; and to extend auxiliary paralleled surfaces for frictional retention. Axial grooves must be parallel to the path of insertion and to each other. They must have form, length, and depth that will give maximal retention but at the same time enable the casting to seat without interference.

Grooves in anterior teeth may be made with taper or straight fissure burs, then shaped labially or buccally with sandpaper disks or files and lingually with smaller burs or files. They should terminate cervically in a flat, beveled seat. A groove running mesio-distally along the incisal edge must be cut so that the labial wall will be of enamel and dentin and approximately twice as wide as the lingual wall.

Incisal grooves provide for metal that may wear or be reduced to simulate wear, give extra protection to the labial enamel, connect the proximal struts, and stiffen the castings. They may be cut with inverted cone burs or stones and should be the same width from one proximal surface to the other.

Auxiliary grooves in posterior teeth can be made with taper or straight fissure burs; they must be parallel to the path of insertion and end in an

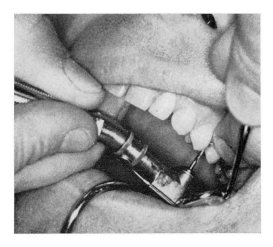

FIGURE 58. Support on incisors is obtained from third finger after second finger was placed at lingual of incisors for more versatile movement of stone or bur.

unbeveled, flat seat. (See Fig. 58.) Such grooves, customarily two or three in number, are of necessity short.

Making Ledges

Ledges, or steps, are cut to support castings under incising pressure, to create surfaces for pinholes, and to give irregularity and strength to thin castings. On the lingual surfaces of anterior teeth they should be at right angles to the long axis of the tooth rather than parallel to the incisal edge. The axial wall of a step should be parallel to the path of insertion or diverge labially from 2 to 5 degrees from the path. The ledge should be at right angles to the path of insertion and of a width calculated to perform the services to be exacted.

Ledges may be cut with cylindrical stones or straight crosscut fissure burs. A straight handpiece, as a rule, will have advantage in control and position.

Making Pinholes

A pinhole is made to accommodate a pin that may make the third leg of a tripod to resist lingual displacement, lifting, torque, or rotation around the long axis. It may be a part of any abutment preparation. The walls of a pinhole are effective as "snubbing" surfaces; also they increase the area of frictional retention.

A pinhole must be parallel to the path of insertion, and if all the retention for the casting accrues from the accumulated pinholes, its depth, and occasionally its diameter, must be increased. If it is being used in conjunction with grooves, the diameter should be large (the size of a No. 702 bur, if circumstances will permit) and from 1.0 to 2.0 mm. in depth. A pinhole for a cast pin may be made with either a taper fissure bur or a drill

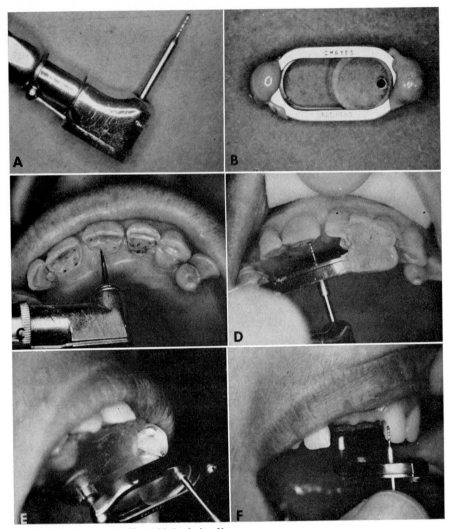

FIGURE 59. *A*, Drill 0.023 inch in diameter.

B, Loma Linda Parallelometer with modeling compound, ready to be attached to teeth for support. Disk in center, holding guiding sleeve, rotates and moves back and forth inside frame. A very effective instrument.

C, Countersinking points of entry for pinholes so that drill will not bounce, and to make the use of Parallelometer easier.

D, Drilling pinholes; lingual path of insertion.

E, Parallelometer attached to baseplate. Holes being drilled for incisal path of insertion.

F, Using Parallelometer and drill to check parallelism of groove with lingual pinholes. Equally effective in partial veneer preparations.

with parallel sides, but a No. ½ or 1 round bur will be suitable for a 24- or 22-gauge wrought wire pin.

Drills for making holes for smaller and more numerous pins have parallel sides. A popular size is 0.023 inch in diameter, but they may be procured up to 0.028 or 0.030 inch.

Section II. USING ACCELERATED TECHNIQUES

It has been established that, with the cutting instruments and equipment available during the past several decades, teeth could be well prepared to receive crowns or to support bridges, and that this could be done without clinical manifestation of any deleterious effects on the pulp. However, some of the designs for retainers and the resultant preparations entailed strenuous effort on the part of the operator, fatigue for the patient. and interminable periods of time.

With the development of rotating cutting instruments which may be used advantageously with augmented speeds,[1, 2] the trauma from many preparations, especially in the fixed partial denture field, has been dramatically reduced. While there is a school of thought which maintains that every phase of most preparations can be realized satisfactorily and safely with the faster techniques of instrumentation, it is generally accepted that the so-called high-speed reduction of tooth structure is an accessory in the correct preparation of a tooth.

At the present time there is considerable controversy as to the necessity for and the methods by which teeth may be lubricated and kept cool,[3] and much research is being done to substantiate the many deductions. The authors have seen excellent results from the "washed field" technique, but have had less experience and have been less favorably impressed with air cooling. Data on clinical cases coming from many practicing dentists suggest that with any technique caution cannot be thrown to the winds, that consideration for living tissue must be paramount, and that in those cases treated most carefully, sensitivity in teeth seldom occurs. Kasloff[4, 5, 6] has demonstrated that some instruments will cause greater checking (at least microscopically) in the enamel than others, although he does not attribute marked clinical significance to this.

An extended observation of preparations executed in what must have been the absolute minimal time would seem to indicate a larger percentage of such teeth exhibiting sensitivity following cementation of bridges,[7, 8] and an increase in the eventual number of candidates for endodontic therapy. There is no apparent advantage in striving for a routine that will eliminate from 30 seconds to 2 minutes in the preparation of a tooth. If, in order to make a preparation with finesse, an additional 5 minutes and more instrument changes are needed, and if there is evidence that because of this extra attention the preparation will be less traumatic for the tooth, the surrounding tissue, and the patient, the authors insist that *more time should be used.* The authors further believe that the suggestion that teeth

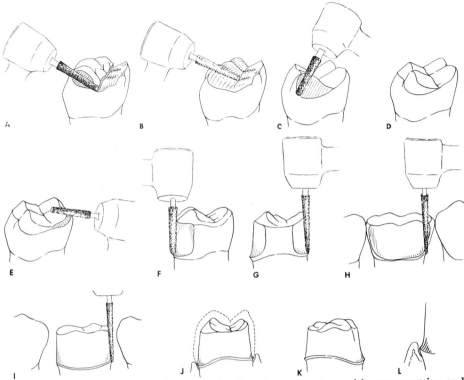

FIGURE 60. *A, B,* Reduction of occlusal surface using stone with square-cutting end. General contour of surface maintained.

  C, D, Reduction of occluding portion of buccal surface.

  E, Reducing lingual portion of lingual cusps.

  F, Cutting down buccal surface. Stone has a round tip.

  G, Lingual reduction. Stone has curved tip, less round than on buccal surface.

  H, I, Cutting through proximal surfaces and establishing cervical margin.

  J, Outline of structure cut away.

  K, L, Chamfered finishing line.

  (These drawings are based on the syllabus written and used by Dr. Harry Lundeen, School of Dentistry, University of Kentucky.)

prepared with accelerated techniques be coated with a cavity liner, such as Copalite,* immediately following the taking of an elastic impression and before the seating of temporary coverings, is worthy of consideration.

A survey conducted to determine the instrumentation for use for full crown, veneered crown, and partial veneer crown preparations showed a wide variety in instruments being used and considerable latitude in the sequence of their use. Predominating was a combination of conventional and accelerated speeds with both standard and very new rotating cutting instruments. In several of the techniques of preparation investigated, parts of the instrumentation were at speeds between 100,000 and 300,000 r.p.m. Those which in the authors' opinions produced the best results employed

---

* Harry J. Bosworth Co., Chicago, Ill.

high acceleration for gross reduction on most surfaces, reverting to speeds of 5000 r.p.m. or less for cutting grooves and pinholes and to less than 1000 r.p.m. for disking groove walls and smoothing preparations.

Included among the questions were requests for the following:

(1) sequence, name, and number of instruments used;

(2) accomplishment with each instrument; and

(3) speed at which each instrument was used.

Five of the returned questionnaires covered almost every routine and contingency.

Tables depicting the stated instrumentation used in the offices of these operators, who are in full-time practice on the east coast, in the midwest, and in the far west, will be included in the chapters on The Full Veneer Gold Crown, The Partial Veneer Crown, and The Veneered Gold Crown. These techniques have been evolved by careful and considerate practitioners who are convinced that everything must be done to safeguard living tissue and the comfort of the patient during the entire period of construction, delivery, and post-cementation.

Each of these techniques has been used by the authors or their associates with end results almost identical to those of the dentists who devel-

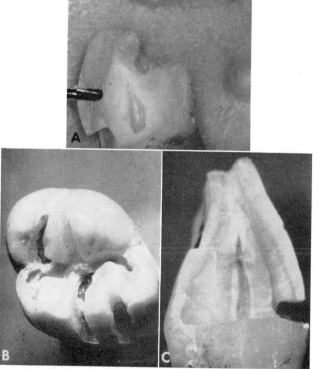

FIGURE 61. Using a bur head to establish a depth gauge for tooth preparation. (Courtesy of Drs. Robert E. Baker and Peter N. Kondon, Tufts University School of Dental Medicine.)

oped them. It is not believed that they are always suitable for use by the undergraduate student except in the final phases of instruction.

FUNDAMENTALS OF RETENTION

The fundamentals of retentive form for a prepared abutment tooth include (1) walls within 5 to 7 degrees of parallel, and grooves or pinholes to resist displacement (except along the path of insertion) and to assure friction or binding between the casting and the tooth; (2) circumferential irregularity to prevent rotation around the long axis of the crown; and (3) reduction to admit a bulk of metal capable of withstanding deformation.

In short teeth, angulation at the occluso-axial angles, as opposed to "rounding of corners," is a basic requirement. A factor not associated with preparation, but one that must be taken into account, is the height of the supporting structure of the abutments in case their long axes are not parallel. The less propitious the crown-root ratio, the more the abutment is prone to movement.[9, 10]

Grooves and pinholes, used to advance mechanical retention, must have both length and depth. Grooves must diverge cervically, and pinholes, if tapered, will ease insertion and withdrawal.

TOOTH FORM AND ITS INFLUENCE ON THE ABUTMENT PREPARATION

Tooth form often influences the choice of retainer and method of stabilization. For instance, on a short clinical crown there will not be competent frictional retention with a standard preparation; it must be supplemented by extra grooves and pinholes. A tooth with a long crown may be prepared with minimal grooving unless it is so positioned that approximate paralleling of the surfaces is impossible. A tooth which is excessively pyramidal or ovoid must be studied carefully so that the pulp will not be traumatized by reduction.[11] One that is small or frail, or one with a large pulp, usually requires extracoronal retention.

REFERENCES

1. Kilpatrick, H. C.: Ultra-speed and auxiliary equipment in fixed partial denture construction. J. Pros. Den., 10:574, May–June 1960.
2. Kilpatrick, H. C.: Recent trends in the management of pain in dentistry—the role of ultra-speed and auxiliary equipment. J. D. Med., 18:113, April 1963.
3. Peyton, F. A.: Effectiveness of water coolants with rotary cutting instruments. J.A.D.A., 56:664, May 1958.

4. Kasloff, Z.: Cracks in tooth structure associated with rotary cutting instruments. J. Den. Res., *40*:769, July–Aug. 1961 (Abstract).
5. Kasloff, Z.: Continuing study of cracks in teeth associated with various rotary cutting instruments. J. Canad. D. A., *28*:244, April 1962.
6. Kasloff, Z., Swartz, M. L., and Phillips, R. W.: In vitro method for demonstrating the effects of various cutting instruments on tooth structure. J. Pros. Den., *12*:1166, Nov.–Dec. 1962.
7. Mosteller, J. H.: The prevention of postoperative thermal sensitivity. D. Clin. North America, Nov. 1963, p. 881.
8. Wilson, H. D.: Hypersensitivity in tooth preparations. D. Survey, *36*:36, Jan. 1960.
9. Pruden, K. C.: Abutments and attachments in fixed partial dentures. J. Pros. Den., *7*:502, July 1957.
10. Adams, J. D.: Planning posterior bridges. J.A.D.A., *53*:647, Dec. 1956.
11. Brotman, I. N.: The roentgenogram as an aid in veneer crown preparation. J. Pros. Den., *4*:349, May 1954.

Kilpatrick, H. C.: High Speed and Ultra High Speed in Dentistry. Equipment and Procedures. Philadelphia, W. B. Saunders Company, 1959.
Leff, A.: Evaluation of high-speed in full coverage preparations. J. Pros. Den., *10*:314, March–April 1960.
Wheeler, R. C.: The implications of full coverage restorative procedures. J. Pros. Den., *5*:848, Nov. 1955.

5

THE FULL VENEER GOLD CROWN

The full veneer gold crown may be used as a single-unit restoration or as a retainer for a bridge. A retainer has been defined as the restoration that rebuilds the prepared abutment tooth and attaches the bridge to the abutment. In fixed partial denture construction the abutment must be reduced to accommodate the metal structure. This should be accomplished in such a way that the restored tooth will not be endangered later by disintegration of the pulp, fracture, or caries. Both the single-unit restoration and the retainer must be biologically and esthetically acceptable. Function and comfort must be introduced or continued with the seating of all restorations.

INDICATIONS

The full veneer gold crown may be placed on any tooth that cannot be returned by other means to an effective working capacity and contour. It should be used as a bridge retainer when the caries index, torque, leverage, or load contraindicates the partial veneer crown, the inlay, or the pinledge. In full mouth reconstruction, on teeth that must be splinted or that are to receive clasps or precision attachments for the support and retention of partial dentures, it is very often the restoration of choice because of its strength, long life, resistance to displacement, protection against caries, and adaptability to changes in form and occlusion. When appearance is an issue, the full veneer gold crown is indicated with a veneer of porcelain or resin. It can be overcontoured to provide maximal masticating efficiency, or undercontoured to curtail stress or to distribute it more evenly over a prosthesis. The preparation, construction, and cementation, although exacting, are not complicated procedures.[1, 2]

74

CONTRAINDICATIONS

If the occlusion is adequate, the gold crown is contraindicated in mouths in which the caries index is low or in which the prosthesis need have less than maximal retention. These conditions make it possible to use less extensive preparations. The full veneer gold crown has some minor disadvantages, such as display of metal, the impossibility of testing vitality,[1] the need for added prophylactic measures to forestall tarnish or corrosion of the metal, and the adverse effect it sometimes has on tissue, even when contoured correctly and extended carefully into the gingival crevice.

PREPARATION OF NONCARIOUS TEETH

The preparation for a full veneer gold crown should cause no harm to the pulp when it is properly done, but it is a dangerous procedure if carelessly performed by an unprincipled operator. Rapid preparation may have grave consequences unless the tooth is lubricated and its temperature controlled. Gingival tissue can be insulted beyond the point of repair, not only during preparation and at the time of its displacement for taking impressions, but also under temporary coverage.

If the crown to be constructed will serve as a bridge retainer, the diagnostic casts should be surveyed with the analyzing rod so that a path of insertion, compatible with all the abutment teeth, can be pictured. A full veneer crown preparation can deviate from the ideal more than other types and still retain the casting. Often, because of long-axis variables of the abutments, it will have walls that converge grossly.

The operator must be adroit when making this preparation so that construction and seating will not be jeopardized by an undercut, which may be formed in one of three ways. When the walls converge cervically toward the path of insertion, the retainer cannot be seated. If the long axis of the preparation diverges from the path of insertion, causing the cervical on the mesial or distal of the preparation to be in an undercut area, the fabricated prosthesis will not go into place even though the proximal walls are parallel or converge occlusally. A third type of undercut could be a depression in a wall surface of the preparation.

A prescribed sequence of steps and a predetermined goal for each step are beneficial in any operation. One method for the full veneer gold crown preparation will be presented at this time.[3] Other plans, utilizing accelerated speeds, are equally effectual[4] and will be outlined.

Mesial and Distal Surfaces.   Step 1 is the reduction of the mesial and distal surfaces. This can be done in a normal situation with diamond or carborundum disks in the straight handpiece. After the demands of the path of insertion have been weighed, these cuts will be started on or just

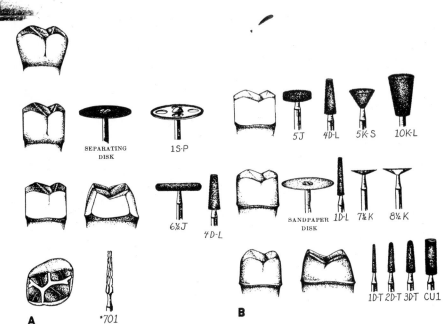

FIGURE 62. Preparation on a molar with cutting instruments suitable for each step. (Numbered stones are Densco diamonds.)

A, Top to bottom: Uncut tooth; proximal slices; facial and lingual reduction; first phase of occlusal reduction.

B, Top to bottom: Occlusal reduction; rounded angles; chamfered finishing line and softened occlusal angles.

inside the marginal ridges on the occlusal surface (Fig. 62*A*) and should extend in a direct line to the gingival crest without producing convexities or concavities in the walls. Although the preparation normally narrows about 5 degrees occlusally along the path of insertion, the long-axis inclination may make more convergence necessary.

Facial and Lingual Surfaces. Step 2 is a reduction of the facial and lingual surfaces. On the buccal surface of both upper and lower teeth and on the lingual of uppers in accurate alignment, it should follow the surface convexities and usually should be made 1.0 mm. deep. The preparation on the lingual surface of mandibular teeth must be congruous with the path of insertion. Buccal and lingual reductions must continue to the gingival line, to the cervical line, or (preferably) cervically to Class V caries or restorations. Tooth position and type may hinder the cervical finishing line on the lingual surface of some lower posterior teeth from going into the gingival crevice.

Occlusal Surface. Steps 3 and 4: The first phase of occlusal reduction is done in the occlusal grooves with a No. 700 or 701 bur and is made 1.0 mm. deep. If caries has penetrated the enamel fold, it must be eliminated. The prepared grooves will regulate the depth of additional cutting on the occlusal surface and also will ensure room for sufficient metal in the central area. If the over-all reduction is 1.0 mm. deep and if it follows the contour of the cusp planes (Fig. 63); the casting will have greater security against movement because there will be broad, semiflat surfaces to oppose forces from many directions.

When the crowned tooth will support a clasp, the marginal ridge under the occlusal rest must be cut down enough to allow depth in the metal for the occlusal rest seat. The area of extra reduction should go about 1.4 mm. in all directions beyond the periphery of the rest seat (Fig. 64).

Cervical Margin. In step 5, the line angles are rounded until the four "corner" cervical areas complement the gingival finishing line (Fig. 62B). All angulation should be removed. This can be done with a coarse sandpaper disk or a long taper diamond stone. With the special "push" and "pull" stones that have been designed for this step, there is often a tendency to overreduce the angles and thus make the preparation too conical.

A chamfer must be developed when a natural chisel-edge does not occur at the cervical finishing line. This concave bevel should be about 0.4 mm. in width and from 0.5 to 1.0 mm. under the gingival margin. It is advantageous if the finishing line can be at the height of contour on both the buccal and lingual surfaces of upper posterior teeth and the buccal surface

FIGURE 63. Proper reduction of buccal and lingual surfaces of a posterior tooth results in relatively parallel surfaces in the cervical one-third. When a preparation follows the anatomical form of the tooth on the occlusal, there will be greater length than can be obtained by making the surface flat. Reduction along line AB would make the preparation unnecessarily short around the periphery and too shallow in the central groove area. If the tooth were reduced to the line CD, the central groove and fossa would be correct in depth, but the over-all preparation would be even shorter and would encroach upon the pulp.

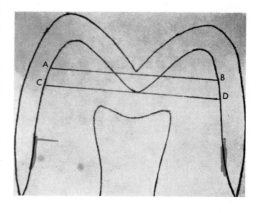

FIGURE 64. Change in occlusal preparation to make space for rest seat.

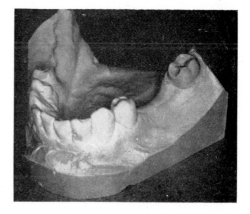

of lowers. However, tooth position and contour, the occluso-cervical length of the clinical crown, gingival recession, or cervical caries may compel a relocation of the cervical margin. The chamfer may be made quickly on the buccal and lingual and at the line angles with a No. 2D-T or 3D diamond stone, while on the proximal surfaces a No. 1D-T diamond stone may be used.

Preparing Teeth with Long, Medium, or Short Crowns

In the preparation of teeth with long crowns, there is an inclination to form cervical undercuts on the distal surfaces. If the handpiece and the disk are not moved cervically simultaneously, the cutting edge of the disk will move in an arc, causing an inward deviation from the path of insertion in the cervical area. This error seldom can be rectified without inordinate reduction of the tooth in the middle and occlusal thirds. The resultant thickness of metal in the crown may provoke sensitivity. The angle at the junction of the occlusal and axial walls should be rounded, since it is not needed to provide stability for the casting.

On crowns of medium length, cuts can be visualized and executed, and line angles rounded easily. Here also the occluso-axial angles should be softened to facilitate taking impressions, fitting and investing patterns, and seating castings, and to make room for more metal in an area susceptible to wear.

Often the crown of the short tooth is conical and the preparation will taper occlusally so much that only slight mechanical retention can be obtained. The occluso-axial angles should be left sharp on such a tooth (Fig. 65). Grooves must be cut on the buccal or lingual surface, parallel with the opposite surface or path of insertion. Using a No. 701 or 702 bur, pinholes 1.5 mm. deep can be placed in the occlusal surface immediately under the cusp tips, or a well can be prepared using the occlusal grooves as a pattern. This should be not less than 1.0 mm. deep and may be made with a No. 558, 559, or 702 bur.

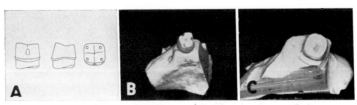

FIGURE 65.   Preparations on medium and short teeth.
A, Occlusal pinholes and axial grooves.
B, Axial grooves.
C, Occlusal well used to increase retention and stability on short teeth.

Preparing Teeth with Gingival Recession

When the cementoenamel junction is exposed, the constriction at the neck of the tooth and predisposition to cervical caries will determine whether the preparation should be moved onto the cementum and into the gingival crevice. This is salutary unless the tooth must be cut so much that some pulp injury may occur.

PREPARATION OF CARIOUS TEETH

When cervical caries is present, the involved structure should be replaced by amalgam or gold (Fig. 66). The final preparation should go cervically beyond the margin of such a restoration, although if this is not feasible because of the eminent dipping of the cervical outline, the margin may rest on the metal.

When a filled or mutilated tooth is to be prepared to receive a full veneer gold crown, the series of steps will differ in some respects from that employed in preparing a sound tooth. All amalgam, gold, cement, and carious tissue should be removed, and the walls and occlusal surface that remain should be prepared in the same way and in the same order as for the noncarious tooth. The tooth is then built to prepared form with amalgam or a gold casting.[5]

The Cast Core

If a casting is to be used, the margins of remaining walls are paralleled or undercuts are removed. Three, four, or five pinholes are placed in the dentin with a taper fissure bur or a drill to a depth of 1.5 or 2.0 mm. The pattern can be carved direct, using wax or plastic pins, or an indirect procedure may be used.

Every effort should be made to have the wax pattern free from distortion and the casting fit with the exactness of an inlay. After it has been cemented, the cervical margin and all other details of the preparation should be perfected. (See Chapter 10.)

The Pin-retained Amalgam Core

Markley[6, 7] has devised an effective method for reinforcing and retaining amalgam cores with threaded steel wire pins (Fig. 67), which has advantages comparable to those of the cast core. By this means also, mutilated or extensively carious vital or pulpless teeth with good root structure can be built to prepared form for either single-unit restorations or bridge retainers. When caries has penetrated close to the pulp,[8] that area should

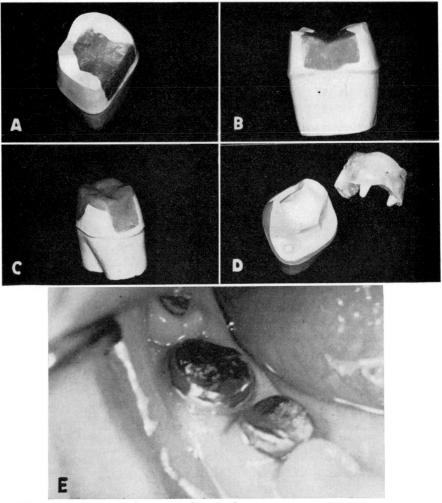

FIGURE 66.   Preparations on carious teeth.

A, Rebuilding tooth to prepared form with amalgam.

B, Preparation should extend, if possible, beyond junction of metal and tooth.

C, Rebuilding tooth to prepared form with gold casting.

D, Casting removed, showing two posts and proximal step.

E, Two teeth rebuilt to prepared form with castings. Remaining tooth structure was exposed by gingivectomy.

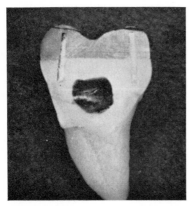

FIGURE 67.   Cross section of molar and two cemented steel pins. Two of eight pins which, through threading and irregular alignment, substantially support and retain alloy restoration.

be insulated against thermal shock with one of the calcium hydroxide-type base materials, a layer of cement, and routinely an application of Copalite cavity varnish.[9] Cement in bulk should be avoided.[10]

Drilling Pinholes. Twist drills,* 0.027 or 0.024 inch in diameter, depending on the size of the tooth, are used in a contra-angle handpiece.

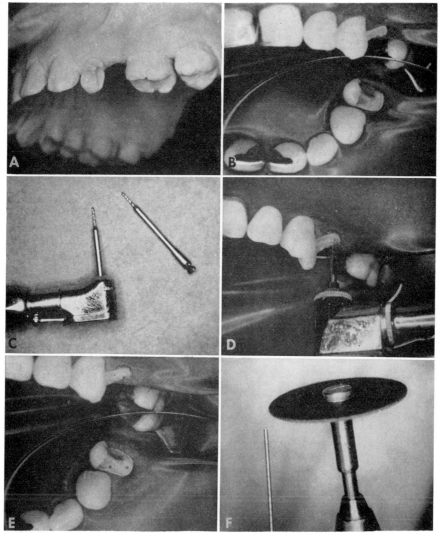

FIGURE 68. *A,* Fractured maxillary bicuspid to be built to prepared form for a veneered gold crown retainer.

B, Tooth explored and caries removed.

C, Twist drills 0.027 inch in diameter.

D, Drilling holes using water and air as a lubricant. Heavy rubber dam in position.

E, Tooth prepared for pins.

F, Wire being squared on end. It was notched irregularly before being cut to length.

---

* Star Dental Mfg. Co., Inc., Philadelphia, Penna.

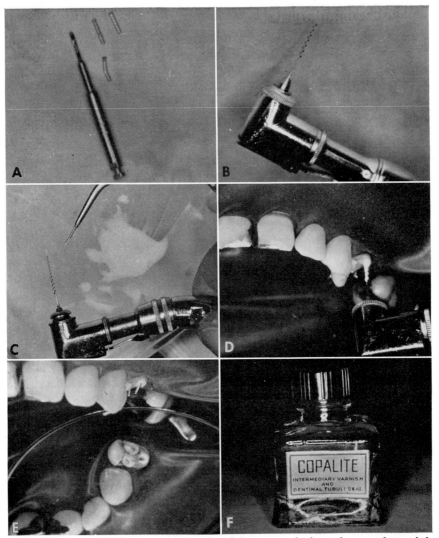

FIGURE 69. *A*, Drill, three cut pins. One is bent to make it conform to the peripheral outline of preparation. Pins protruding through the amalgam are not easily smoothed to surface of preparation.

B, Spiral for carrying cement into pinhole.

C, Spiral and pin, each carrying cement. Pin is held with grooved pliers.

D, Spinning cement into hole.

E, Pins cemented. Excess will be broken off.

F, Copalite varnish used on exposed dentin.

The holes, carefully located by viewing radiographs and with a knowledge of tooth anatomy to avoid the pulp or perforation of the outside root surface or bifurcation walls, are drilled from 2.0 to 4.0 mm. into the dentin. The holes need not be parallel; in fact, the pins will be more retentive if they are not. A speed of not more than 1000 r.p.m. is recommended, with a stream of air as a coolant. The drill should be removed from the hole frequently to clean out the debris (Fig. 68).

Preparing Pins.   Threaded stainless steel wire* 0.025 to 0.022 inch in diameter, is used for the pins. The end of the wire is made square, the edge rounded, and is then cut to correct length for the individual hole. When pins have been seated in the several holes (from 5 to 9), some may require bending to conform to the periphery of the prepared form anticipated. Cotton plier beaks may be grooved to make handling easier.

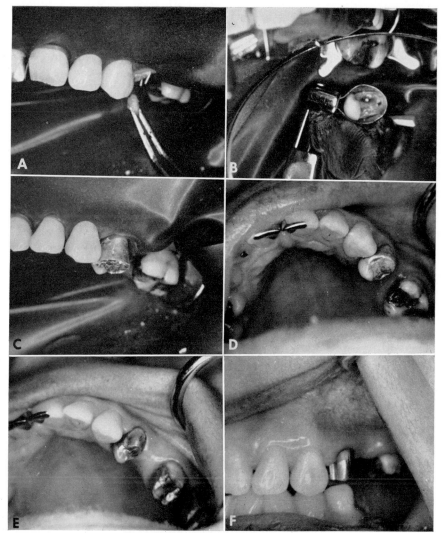

FIGURE 70.   *A,* Applying Copalite to exposed cut surface.

B, Adapting band and supporting modeling compound. Steel band must be well stabilized.

C, Rebuilt tooth after matrix was removed.

D, Alloy trimmed.

E, F, Tooth prepared.

* K and R Dental Products Co., Blue Island, Ill.

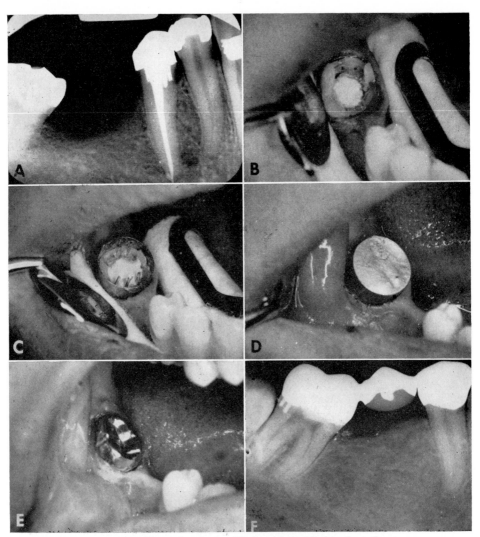

FIGURE 71. *A*, Radiograph of mandibular bicuspid showing pins.
B, Mandibular molar showing five pinholes.
C, Copper band fitted—rubber dam and modeling compound reinforcement were used.
D, Compound and dam removed. Band still in place.
E, Tooth prepared.
F, Radiograph of bridge.
(Illustrations *B*, *C*, *D*, *E*, and *F* through the courtesy of Dr. William Hohlt.)

Cementing Pins. A shortened lentulo-spiral, designed for filling root canals with medicaments, should be used to carry cement into the pinholes (Fig. 69*B*). Mixing should be on a cold slab. One pin at a time is removed, and the cement is carried into the pinhole with the revolving spiral while an assistant coats the pin with cement. The pin, held by the grooved pliers, is repositioned in the hole. If air is trapped and the pin fails to seat, the process is repeated. Excess cement is removed after setting.

The Matrix. A heavy rubber dam is placed on the tooth. The matrix may be a copper band or adjusted steel band contoured to a snug fit around the cervical of the remaining tooth structure and competently supported by modeling compound (Fig. 70*B*).

Condensing the Amalgam. Small condensers, 1.0 mm. or less in diameter (Wesco-Mortenson #2), should be used to insert the amalgam. This phase must be done *thoroughly*, to eliminate any voids. Several mixes

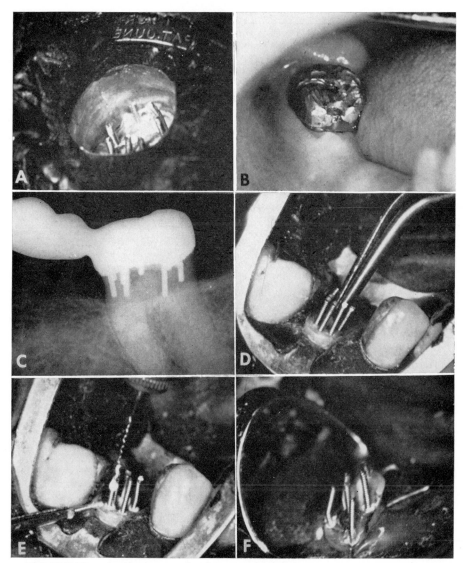

FIGURE 72. *A*, Pins cemented prior to packing.
B, Rebuilt tooth.
C, Radiograph of abutment.
D, Pins fitted prior to cementing.
E, Cementing pins.
F, Pins cemented and contoured to dimension of finished preparation.
(These illustrations through the courtesy of Drs. Markley and Going.)

of amalgam will be required for bulk and consistency. After placing the alloy, the compound and matrix are removed.

Completing the Preparation

Markley recommends shaping the tooth to prepared form immediately, but the authors have found that final preparation of the tooth is facilitated if the alloy is given time to set. This may take place under any kind of temporary covering, which is positioned and trimmed to push away the gingival tissue slightly, in order to afford better access for establishing the cervical margin and finishing the preparation with either diamonds, carbides, or disks.[11]

Smith[12] has designed a set of self-limiting diamond cutting instruments that make it possible to displace the gingival tissue and extend the full veneer gold crown preparation evenly into the gingival crevice. Stones may be obtained for either the chisel-edge or chamfer finishing line. (See CU series, Fig. 40, Chapter 3.)

ROUTINES FOR PREPARATIONS AT ACCELERATED SPEEDS

There are many widely accepted routines for preparing teeth for full veneer gold crowns that include accelerated speeds. Several of these, frequently used by the authors, will be listed in table form.

POSTERIOR TEETH

Table 1

INSTRUMENT	TO BE ACCOMPLISHED	R.P.M.
71L Premier "Ela" carbide	Complete axial and occlusal reduction. Location and contour of cervical margin.	150,000
70L Premier "Ela" carbide	(When there is an approximating tooth, a 70L premier "Ela" carbide is used to cut from either buccal or lingual to break the contact and simultaneously reduce the proximal surface.)	150,000
4D Densco diamond	Irregularities smoothed and sharp angles rounded.	8,000 to 10,000
Note: Round burs, steel fissure burs, spoon excavators, hatchets, chisels	Removal of caries, if present. Cement or amalgam smoothed if used to build tooth to prepared form.	Slow speeds

Table 2

INSTRUMENT	TO BE ACCOMPLISHED	R.P.M.
701L R&R carbide	Gross buccal, lingual, and occlusal reduction.	150,000
700L R&R carbide	Proximal surface reduction.	150,000
Safe-side disk (any brand)	Proximal surface reduction (when a 700L carbide cannot be used).	6,000
1D-T Densco diamond	Location and contour of cervical margin.	150,000
Sandpaper disks (any brand)	Irregularities smoothed and sharp angles rounded.	Slow speeds

Table 3

INSTRUMENT	TO BE ACCOMPLISHED	R.P.M.
2D Densco diamond	Complete axial reduction.	200,000 (approx.)
¾D Densco diamond	(When there is an approximating tooth, a ¾D Densco diamond is used to cut from either buccal or lingual to break the contact and simultaneously reduce the proximal surface.)	200,000
123 SSW diamond	Occlusal reduction.	200,000
116 SSW diamond	Location and contour of cervical margin.	200,000
1D-T Densco diamond (worn) or 44 SSW carborundum stone	Irregularities smoothed.	200,000 or 3,000

Table 4

INSTRUMENT	TO BE ACCOMPLISHED	R.P.M.
701 R&R carbide	Buccal, lingual, and occlusal reduction.	150,000
700 or 699 R&R carbide	Proximal surface reduction.	150,000
1D-T or 1D-C Densco diamond	Peripheral finish and location and contour of cervical margin.	150,000

Table 5

INSTRUMENT	TO BE ACCOMPLISHED	R.P.M.
701 or 701-L Densco carbide	Complete axial and occlusal reduction. Location and preparation of cervical shoulder.	150,000 to 200,000
1D Densco diamond	Irregularities smoothed and shoulder finished.	150,000 to 200,000
Sandpaper disks (any brand)	Irregularities smoothed and sharp angles rounded.	500 to 1,000

Before the prepared teeth are covered, impressions for the working casts, a face-bow registration, and an occlusion registration must be taken. These are discussed in Chapter 10, The Working Cast.

TEMPORARY PROTECTION

A vital tooth that has been prepared for a full veneer gold crown must be shielded at all times (Fig. 73). The temporary covering must keep it free from contact with saliva and food debris and must be contoured to block extrusion or lateral movement.

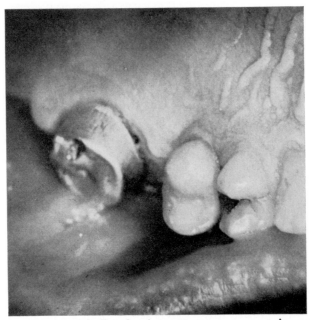

FIGURE 73.   Aluminum shell and resin temporary crown covering prepared teeth.

Aluminum Shells and Resin Crown Forms

An aluminum shell, slightly larger in circumference than the cervical of the preparation, should be trimmed to conform to the contour of the gingival margin and to rest on the occlusal surface of the preparation without displacement of, and about 0.5 mm. short of, the gingival tissue. Aluminum shells are pliable and can be manipulated or ground to integrate with the opposing teeth. When a resin crown form is in position, it should be in alignment without displacing the soft tissue.

Temporary stopping, when used inside either an aluminum shell or a resin crown form, serves well as a protective cover for a prepared tooth. The shell, filled with heated stopping, must be forced onto the tooth far enough for the preparation to be covered and for the occlusion to be comfortable.

The shell is removed, and after the cervical excess of stopping has been trimmed so that no blanching of the soft tissue will occur, the temporary covering is replaced and the stopping going into the gingival crevice is smoothed and adapted to the tooth with a warm instrument. The crown is removed and the inside is cleaned, dried, and moistened with eugenol or a cavity varnish before being returned to the isolated and dried tooth. If the period of construction is not overlong, the temporary crown will safeguard the tooth and keep it in position. Zinc oxide and eugenol paste is used instead of stopping, and probably more often, but it does not displace tissue.

Temporary crowns can also be constructed with a self-curing tooth-colored resin. These should be considered particularly for use on bicuspids or anteriors. Resin crowns may be sealed with zinc oxide and eugenol or cavity varnish. However, on teeth with limited retention, zinc phosphate cement can be more effective.

Construction of a Temporary Resin Crown or Bridge

Adequate temporary resin crowns can be made over a stone die or on the prepared tooth. In either instance the stump should be lubricated. Before the preparation was made, an alginate or rubber impression (of the tooth, quadrant, or arch, as the case may be) should have been taken and stored in a humidifier. The areas in the impression covering the teeth that have been prepared are filled with self-curing resin, and the impression is reseated in the mouth or on the cast. Before the resin has polymerized beyond the semiplastic stage, the impression and resin must be taken from the mouth or cast and the resin lifted from the impression or removed from the teeth. The rough, temporary crown can then be trimmed, shaped, and adjusted for occlusion. Polishing can be done after seating with a temporary luting material. (See Figs. 74 and 75.)

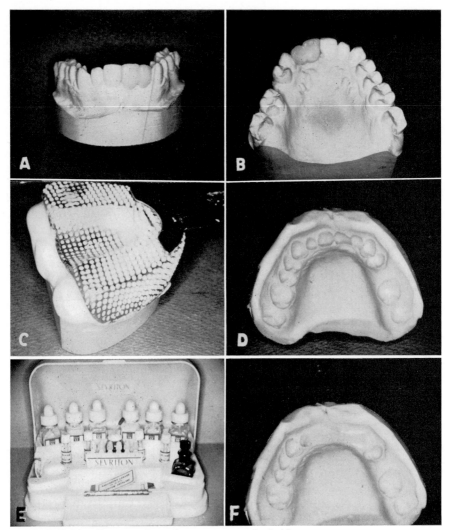

FIGURE 74.   Construction of temporary resin bridge or crown.
A, B, Diagnostic cast with pontics in wax.
C, D, Impression of cast.
E, Material used for temporary bridge.
F, Resin placed in impression.

A temporary resin crown may be built in advance over a simulated preparation made on the stone diagnostic cast. Before seating it must be machined inside and either trimmed or, with added resin, recontoured to length.

For an edentulous space, wax pontics should be built on the diagnostic cast and an alginate impression taken over the stone and wax. The temporary bridge is then constructed by filling the prepared teeth and pontic areas with self-curing resin and seating the impression on a duplicate or simulated plaster cast of the prepared arch.[13, 14] Removal, trimming, and polishing follow the technique employed for the temporary single unit.[15, 16]

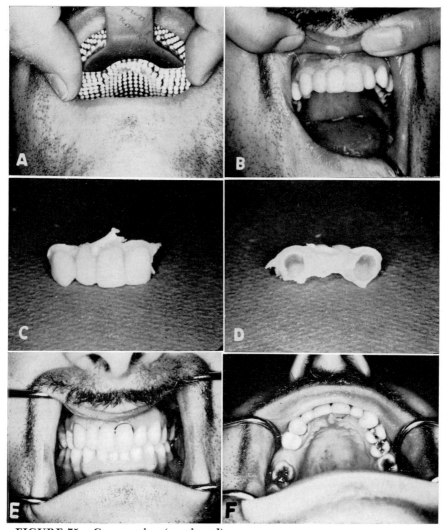

FIGURE 75. Construction (continued).

A, Filled impression seated in mouth. Abutments were lubricated. There is slightly more difficulty in correctly seating impression in mouth but time is saved. Heat generated by most materials suitable for temporary bridges does not seem to overstimulate the pulp.

B, Before removal for trimming.

C, *D*, Bridge removed.

E, *F*, Temporary bridge trimmed and seated with temporary cement over lightly lubricated teeth.

THE WAX OCCLUSION REGISTRATION

Before placing the covering on the tooth, an occlusion registration is sometimes made by using softened inlay wax to cover the occlusal, mesial, and distal surfaces and partially to cover the buccal or lingual of the preparation. When this has been placed on the occlusal surface, the patient should be asked to close in centric occlusion and to open immediately.

After compressing the wax against the occlusal, buccal, and lingual surfaces, the patient is instructed to close again and to hold this position until the wax has become rigid. The wax registration, which is better made on the working cast, will furnish a pattern on the die for occlusal carving and for thickness in the contact area between the preparation and the approximating tooth. Adding wax to the "bite" to build the pattern to contour must be done meticulously, or the finished casting will have flaws and potentially weak areas.

The die and working cast should be constructed by the methods described in Chapter 10, The Working Cast.

REFERENCES

1. Smith, G. P.: What is the place of the full crown in restorative dentistry? Am. J. Orthodont. &. Oral Surg., *33:*471, June 1947.
2. Wheeler, R. C.: The implications of full coverage restorative procedures. J. Pros. Den., *5:*848, Nov. 1955.
3. Thom, L. W.: Principles of cavity preparation in crown and bridge prosthesis. I. The full crown. J.A.D.A., *41:*284, Sept. 1950.
4. Barker, B. C. W.: Restoration of nonvital teeth with crowns. Austral. D. J., *8:*191, June 1963.
5. Kuratli, J.: Restoration of broken-down vital teeth for fixed partial denture abutments. J. Pros. Den., *8:*504, May 1958.
6. Markley, M. R.: Pin reinforcement and retention of amalgam foundations and restorations. J.A.D.A., *56:*675, May 1958.
7. Markley, M. R.: Restorations of silver amalgam. J.A.D.A., *43:*133, Aug. 1951.
8. Silberkweit, M., Massler, M., Schour, I., and Weinmann, J. P.: Effects of filling materials on the pulp. J. D. Res., *34:*854, Dec. 1955.
9. Going, R. E., and Massler, M.: Influence of cavity liners under amalgam restorations on penetration by radioactive isotopes. J. Pros. Den., *11:*298, March–April 1961.
10. Volland, R., et al.: Zinc phosphate cement. J.A.D.A., *22:*1281, Aug. 1935.
11. Wheeler, R. C.: Complete crown form and the periodontium. J. Pros. Den., *11:*722, July–Aug. 1961.
12. Smith, G. P.: The marginal fit of the full cast shoulderless crown. J. Pros. Den., *7:*231, March 1957.
13. Freese, A. S.: Impressions for temporary acrylic resin jacket crowns. J. Pros. Den., *7:*99, Jan. 1957.
14. Rubinstein, M. N.: Immediate acrylic temporary crown and bridge. D. Digest, *60:*12, Jan. 1954.
15. Segat, L.: Protection of prepared abutments between appointments in crown and bridge prosthodontics. J. Michigan D. A., *44:*32, Feb. 1962.
16. Taylor, A. G.: Temporary protection of prepared abutment teeth. Roy. Canad. D. Corps Quar., *2:*8, Oct. 1961.

Caplan, J.: Maintenance of full coverage fixed-abutment bridges. J. Pros. Den., *5:*852, Nov. 1955.
Hoffman, J. M.: Common problems in the construction of the full cast crown. J.A.D.A., *48:*272, March 1954.
Kilpatrick, H. C.: Ultra-speed and auxiliary equipment in fixed partial denture construction. J. Pros. Den., *10:*574, May–June 1960.

Lyon, D. M.: Abutments in fixed prosthesis. Arkansas D. J., *24*:6, Dec. 1953.

McCabe, D. J., and Rinne, V. W.: Treatment of carious teeth. Disadvantages of full coverage. D. Clin. North America, Nov. 1960, p. 639.

Murto, C. B.: Modern bridge retainers. J. Ontario D. A., *33*:15, Feb. 1956.

Shooshan, E. D.: Full veneer cast crown. J. South. California D. A., *23*:27, Sept. 1955.

Smith, G. P.: Full crown preparation. New York J. Den., *26*:307, Oct. 1956.

Stone, E.: Gingivectomy and crown preparation in occluso-rehabilitation. J. Pros. Den., *8*:640, July 1958.

Tanner, H.: Ideal and modified inlay and veneer crown preparations. Illinois D. J.. *26*:240, April 1957.

6

THE PARTIAL VENEER CROWN

The partial veneer, or three-quarter crown, is used primarily as a bridge retainer but may be used, in combination with resin or silicate cement, as a single-unit restoration on a fractured tooth. It normally covers the proximal, lingual, and occlusal surfaces or incisal edge of the tooth, with the buccal or labial surface being untouched except along the bucco-occlusal or labio-incisal margin. (See Fig. 5.) When conditions permit minimal buccal or labial extension, the esthetic result will be in accord with the most discriminating taste.[1-4]

INDICATIONS AND CONTRAINDICATIONS

This retainer, which demands far less cutting of the tooth than the veneered gold crown, will provide retention for the fixed prosthesis when there is a good axial relationship to the path of insertion, when the clinical crown of the tooth is of average length, and when there is dentin connecting the tooth walls. If an abutment tooth is well supported and if the crown is long and sturdy, the partial veneer crown can be used on the anterior end of a prosthesis supplying as many as three posterior teeth.

It is indicated particularly on maxillary centrals, cuspids, and bicuspids, and on mandibular cuspids and second bicuspids. Usually these teeth have proximal surfaces that can be reduced to assure ample thickness in the casting to resist deformation from the occlusion, and grooved to assure retention of the bridge. The metal over the reduced lingual surfaces will have irregular form and rigidity.

Occasionally it is possible to restore a broken-down vital upper cuspid to prepared form with a pin-retained casting and, using another path of seating, to place a partial veneer crown over the reconstructed tooth. This

94

infrequent preparation can be employed after caries has occurred around and under some other kind of retainer, resulting in a weakened labial wall with too little bulk for a veneered gold crown.

Square tooth form is a requisite to the most satisfactory application of this retainer. Gold is most often seen when the partial veneer crown preparation is made on teeth that are ovoid, tapered, or conical, and on anterior teeth with proximal caries, but generally this can be avoided. Some patients do not object, but if there will be an unsightly exhibition of metal, the veneered gold crown should be considered instead.

The partial veneer crown cannot routinely be adapted as successfully to lower first bicuspids and to upper lateral incisors and first molars. Crown forms of mandibular first bicuspids are often unfavorable for preparations that will furnish retention without an obvious show of metal. Pleasing appearance on many maxillary lateral incisors cannot be attained without very deep linguo-proximal reduction. The marginal line of the partial veneer crown on the maxillary first molar is very long and the form of the pattern makes casting critical. Since this tooth is not often noticeable, a less complicated retainer should be built. It may be used on mandibular molars which, owing to malrelationship with the approximating teeth, are not suitable for the full veneer gold crown preparation. While mandibular incisors will accept this preparation, many times the lingual surface of the retainer must be overcontoured.

Partial veneer crowns are contraindicated on (1) short teeth, teeth grossly carious, and (excepting lower molars) those which have a poor long-axis relationship with the path of insertion; (2) upper cuspids that have long incisal arms, contact areas at the gingival margin, and very short mesial and distal surfaces (because grooves in such surfaces will not hold the prosthesis); (3) teeth too small or thin for accurate positioning and cutting of the proximal grooves; (4) teeth in which there is extensive cervical caries, since the grooves would extend into partially disintegrated tooth structure; and (5), because of the long marginal line, in mouths in which the caries index is high. The partial veneer crown cannot be used advantageously on many of the extreme forms of upper lateral incisors because of the difficulty in making or paralleling grooves.

PREPARATION OF A MAXILLARY CENTRAL INCISOR

A preparation that affords greater potentialities and the expectation of fewer corrections can be accomplished in shorter time if the sequence of steps and the instrumentation are standardized. The principles and procedures that will be described first in this chapter have been used for years and have been discussed by many authors.[5-8] Other designs and approaches to partial veneer preparations, which are equally meritorious and have essentially the same principles of retention and fixation, will be included.

After a survey of the diagnostic cast has determined the most logical path of insertion for the involved teeth, the labial outlines of the proximal cuts, paralleling the path of insertion, should be drawn on the central incisor of the cast. The exposure of metal on the labial surface will depend to some degree on the lingual convergence of the proximal surfaces, proximal caries, if present, the contour of the labial surface, and the amount of metal necessary to prevent deformation.

With this picture in mind, the tooth can be prepared in the following manner:

(1) reduction of the mesial and distal surfaces;

(2) reduction of the lingual surface from the middle of the cingulum to the incisal edge of the tooth;

(3) beveling the incisal edge and cutting the incisal groove;

(4) penciling the mesial and distal grooves parallel to the previously planned path of insertion;

(5) cutting the mesial and distal grooves;

(6) reduction of the cingulum area;

(7) beveling the labial walls of the mesial, distal, and incisal grooves;

(8) rounding the lingual walls of the mesial and distal grooves and finishing the cervical margin; and

(9) sinking a pinhole in the cingulum, parallel to the proximal grooves.

Mesial and Distal Surfaces

The proximal cuts can be made using a disk in a straight handpiece (Fig. 76). These should converge lingually a little more than the mesial and distal surfaces and should extend from the incisal edge to the gingival line unless the tooth is too angular or the gingiva has receded beyond the cementoenamel junction. The preparation should not continue beyond the line angles on the labial.* On any surface made more prominent through rotation, the labial margin must be kept to the lingual so that the finished casting will be inconspicuous. Often adjacent teeth must be separated and a thin steel disk used to prevent the labial surface from being cut beyond the desired point.

Lingual Surface

By using a No. 2½J diamond stone in the straight handpiece, the lingual surface should be reduced uniformly to a depth of 0.7 mm., from

---

* The labial "line angle" is assumed to be the junction of the labial and proximal surfaces. It is an imaginary line slightly to the labial of the contact area, following the height of convexity produced by the merging of the labial and proximal surfaces.

the crest of the cingulum to the incisal edge. Where contact is made with opposing teeth, in centric closure and along the paths of eccentric excursions, the depth should be at least 1.0 mm.

Incisal Bevel and Groove

The bevel on the incisal edge may be made with the same instrument used on the lingual or with a No. 5J-T flat-edge wheel. It should be approximately at right angles to the line of force against the linguo-incisal of the tooth, the same width from mesial to distal, and have a clearance of 1.0 mm. at the lingual margin and 0.25 mm. at the labial margin of the bevel. The labial margin of the bevel should simulate the uncut incisal edge of the tooth.

The incisal groove can be cut using a No. 37 inverted cone bur in a straight handpiece. The labial wall should be twice as wide as the lingual wall in order to throw the apex of the groove toward the lingual surface of the tooth, leaving dentin to support the labial wall of enamel. This will avert discoloration of the tooth when the casting is cemented. When the incisal edge has been abraded markedly, because of powerful thrusts from opposing teeth, a deeper groove is required.

The incisal groove is an integral feature of this preparation. It makes room for metal, which will add to the rigidity of the casting and impede its springing away from the proximals, and furnishes gold for future incisal equilibration.

Proximal Grooves

The directional line of the parallel proximal grooves, coordinated with the plane of the incisal two-thirds of the labial surface, should be penciled on the tooth. In a majority of instances, the grooves can be so placed and thus can be longer, can terminate in cleansable areas, will institute more circumferential retention against lingual displacement, and will exact the least reduction of the labial enamel.

Using a No. 700 taper fissure bur, an indentation is made in the proximal surface at the incisal groove. With this as a point of stabilization, the groove is cut along the pencil line to a depth matching the greatest diameter of the bur. Often it will be impossible for the groove to reach the gingival crevice without excessive cutting. Parallelism to the path of insertion will be expedited if the first groove is cut on the surface next to the edentulous area (see Fig. 76B).

Cingulum

The cingulum must be decreased about 1.0 mm. by use of a cylindrical

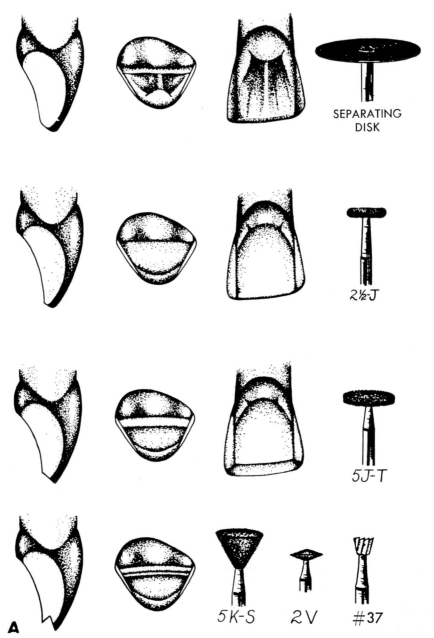

SEPARATING
DISK

2½-J

5J-T

5K-S   2V   #37

A

FIGURE 76.   Preparation on a maxillary central incisor with cutting instruments suitable for each step. (Numbered stones are Densco diamonds.)

A, Top to bottom: Proximal slices; lingual surface; incisal bevel; incisal groove.

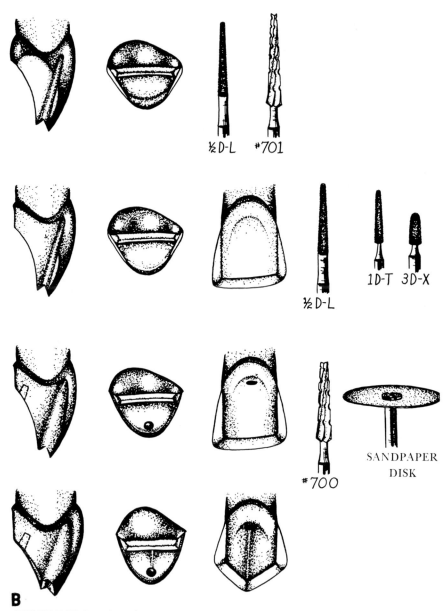

FIGURE 76 (*continued*).   *B*, Top to bottom: Proximal grooves; cingulum reduction; beveling labial walls of all grooves; cervical finishing line and pinhole in cingulum. Preparation on maxillary cuspid.

or tapered round-tip stone in the contra-angle handpiece. Theoretically, the lingual wall should be parallel to the proximal grooves, but this creates a lingual shoulder, which should be avoided.

Bevel and Finishing Line

Using sandpaper disks in a straight handpiece, the labial wall of the incisal groove should be made smooth, being certain that the mesio- and disto-incisal angles are beveled so that the casting will protect them. The labial walls of the proximal grooves should be projected on a flat plane from the deepest part of the groove to the buccal margin of the preparation, eliminating all of the proximal cut. The groove length should not be increased, nor should the end of the groove be scarred at this time.

The cervical finishing line is made with a No. ½D-L, 1D-T, or 3D-X diamond stone in the contra-angle handpiece. In this step the critical portions are on the proximal surfaces between the mesial and distal grooves and the cingulum reduction. These sections can be prepared 0.5 mm. in depth at the same time that the finishing line is made and the linguals of the proximal grooves are rounded. Using a No. 56 bur, the grooves should be recut pulpally until they are at least 0.75 mm. deep.

Pinhole

A pinhole should be made in the cingulum with a No. 701 or 702 taper fissure bur. It should be 1.25 mm. deep and parallel to the proximal grooves. It must be placed a little to the mesial or distal of the center of the cingulum so that any lingual pulp horn may be skirted. The pin of the casting will form a tripod with the struts in the proximal grooves, immobilizing the casting. Also, the frictional retention will be increased and there can be no movement except in reverse along the path of insertion. For these reasons, the pinhole is a fundamental part of the partial veneer preparation on any anterior tooth.

MODIFIED PREPARATION FOR A MAXILLARY CENTRAL INCISOR

Willey[1] has described a slightly different concept of the anterior partial veneer crown preparation. The basic differences are (1) less labial extension, especially on the mesio-proximal; (2) more axial reduction of the cingulum, both proximally and lingually (the resultant bulk of metal adds rigidity to the casting and reduces any tendency to deformation at the cervical); (3) an incisal offset rather than a groove; (4) labial walls of proximal grooves and incisal offset convex instead of flat; and (5) no pinhole in the cingulum (Fig. 77).

The labial extension is better controlled and restricted because proximal cutting is done with a long, small taper stone or bur. It is started from the lingual and brought labially only to the center of the contact area. A fine sandpaper disk or a chisel is used to bring the margin labially as far as is esthetically desirable, with a slightly convex rather than a flat surface. The finished proximal groove is less deep but the casting is bulkier. If the facings were selected, contoured, and aligned on the diagnostic cast prior to preparing the teeth, they can be used to help establish the margin of the preparation (Fig. 78).

FIGURE 77. Figure on right shows proximal view of maxillary anterior PV preparation as taught by the authors. Figure on left shows concept of maxillary anterior PV preparation as advocated by Smith and Willey. Pinhole has been placed in cingulum because authors consider this one of the fundamentals of this preparation.

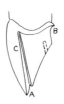
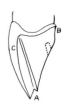

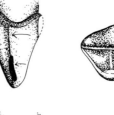
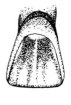

FIGURE 78. Top to bottom: Reduction of cingulum and proximals; reduction of lingual; incisal groove or offset; proximal grooves. (Smith and Willey.)

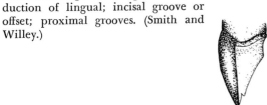
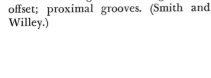

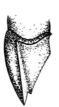

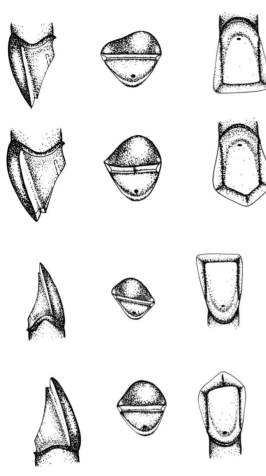

FIGURE 79. Top to bottom: Finished preparation, maxillary central; finished preparation, maxillary cuspid; finished preparation, mandibular incisor; finished preparation, mandibular cuspid. (Smith and Willey.)

The form given to the cingulum will show a much heavier chamfer or shoulder on the lingual and a wall parallel or almost parallel to the proximal grooves. The added bulk of metal increases the rigidity and stability of the casting and lessens the probability of deformation through prolonged use. In theory, this supersedes using a pin in the cingulum (Figs. 79 and 80).

In form the incisal offset is more shallow than the incisal groove described earlier, going a little farther onto the lingual surface. With increased bulk in the labial wall, it can be made convex, which is believed to throw back light rays in a favorable direction. This is an empirical assumption, but the end result, using this concept, is very gratifying.

Because of the limited labial extension of this preparation, it is difficult to reproduce with an elastic impression material. Direct wax pattern carving is recommended.

The castings should be fitted and equilibrated in the mouth. If the pontics are completed and aligned on the diagnostic cast and then transferred to the mouth on a baseplate, assembly of the bridge can be

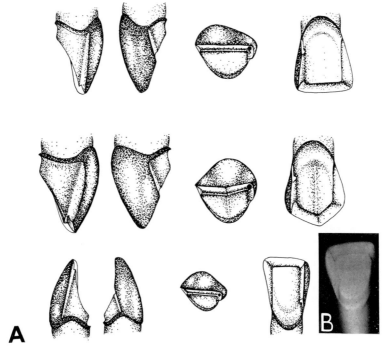

FIGURE 80. *A*, Preparations involving only one contact area: Top, maxillary central incisor; center, maxillary cuspid; bottom, mandibular incisor. (Smith and Willey.)

B, Maxillary central. Groove on proximal at right of cingulum prepared as usual. Short groove to lingual of contact on left. Preparation crosses left marginal ridge. Lingual reduced. Incisal groove ends in pinhole inside left marginal ridge. (Smith and Willey.)

accomplished without a working cast and the final two solder joints may be done singly, thus checking each step. Such a procedure does require considerably more chair time.

PREPARATION OF A MAXILLARY CUSPID

The partial veneer crown preparation on the upper cuspid is virtually the same as that on the central incisor. The chief difference is in the incisal groove, which may be divided and sharp-cornered since it must follow the cusp arms. Frequently, too, the preparation must be deeper so that the casting may withstand greater torque. When the mesial and distal surfaces are short inciso-cervically, it will be mandatory to supplement the retention with two additional pinholes in the lingual surface, placed at points close to the mesial and distal margins and 0.7 mm. from the incisal groove. Either a No. 700 or 701 taper fissure bur may be used to prepare these pinholes. This mode of auxiliary retention can be made a part of any anterior partial veneer preparation. (See Fig. 76B.) If the incisal cusp arms end mesially and distally in contact areas that are on a level with the

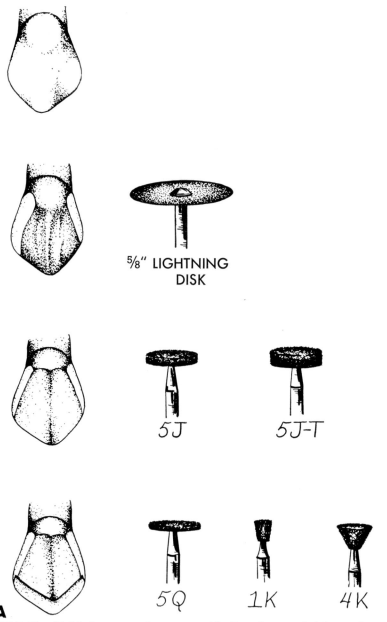

FIGURE 81. Vedder's preparation on cuspid. (Drawings copied from photographs of Dr. Vedder's models.)

A, Top to bottom: Uncut tooth; proximal slices; lingual reduction; incisal groove or ledge.

B, Top to bottom: Proximal grooves; finish of cingulum and groove walls; preparation on central incisor; pinholes preliminary to cutting proximal grooves when insufficient space exists between surface and approximating tooth to allow placement of No. 700 bur.

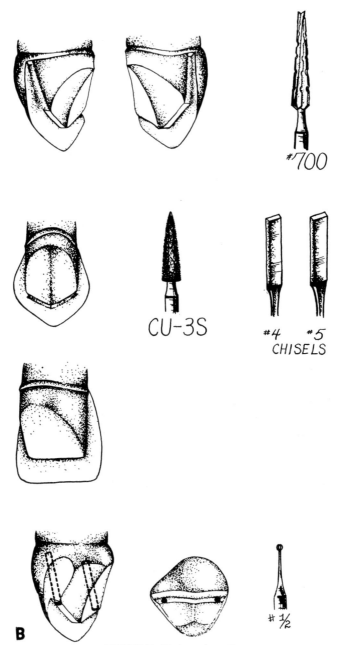

FIGURE 81 (*continued*).

gingival crest, it may be unwise to use a partial veneer crown unless supplementary retention can be gained from lingual pins. There must be enough proximal surface showing for grooves to be formed and a solder joint to be placed. Re-forming the silhouette of such a tooth with a partial veneer crown creates an unsightly restoration.

Indications, other contraindications, steps of preparation, and instrumentation are the same as for a central incisor.

MODIFIED PREPARATION FOR A MAXILLARY CUSPID

Vedder[2] advocated and used a preparation (Fig. 81*A*) on upper incisors and cuspids which results in maximal esthetics. The proximal cuts are made with a 5/8 inch Lightning disk,* converging sharply to the lingual and extending labially just past the labial margin of the contact area. These cuts should be very shallow. If there is an adjacent tooth, it may be necessary to use mechanical separation in order to provide sufficient space for the disk.

The lingual surface is reduced with a Densco 5J or 5J-T stone,† from the middle of the cingulum to the crest of the incisal edge. This cut will vary in depth from 0.5 to 1.0 mm., depending on the load and occlusion. The incisal groove or ledge terminates labially at the crest of the incisal edge, or it may be lingually and cervically to that position. The labial wall of the groove is parallel to the path of insertion or slopes to the labial only a few degrees. It is prepared with a Densco 5Q diamond stone, followed by a Densco 1K or 4K.

The proximal grooves, made with a No. 700 bur, begin at the mesial and distal ends of the incisal groove and are made parallel to the path of insertion. They are given maximal depth pulpally and are cut at right angles to the labio-lingual plane of the tooth. The cervical seats are made flat. The labial walls are planed with No. 4 and 5 chisels. The lingual walls will provide a secure gripping surface for the casting (Fig. 81*B*).

Frequently the amount of proximal reduction will not be great enough to allow the introduction of a No. 700 bur into the proximal space without mutilation of an adjacent tooth. If this is the case, the proximal groove can be made with a No. ½ round bur. The incisal termination of the groove is located and marked with a pencil. Starting at this point and continuing in a straight line to the cervical termination, a "pinhole"-type cut is produced. The handpiece must be held parallel to the exact direction of the proposed groove in both the labio-lingual and mesio-distal aspects, after which a No. 700 bur is inserted into this hole and brought out to the proximal to complete the proximal groove. The lingual cingulum wall is prepared with a Densco CU-3S diamond stone and the reduction is extended mesio- and disto-labially to connect with the initial proximal cuts.

The cervical finishing line may or may not require chamfering, depending on the form of the tooth. Vedder did not recommend universal use of a pin in the cingulum.

This preparation should be in the repertory of every dentist who builds maxillary anterior bridges.

---

* The J. Bird Moyer Co., Inc., Philadelphia, Penna.

† Densco, Inc., Denver, Colo.

OTHER SYSTEMS OF INSTRUMENTATION

The authors have employed the following patterns of instrumentation with success. These were suggested by the same operators referred to in Chapter 5, The Full Veneer Gold Crown. Essentially the same "prepared form" can and should be obtained with them as with the standard sequence of steps outlined earlier in this chapter.

ANTERIOR TEETH

Table 6

INSTRUMENT	TO BE ACCOMPLISHED	R.P.M.
⅞" steel "Lightning" separating disk	Proximal contact reduction.	3,000
70L Premier "Ela" carbide	Placement of proximal grooves. Reduction of periphery of cingulum. Location and contour of cervical margin.	150,000
3½J Densco diamond	Lingual surface reduction.	10,000
4D Densco diamond	Incisal beveled.	8,000
36 or 37 steel bur (any brand)	Placement of incisal groove.	500 to 1,000
701 or 702 steel bur (any brand)	Placement of cingulum pinhole.	1,000
Sandpaper disks (any brand)	Axial walls and cavo-surface angle smoothed.	500

Table 7

INSTRUMENT	TO BE ACCOMPLISHED	R.P.M.
701 R&R carbide	Incisal reduction.	150,000
700 R&R carbide	Proximal surface reduction.	150,000
5J-T Densco diamond	Lingual surface reduction.	6,000
701 R&R carbide	Reduction of cingulum periphery. Location and contour of cervical margin.	150,000
700 or 701 steel bur (any brand)	Placement of proximal grooves and cingulum pinhole.	6,000
35, 36, or 37 steel bur (any brand)	Placement of incisal groove.	1,000
Sandpaper disks (any brand)	Axial walls and cavo-surface angle smoothed.	500

Table 8

INSTRUMENT	TO BE ACCOMPLISHED	R.P.M.
1D Densco diamond *or* ⅞″ steel "Lightning" separating disk or carborundum disk	Proximal surface reduction. (When there is an approximating tooth, a disk is used to open contact.)	200,000 6,000
123 SSW diamond	Lingual surface reduction.	200,000
1D Densco diamond	Reduction of cingulum periphery. Location and contour of cervical margin. Incisal reduction.	200,000
½D Densco diamond	Proximal grooves started.	200,000
700 R&R steel bur	Proximal grooves finished.	3,000
37 SSW carbide	Placement of incisal groove.	200,000
701 R&R steel bur	Placement of cingulum pinhole.	3,000
Sandpaper disks (any brand)	Axial walls, grooves, and cavo-surface angle smoothed.	500

Table 9

INSTRUMENT	TO BE ACCOMPLISHED	R.P.M.
170 SSW carbide	Incisal reduction.	200,000
1D-C Densco diamond	Reduction of cingulum periphery.	200,000
2½J Densco diamond	Lingual surface reduction.	200,000
170L SSW carbide	Proximal grooves started.	200,000
700 SSW steel bur	Proximal grooves finished. Interproximal cervical reduction.	5,000
35, 36, or 37 SSW steel bur	Placement of incisal groove.	5,000
1D-T Densco diamond	Location and contour of cervical margin. Preparation smoothed.	200,000
701 SSW steel bur	Placement of cingulum pinhole.	5,000

Table 10

INSTRUMENT	TO BE ACCOMPLISHED	R.P.M.
2T Densco diamond	Proximal surface reduction.	4,000
701-L Densco carbide	Reduction of cingulum periphery. Placement of proximal grooves. Location and contour of cervical margin.	200,000
1½J Densco diamond	Lingual surface and incisal reduction.	10,000
1K Densco diamond	Placement of incisal groove.	6,000
Sandpaper disks (any brand)	Axial walls and cavo-surface angle smoothed.	500

ANTERIOR PATTERNS

If it is desirable to carve an anterior partial veneer pattern directly on the prepared tooth, a circular matrix is so shaped that there will be at least 1.0 mm. clearance in the areas of the lingual line angles. The cervical of the band is trimmed to conform to the cervical outline of the preparation, and the linguo-incisal portion is cut away so that the teeth can be occluded. The inside of the band is coated with Microfilm,* the band is filled with soft wax, the cavity surface is resoftened, and the band is held in position against the labial surface and is forced to place on the tooth with the finger being held over the top of the band. In this way wax is forced ahead of the band to insure an excess of wax around the margins of the preparation. When the band is partially seated, or when it appears that the preparation is filled and covered with wax, the finger is removed and the band is completely seated. The patient is asked to close so that the posterior teeth are in full contact, and then to open. Light pressure with the finger is applied to the lingual surface to readapt the wax in the incisal area.

A heated root canal plugger or a Pinwaxer† is inserted into the cingulum pinhole. This process is repeated, and the wax is permitted to solidify without chilling with cold water. The excess around the lingual and cervical of the band is trimmed off and the band is removed, meanwhile holding the wax in position on the tooth. The pattern must be held on the tooth *at all times* while carving. Form may be produced with a variety of instruments, such as the Tarno No. 4 plastic instrument,‡ a discoid excavator, a Wagner instrument,§ and S. S. White No. 5 and No. 23 explorers.

A No. 12 Crenshaw scaler is helpful in trimming the cervical (Fig. 82).‖ An Ash England No. 5** or S. S. White Tarno No. 5 may be used in spots. The finished pattern is polished with wet cotton, and the pattern is removed with two explorers, one on each proximal surface.

SPRUING

The sprue pin is attached on the contact area, in a direction that will guide the molten metal along the lingual surface. Dressel[9] and Paul[10], among other authorities, advocate attaching the sprue pin while the

---

* Kerr Mfg. Company, Detroit, Mich.
† The S. S. White Dental Mfg. Co., Philadelphia, Penna. (Designed by E. E. and L. L. Kraus, Milwaukee, Wis.)
‡ The S. S. White Dental Mfg. Co., Philadelphia, Penna.
§ Dr. Wagner's Dental Specialties, Janesville, Wis.
‖ J. W. Ivory, Inc., Philadelphia, Penna.
** Claudius Ash, Sons & Co., Inc., Niagara Falls, N. Y.

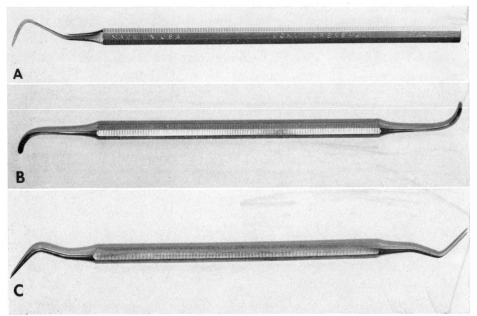

FIGURE 82. *A,* Crenshaw scaler.
B, Ash instrument.
C, Wagner instrument.

pattern is on the tooth. A small excess of wax is placed just to the lingual of the incisal edge, and the heated pin is attached parallel to the proximal grooves of the preparation. When the pin and wax have cooled, the pattern is removed, using the pin as a handle.

Proponents of this technique state that no pattern distortion results. In the hands of the authors and their students, many margins have been distorted by this method in the incisal area nearest to the point where the pin was attached. If pins are attached in the mouth, any movement of the attached pin must be avoided. As always, the pattern should be invested immediately.

Starr[11] has a unique and very good method for adapting a semicarved partial veneer pattern to the tooth. He opens the contact area just enough to permit binding tape or a strip of rubber dam to be slipped into the proximal space. The ends are then drawn together on the buccal or labial until pressure is exerted on all areas of the pattern except the center of the incisal edge or occlusal surface. The tape is removed and the margins are checked and, if necessary, recarved to the surface of the tooth. The pattern is removed (Fig. 83) and the sprue pin is attached on the contact area previously reduced. If the pattern is for an anterior tooth, the pin should be pointed in a plane continuous with the lingual surface; if a posterior pattern, toward the opposite cervical margin. (See Chapter 13, Spruing, Investing, and Casting.)

FIGURE 83. Removal and spruing of pattern.

MAXILLARY BICUSPIDS: INDICATIONS AND CONTRAINDICATIONS

This retainer can support posterior bridges supplying one, two, or three teeth, and anterior bridges replacing the cuspid or the cuspid and lateral. When splinted, it may be used on longer anterior prostheses. It has merit, also, on intermediate abutments. The partial veneer crown may be placed on rotated or tipped bicuspids if the latter eccentricity is not too pronounced. It can be applied when the lingual cusp has been fractured or where most of the supporting dentin under the lingual cusp has been destroyed. If such teeth were prepared for veneered gold crowns, the remaining tooth structure would not stand up against the forces sometimes transmitted through the bridge.

The partial veneer crown is contraindicated on a short bicuspid when it is to be used alone on one end of a bridge, but it may serve well on this type of tooth when used as a segment of a multiple retainer. Brooks[12] says: "Where there is extensive loss of tooth structure, a large restoration with resultant weakened tooth walls, or multiple active carious areas in the abutment tooth, a full veneer crown should be considered rather than the partial veneer retainer."

When the diagnostic cast is surveyed, the path of insertion should be marked on the buccal surface to pilot the proximal slices and the buccal margins of the preparation. When the long-axis directions of the bicuspid and the other abutments are identical (Fig. 84), both proximal cuts can closely parallel the path of insertion. When there is a discrepancy in the long-axis relationship between the abutment teeth, the bicuspid frequently will receive a near-classic preparation.

If the bicuspid partial veneer crown is to be the anterior retainer, most of the deviations must be in the preparation of the molar tooth. For example, with the bicuspid position upright and the molar tipped to the distal and the buccal, the mesial of the bicuspid and the distal and buccal of the molar must be made parallel or be prepared so they approach each other slightly toward the occlusal. In this case, due to the long-axis relationship of these two teeth, the distal of the bicuspid and the mesial of the molar could not be paralleled but would diverge occlusally. The major retention for this bridge, then, would come from the mesial of the bicuspid and the distal of the molar. Here, the associated angulation

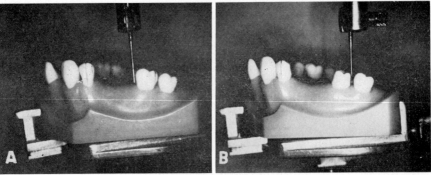

FIGURE 84. Survey of diagnostic cast and check on preparation.

A, Path of insertion drawn on buccal of bicuspid abutment; buccal extension of distal proximal slices on bicuspid and molar. Analyzing rod shows that minimal cutting will be needed on mesial of molar.

B, Teeth prepared to marked path of insertion which is parallel to analyzing rod.

of the walls could be calculated on the diagnostic cast with the analyzing rod of the surveyor. If the bicuspid is the posterior abutment, the partial veneer crown probably could not be relied on if the long-axis relationship with the anterior abutment were distinctly abnormal.

PREPARATION OF A MAXILLARY BICUSPID

The partial veneer, or three-quarter crown, preparation on the upper bicuspid might be termed a combination of the MOD inlay and full veneer gold crown preparations. All of the occlusal surface must be covered with this retainer. The reduction of the lingual surface follows its contour and may have a chamfer finishing line. If the crown is long occluso-cervically and if dentin remains buccally and lingually, the lingual margin may be short of the gingival crevice. The proximal surfaces are prepared in inlay form, although more shallow pulpally and more narrow bucco-lingually.[13]

The routine for this preparation is:

(1) reduction of the mesial and distal surfaces,

(2) reduction of the occlusal surface, and

(3) reduction of the lingual surface;

(4) cutting the mesial and distal boxes;

(5) flaring the buccal walls of the mesial and distal boxes;

(6) establishing the cervical finishing line; and

(7) beveling the bucco-occlusal margin.

Mesial and Distal Surfaces

The mesial and distal surfaces are flattened with a separating disk in the straight handpiece, starting on or inside the marginal ridge and ending at the gingival line or the cementoenamel junction (Fig. 85*A*). One proximal cut must be parallel to the path of insertion or converge only a few degrees occlusally. The other proximal surface should be prepared, as nearly as conditions will permit, parallel to the first cut or barely inclined toward the center of the occlusal.

Bucco-lingually, the width of the lingual embrasures will be increased; thus there will be access for the preparation of the cervical finishing line. On the disto-buccal, the margin should stop at the line angle, and on the mesial, to enhance esthetics, it may be just to the buccal of the contact area.

Occlusal Surface

The groove pattern may be prepared with a bur in order that space for metal will be guaranteed. The occlusal is shortened 1.0 mm. in all other sections, using wheel-shaped and inverted cone stones. To check clearance, the patient should be asked to close on articulating paper (folded to eight thicknesses) and to move the mandible in lateral and protrusive excursions.

Lingual Surface

The lingual preparation, following the normal contour from cusp tip to cervical, can be made with wheel-shaped and tapered round-end stones. If the tooth is in normal alignment, the depth should be approximately 1.0 mm. except in the occluding area. Here it should be slightly deeper.

Boxes

The proximal boxes should parallel each other and the path of insertion (Fig. 85*B*). Best produced with a No. 557 or 556 bur, they should be in the buccal half of the tooth and twice as wide as the diameter of the bur used. In depth, pulpally, they should be one-half the diameter of the same bur. The beveled cervical margin of the box should be in the gingival crevice, although recession may make this infeasible.

The buccal walls of the proximal boxes should be angled from the pulpal wall to the buccal margin, obliterating the original cuts on the proximal surfaces. While this can be effectuated with hand instruments, it will be more perfect mechanically if done with a sandpaper disk.

Finishing Line and Bevel

The cervical finishing line is begun by beveling the cervical seats of

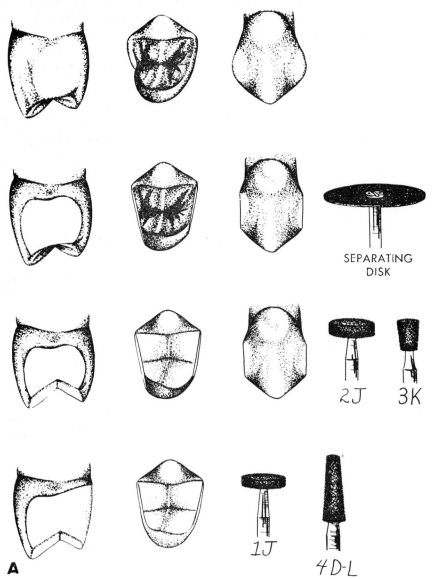

SEPARATING DISK

2J   3K

1J

4D-L

A

FIGURE 85. *A*, Top to bottom: Uncut tooth; proximal slices; occlusal reduction; lingual reduction.

B, Top to bottom: Proximal boxes; buccal walls of boxes angled to buccal line angle and cervical finishing line; buccal chamfer on carious tooth.

the proximal boxes with any cervical margin trimmer. The remainder of the cervical finishing line may be chamfered with a No. 1D-T tapered round-end stone in the contra-angle handpiece.

A bevel 0.5 mm. wide is placed on the buccal surface at the bucco-occlusal margin. It should be at such an angle that the seated casting

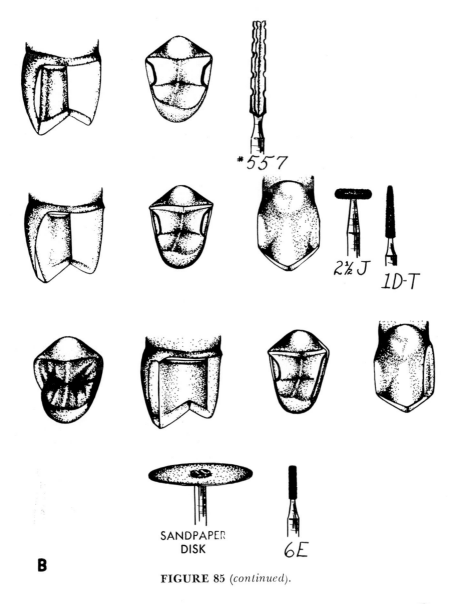

*557

2½ J

1D-T

SANDPAPER
DISK

6E

B

FIGURE 85 (*continued*).

FIGURE 86. Preparation on maxillary bicuspid not covering all of buccal cusp is used only on teeth with long crowns when minimal display of gold is imperative. Teeth so prepared seem to be more susceptible to splitting; also, the retainers loosen more often.

will engage the buccal surface when forces on the casting are toward the lingual.

Willey[1] advocates proximal grooves instead of boxes and he deepens

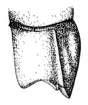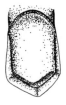

FIGURE 87. (Smith and Willey.)

the reduction of the lingual half of the tooth (see Fig. 87). The greater bulk of metal increases the rigidity of the casting. Also, he recommends less extension at the bucco-proximal and bucco-occlusal angles. However, the authors feel that the shorter the teeth, the greater the indication for proximal boxes.

OTHER SYSTEMS OF INSTRUMENTATION

The following plans for instrumentation have all proved satisfactory in the authors' hands and are applicable also to molars.

BICUSPIDS

Table 11

INSTRUMENT	TO BE ACCOMPLISHED	R.P.M.
70L Premier "Ela" carbide	Complete axial and occlusal reduction. Placement of proximal boxes.	150,000
1D Densco diamond	Location and contour of cervical margin. Irregularities smoothed. Buccal cusp contrabeveled.	10,000
700 R&R steel bur	Refinement of proximal boxes.	5,000

Table 12

INSTRUMENT	TO BE ACCOMPLISHED	R.P.M.
⅛″ carborundum disk (any brand)	Proximal reduction.	6,000
701 R&R carbide	Lingual and occlusal reduction. Buccal cusp contrabeveled.	150,000
701 R&R carbide	Location and contour of cervical margin.	6,000
700 or 701 steel bur (any brand)	Placement of proximal boxes.	6,000
Cervical trimmers	Beveling of proximal box cervical margin.	Hand
Sandpaper disks (any brand)	Axial walls and cavo-surface angle smoothed.	1,000

Table 13

INSTRUMENT	TO BE ACCOMPLISHED	R.P.M.
1D Densco diamond	Complete axial and occlusal reduction. Buccal cusp contrabeveled. Location and contour of cervical margin.	200,000
½D Densco diamond	Placement of proximal boxes.	200,000
1D-T Densco diamond (worn) or	Preparation smoothed.	200,000
44 SSW carborundum stone		3,000
701 R&R carbide	Cervical seat of boxes made square.	8,000
700 R&R steel bur	Refinement of proximal boxes.	3,000

Table 14

INSTRUMENT	TO BE ACCOMPLISHED	R.P.M.
701 R&R carbide or 701 SSW carbide	Occlusal and lingual reduction.	200,000
700 SSW carbide or 699 Densco carbide	Placement of proximal boxes.	200,000
700 SSW steel bur	Refinement of proximal boxes.	5,000
⅝″ Moore garnet disk	Finish and flare of proximal boxes.	5,000
F, 1D-T, or 1D-C Densco diamond	Completion of proximal reduction. Location and contour of cervical margin. Preparation smoothed.	200,000
170 SSW carbide	Buccal cusp contrabeveled.	200,000

Table 15

INSTRUMENT	TO BE ACCOMPLISHED	R.P.M.
701 or 701-L Densco carbide	Complete axial and occlusal reduction. Placement of cervical shoulder. Placement of proximal boxes.	200,000
¾D Densco diamond	Irregularities smoothed. Refinement of cervical shoulder. Buccal cusp contrabeveled.	200,000
Sandpaper disks (any brand)	Axial walls and cavo-surface angle smoothed.	500

PREPARATION OF A MAXILLARY FIRST MOLAR

The partial veneer crown should be used on the upper first molar only when the mouth is relatively caries-free, when the crown is long

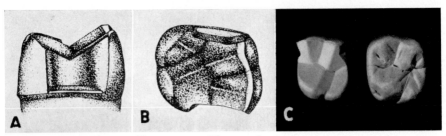

FIGURE 88.   Preparations on maxillary molar.
A, B, With boxes. When molars are short and a partial veneer crown is indicated, boxes provide more stability.
C, With grooves.

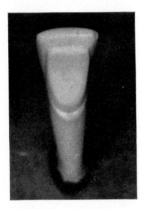

FIGURE 89.   Preparation on mandibular incisor without cingulum pinhole. (Smith and Willey.)

occluso-cervically, and when the mesio-buccal area of the tooth is exposed as the patient talks or smiles. Otherwise, because of difficulty of construction, it is contraindicated in favor of the full veneer gold crown.

The preparation on the upper first molar differs from that on the bicuspid in two ways. To attain a circumferential hold on the tooth, its mesial and distal surfaces should approach each other toward the buccal instead of the lingual. Proximal retention is increased by cutting wide grooves, instead of boxes, in the buccal one-third. If the crown is long, the finishing line on the lingual surface can be placed 1.5 to 2.0 mm. occlusally to the gingival line.

The steps and the instruments used in this preparation are the same as for the bicuspid except that the proximal grooves are cut with a No. 702 taper fissure bur (Fig. 88).

PREPARATION OF A MANDIBULAR INCISOR

The mandibular incisor is not well adapted to a partial veneer crown preparation. The long established routine, which begins with proximal slices, does not satisfy all esthetic demands even though retention may be adequate.

For the most gratifying result, carbide burs should be used (Fig. 89), for both proximal and cingulum reduction, at a rotational speed best suited to the operator. Cutting should be started on the cingulum, with the instrument parallel to the intended path of insertion, and should proceed around the tooth and onto the proximal surface. Depth on the proximal must be enough to avoid contact with an approximating tooth. Reduction should stop just labially to the center of the contact area but short of the labial line angle. Cervically, when possible, the preparation on the proximals should be 0.25 mm. below the gingival crest. Lingually, gingival recession can make it impracticable to place the margin in the crevice.

The lingual surface is not reduced except where the linguo-incisal offset, or groove, is cut from proximal surface to proximal surface. The offset is 1.0 to 1.5 mm. below the incisal edge. Its pulpal wall should be made convex and be extended just beyond the linguo-incisal angle. The proximal grooves are made with a long and small carbide bur or with a No. 700 steel bur. As a rule the direction is the same as for other anterior teeth, although the depth may be less. The labial walls of the proximal grooves, shaped with either disks or chisels, are also convex. A pinhole 1.0 mm. deep is placed in the cingulum. The depth of the preparation should be sufficient to create a discernible and helpful finishing line.

It can be difficult to reproduce the partial veneer crown preparation on a mandibular incisor with an elastic impression unless it is made too deep and is overextended. The sharp labial margins and the direction of the grooves make withdrawal precarious and often cause tearing or cutting of the impression material. Direct pattern carving is suggested.

PREPARATION OF A MANDIBULAR CUSPID

When the partial veneer crown is planned for the lower cuspid, there should be a comprehensive evaluation of the occlusion of the incisal third of the labial surface with the linguals and incisals of the opposing teeth. In many cases, the linguo-incisal groove must be omitted, with a step across the labio-incisal being substituted. The metal covering this

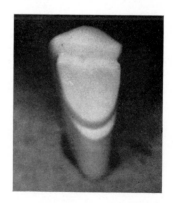

FIGURE 90. Preparation on mandibular cuspid. (Smith and Willey.)

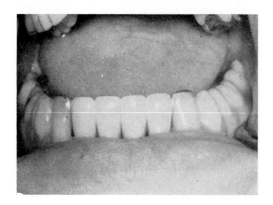

FIGURE 91. Mandibular anterior bridge with partial veneer crown retainers on cuspid abutments.

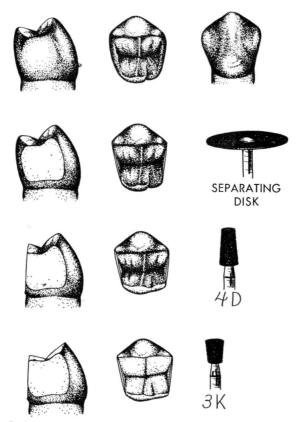

SEPARATING DISK

4D

3K

A

FIGURE 92.   Preparation on mandibular bicuspid.

A, Top to bottom: Uncut tooth; proximal slices; lingual aligned to path of insertion; occlusal reduced.

B, Top to bottom: Proximal grooves; buccal bevel; buccal chamfer; cervical finishing line; bucco-occlusal bevel.

area will curb lingual movement of the casting, will receive and dissipate the incising and masticating forces, and can be contoured to support occlusion. When it is essential to eliminate any display of metal and the tooth is long, a lingual offset, sometimes as much as 2.0 mm. below the

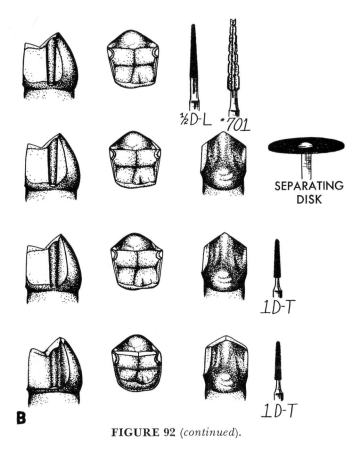

½D-L *701

SEPARATING
DISK

1D-T

1D-T

B

FIGURE 92 (*continued*).

incisal edge, may be used. The proximal grooves should follow the plane of the labial surface but can be made to parallel the long axis of the tooth. Sometimes, before a pinhole can be made, a ledge or an indentation must be cut on the lingual surface at the cervical. (See Fig. 91.)

The partial veneer crown can be a competent retainer on the mandibular cuspid if (1) the preparation will control lingual displacement; (2) the reduction on the proximal surfaces and across the incisal can be deep enough for a strong, rigid casting; (3) the cervical pin is employed; (4) an adjacent tooth will not interfere with seating the bridge or it can be changed in form to nullify interference; (5) the long-axis relationship with the other abutment teeth will allow substantial proximal grooving; (6) the caries rate seems to be low; (7) extra lingual pins are placed to supplement the retention from the proximal grooves when the labio-incisal ledge is not used; and (8) if the long axes are parallel.

When the mouth is being prepared for a removable partial denture, the cingulum of the partial veneer crown can be shaped to support the denture and on the distal and lingual it can be flattened to receive the lingual arm of a clasp and to form guiding planes. It will retain a six-unit anterior bridge, and unilaterally, alone or splinted, a posterior bridge supplying one or two, and occasionally three, teeth.

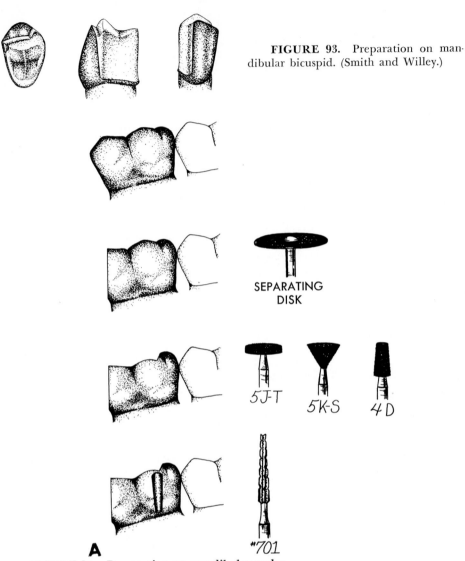

FIGURE 93. Preparation on mandibular bicuspid. (Smith and Willey.)

SEPARATING DISK

5J-T   5K-S   4D

A   #701

FIGURE 94. Preparation on mandibular molar.

A, Top to bottom: Uncut tipped tooth; proximal cut; occlusal reduced; buccal and lingual grooves.

B, Top to bottom: Grooves connected to proximal by reducing buccal and lingual; cervical finishing line and pinholes; occlusal view.

For maximal esthetics, the preparation can be made following the same technique advocated for the lower incisor.

PREPARATION OF A MANDIBULAR BICUSPID

Many times the partial veneer crown is contraindicated on the lower first bicuspid. The lingual slant of the crown and the extremely short

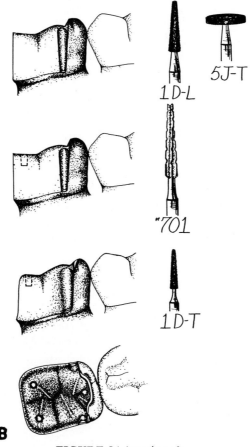

FIGURE 94 (*continued*).

lingual cusp often will make a retentive preparation doubtful unless the preparation can be extended so far cervically on the buccal surface that it shows as much metal as the full veneer gold crown. In such a case, its esthetic characteristics are ruined. (See Fig. 92*A*.)

The mandibular second bicuspid is better suited to this preparation,[14] because the crown has less lingual angulation, a longer lingual cusp, and is more nearly square when viewed from the occlusal. Frequently it may be prepared in a manner corresponding to the maxillary bicuspid, except that proximal grooves are used instead of boxes, and by means of a bevel or a step the preparation covers the occluding portion of the buccal surface so that only the casting will contact the opposing teeth in all excursions.

Retention will be increased by a bevel 1.0 mm. wide on the buccal surface along the disto-buccal margin (Fig. 93). Since it will not be parallel to the path of insertion, it should go as far cervically as the convexity of the tooth will tolerate. The bevel should be 0.7 mm. deep at the junction of the buccal surface and distal cut, and with a small cylindrical stone should be made concave, in the form of a chamfer. This concavity will improve the finishing line at the buccal margin of the bevel and also will increase the strength of the lip of metal coming around onto the disto-buccal surface. Two pinholes, 1.0 mm. deep, may be placed in the occlusal surface at the tips of the cusps, to augment the stability and holding power of the retainer. They should be made with No. 701 or 702 taper fissure burs. The finishing line on the lower bicuspid may be a chamfer, but usually the mesial, distal, and lingual walls will end at a chisel-edge margin, which suffices (Fig. 92B).

Partial veneer crowns on lower bicuspids are satisfactory when splinted to each other or to a retainer on the cuspid.

PREPARATION OF A MANDIBULAR MOLAR

The partial veneer crown is not indicated on a lower molar except under one peculiar condition. When the molar is tipped mesially so much that the path of insertion cannot be accommodated to a distal approximating tooth, this retainer may function admirably. With the mesial contact area of the distal tooth anterior to the distal gingival line of the abutment, placement or removal could not be effected without radically altering the path of insertion, which may be impractical, or reshaping the mesial of the overhanging tooth with another restoration.

The preparation should be started by slicing off the mesial of the abutment along the plane of the path of insertion (Fig. 94A). The occlusal is then cut distally to the marginal ridge. From this line, grooves are made in the buccal and lingual surfaces, parallel to the path of insertion, and as far cervically as form and lingual inclination will allow. These two surfaces are then connected with the mesial reduction, after which the buccal and lingual grooves are made deeper to ensure a horseshoe grip on the tooth. Using a No. 702 taper fissure bur, three pinholes, from 1.0 to 1.5 mm. deep and parallel to the path of insertion, are placed in the occlusal surface. One is near the disto-occlusal margin, midway between the buccal and lingual surfaces; the others are placed in the mesial cusps. The cervical finishing line will be either a chamfer or a chisel-edge, depending on tooth position and contour (Fig. 94B).

This retainer should never be used if caries is active. Instead, the abutment tooth should be prepared for a full veneer gold crown and the tooth to the distal recontoured and restored.

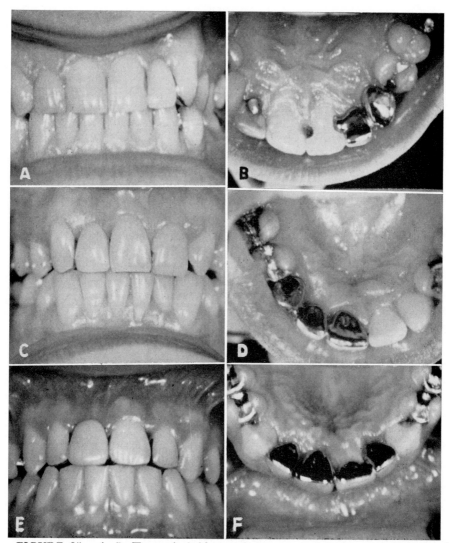

FIGURE 95. *A, B,* Two-unit bridge replacing upper left lateral incisor. Partial veneer crown retainer on cuspid abutment with a lingual rest in rest seat prepared in gold foil restoration in disto-lingual of central incisor.

C, D, Three-unit bridge replacing upper right lateral incisor. Two partial veneer crown retainers. Mesio-incisal angle of cuspid preparation should have been rounded slightly.

E, F, Three-unit bridge replacing upper right central incisor. Partial veneer crown retainers and a third partial veneer crown, a single-unit restoration, on left lateral. Lingual extension of pontic was reduced to a minimum because of chronic irritation of the palatal mucous membrane.

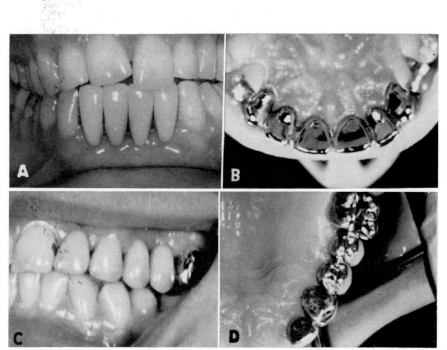

FIGURE 96.   *A*, Lower six-unit bridge retained by partial veneer crowns on cuspids.
B, Lingual view of six-unit upper anterior bridge supported by partial veneer crown retainers on the cuspids and lateral incisors.

C, D, Five-unit upper posterior bridge with a cantilever lateral incisor pontic. Partial veneer crown retainer on the cuspid abutment.

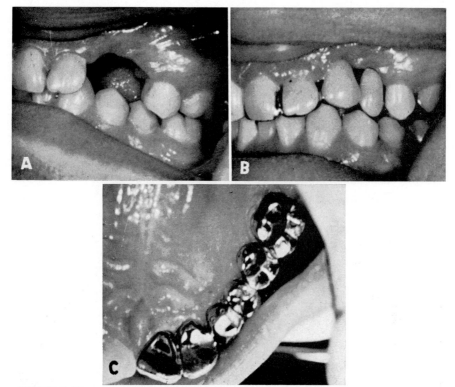

FIGURE 97.   *A,* Edentulous area with cuspid and first bicuspid missing. The proposed abutment teeth are quite short. The vertical overlap is more than 50 per cent.

B, C, Six-unit bridge constructed to restore space (*A*). Four partial veneer crown retainers were used on the central and lateral incisors, second bicuspid, and first molar abutments. Short crowns and lever arm made this necessary.

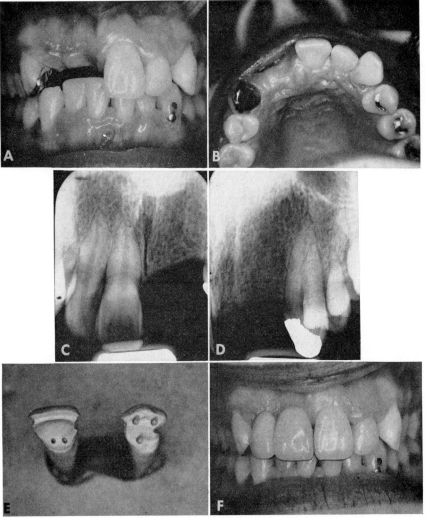

FIGURE 98.   *A*, *B*, Maxillary anterior space.
C, *D*, Radiographs of abutments. Incisor very thin.
E, Dies of prepared abutments.
F, Cemented bridge.

REFERENCES

1. Willey, R. E.: Preparation of abutments for veneer retainers. J.A.D.A., *53*:141, Aug. 1956.
2. Vedder, F. B.: Personal communication.
3. Grubb, H. D.: Fixed bridgework. J. Pros. Den., *3*:121, Jan. 1953.
4. Cowger, G. T.: Retention, resistance and esthetics of the anterior three-quarter crown. J.A.D.A., *62*:167, Feb. 1961.
5. Thom, L. W.: Principles of cavity preparation in crown and bridge prosthesis. II. The three-quarter crown. J.A.D.A., *41*:443, Oct. 1950.
6. Ante, I. H.: Abutments. J. Canad. D. A., *2*:249, 1936.
7. Guyer, S. E.: Partial veneer crowns: preparation alignment. Washington Univ. D. J., *26*:72, May 1960.
8. Tinker, H. A.: Three-quarter crowns in fixed bridgework. J. Canad. D. A., *16*:125, March 1950.
9. Dressel, R. P.: Anterior fixed bridges. Paper read before Indiana Univ. School Den. Symposium, April 1955.
10. Paul, F. K.: Personal communication.
11. Starr, F.: Crown and bridge postgraduate course, Ohio State Univ. School Den., 1948.
12. Brooks, E. C.: A practical approach for crown and bridge construction. Paper read before Kentucky State D. A., April 1955.
13. Murto, C. B.: Modern bridge retainers. J. Ontario D. A., *33*:15, Feb. 1956.
14. Lyon, D. M.: Abutments in fixed prosthesis. Arkansas D. J., *24*:6, Dec. 1953.

Berridge, C. M., and Bogdonoff, C. M.: Surface of the cavity preparation after instrumentation. Georgetown D. J., *29*:19, June 1963.
Moulton, G. H.: Esthetics in anterior fixed bridge prosthodontics. J.A.D.A., *52*:36, Jan. 1956.
Simpson, D. H.: Considerations for abutments. J. Pros. Den., *5*:375, May 1955.

7

THE PINLEDGE RETAINER

In the field of anterior fixed partial dentures, stability and esthetics deserve equal consideration. Stability can be obtained with partial veneer and veneered gold crowns and the MacBoyle retainer, even though constructed without finesse. However, to achieve a wholly satisfactory esthetic result with the partial veneer crown, alterations which might lessen both retention and stability may have to be made in the standard preparation.[1,2] The veneered gold crown poses the problems of trauma, contour, masking, and shading. The MacBoyle retainer usually leaves much to be desired esthetically.

Preservation of unblemished labial enamel is always an asset to appearance.[3] A correctly designed and well-made pinledge displays minimal metal and requires the least cutting of tooth structure of any of the anterior retainers. It is unexcelled if used in mouths where the caries index is low or where it has been controlled, if used on caries-free teeth or those which have been restored with gold foil, and if used on teeth with some bulk in the incisal one-third. With meticulous application, when the occlusion is favorable, it can be placed on thin teeth; and if the patient and operator will cooperate in observing the mouth closely in the future, it can be placed over exposed proximal silicate or resin restorations.

There has been much progress during the past five years in the indirect construction of the pinledge retainer. New techniques in preparation of the abutment tooth and methods of obtaining the die and casting have given the profession a retainer with esthetics equal to that produced by the direct technique heretofore used, and with retention or stability seemingly equal to the partial veneer crown and many of the veneered crowns that are built over the omnipresent tapered preparation.

The use of drills that are small in diameter has made it possible

130

to place pinholes more strategically and thus to make them deeper without heightening the danger of pulpal trauma. The facts that these holes have parallel walls and the castings made to fit into them have closely fitting parallel sides are all-important in augmenting resistance to displacement. The cast pins are small enough to enable them to be covered by a layer of dentin behind the labial enamel. There may be an occasional exception when the 24-gauge wire pin would be more acceptable esthetically, but such a situation is very rare.

A great majority of operators can prepare teeth for the pinledge, provided that a paralleling device is employed while drilling the pinholes. Several such instruments are available.* [4, 5]

It is highly recommended that a diagnostic cast of the arch to receive the fixed prosthesis be mounted on a surveying table, so that by using an analyzing rod the most logical mechanical path of insertion may be determined, although information from radiographs may suggest some modification.

There must be no stress on the teeth when seating a pinledge bridge. It must fit precisely and it must slip into place without interference, or the bridge must be reassembled. In an end-to-end occlusion the casting must provide incisal protection or the path of insertion must be from the lingual. Even here incisal coverage is safer. All joints must be rigid.

INDICATIONS

Formerly the pinledge bridge was used only where moderate torque would be generated and where the lever arm was short or broken by intermediate abutments. Now, however, retention has been greatly increased and seems to compare favorably with more extensive retainers. When used on multiple splinted abutments, resistance to displacement is notable.[6, 7]

Maxillary Arch

In the maxillary arch the pinledge can be used in the following circumstances:

(1) on the central and lateral incisors when replacing a central;

(2) on the cuspid and central when the lateral is missing;

(3) on the central and cuspid when replacing an approximating central and lateral;

(4) for older persons, on the lateral incisor, or on both the lateral and central, with an inlay or partial veneer crown on the first bicuspid when the cuspid has been lost;

---

* Loma Linda Parallelometer, Chayes Dental Instrument Corp., Danbury, Conn.
  Pontistructor, J. F. Jelenko & Co., Inc., New Rochelle, N. Y.
  Jermyn Parallaid, Williams Gold Refining Co., Inc., Buffalo, N. Y.

(5) if cusp angles are flat, on the cuspid, with an inlay or partial veneer crown on the second bicuspid, when the first bicuspid space is to be filled;

(6) on the two cuspids and lateral when both centrals and a lateral have been lost; and

(7) on the cuspid, central, and lateral when replacing the left lateral and right central.[8]

On maxillary cuspids with long mesio- and disto-incisal arms and short mesial and distal surfaces, the pinledge, when made with cast pins, has more retention than a partial veneer crown. It is an efficient splinting restoration on upper anteriors, and it may be used to recontour lingual occluding surfaces in oral reconstruction.

Mandibular Arch

In the mandibular arch, when the abutments are caries-free, the pinledge is the retainer of choice when one or two central incisors or one lateral must be inserted. By using a partial veneer crown or pinledge on the cuspid, and pinledges on the central and lateral abutments, a bridge replacing an approximating central and lateral will cause a minimum of mutilation to the abutments. It makes an ideal splinting attachment for slightly mobile mandibular anteriors, and it may be used to recontour lingual surfaces of cuspids or incisors for the support and retention of partial dentures.[9]

PREPARATION

A pinledge preparation is best done at moderate speeds and with a variety of stones and burs. It is a delicate preparation and must be planned from surveyed diagnostic casts and bite-wing radiographs so that the pinholes can be placed to the mesial, distal, and lingual of the pulp without danger of injury.

The operation on a maxillary central incisor should proceed in the following sequence of steps:

(1) reduction of the marginal ridge and contact area adjacent to the space, and

(2) reduction of the lingual surface;

(3) locating and placing ledges;

(4) making indentations;

(5) sinking pinholes;

(6) creating the finishing line; and

(7) beveling the prepared incisal edge and incisal angle.

Proximal Surface.   The marginal ridge (Fig. 99*A*) is reduced with a disk in the straight handpiece. This cut, compatible with the path of insertion, extends from midway on the cingulum to the incisal edge, covers the contact area, and reaches the labial surface at this point only. It is made at an angle of 45 degrees from the plane of the lingual surface and may or may not go through the enamel.

Lingual Surface. Using a small wheel stone with a round edge, the lingual surface is reduced evenly to a depth of 0.5 mm., starting from the original cut and extending to and frequently onto the remaining marginal ridge. Inciso-cervically this will include about three-fourths of the incisal edge and one-half or two-thirds of the cingulum. When the maxillary teeth are thin, with a long vertical overlap and little overjet, a compromise in depth may be necessary, with some space being procured by grinding the incisal edges and upper labial surfaces of the mandibular teeth. On an upper, when the bite is open, and on a lower incisor, less cutting should be done on the lingual, even though the casting will increase the over-all thickness of the tooth; however, a discernible finishing line must be produced.

Ledges and Indentations. Two supporting ledges, as a rule perpendicular to the long axis of the tooth, must be cut on the lingual surface. Exceptions are the maxillary cuspid or an abraded incisor, when the incisal ledge can conform to the outline of the incisal edge of the tooth. The prepared portion of the lingual surface is divided into fourths, and one ledge is made on the line between the incisal and second sections. The other is cut on a new line made by bisecting the prepared cervical fourth incisocervically.

These ledges must completely cross the prepared lingual surface. Linguo-labially they should be uniformly as wide as half the diameter of the bur used, with the pulpal wall being parallel to the path of insertion. They should be made with a No. 557 or 57 bur, or a small cylindrical stone. If the tooth is thin, a No. 556 or 56 bur may be substituted. A straight handpiece is advised for upper preparations, a contra-angle for lowers.

Before making the indentations, bite-wing or apical radiographs should be re-examined to verify the exact position of the pulp and the proximal dentinoenamel junctions. The incisal indentations must be *just inside* the marginal ridges between the dentinoenamel junctions and the pulp horns, and the one at the cervical *slightly off center* toward the space. The wider their triangular spread, the greater is the stability of the casting. Using either a No. 557 or 56 bur, the indentations are cut as deep as half of the diameter of the bur and should be parallel to the path of insertion.

Pinholes. Pinholes may be made with No. 700 or 701 taper fissure burs, with a No. 1/2 round bur, or with 0.023 inch drills. This phase of the preparation may be done freehand with a straight handpiece on upper teeth and a contra-angle on lowers. (See Fig. 99*B*.) The holes must be parallel

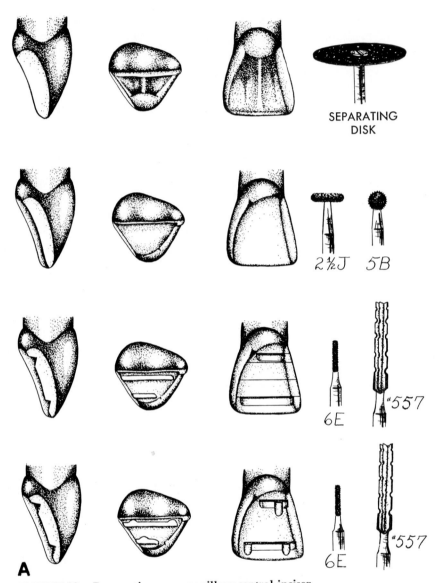

SEPARATING
DISK

2½J   5B

6E   #557

6E   #557

A

FIGURE 99.   Preparation on a maxillary central incisor.

A, Top to bottom: Reduction of marginal ridge and contact area; reduction of lingual surface; ledges cut; indentations prepared.

B, Top to bottom: Pinholes and chamfered finishing line on lingual; pins in position; usual area of solder joint (left) and notch cut to facilitate seating in a plaster impression.

to the path of insertion, 2.0 to 2.25 mm. deep, and should start from the center of the indentation. When using No. 700 or 701 burs, a pilot hole may be made first with a No. ½ round bur, then enlarged with the taper bur.

When made with drills, it is recommended that a paralleling device

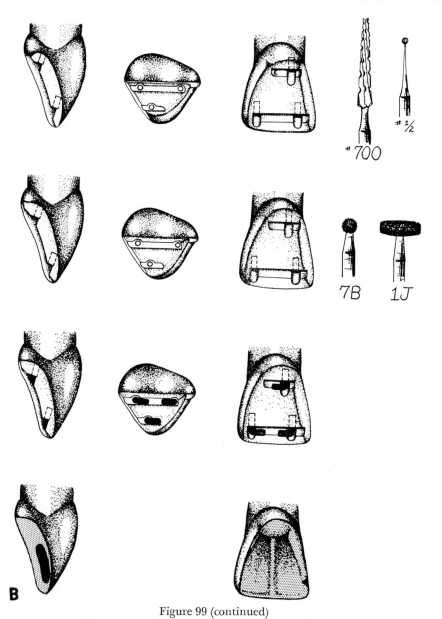

#700   #1/2

7B   1J

B

Figure 99 (continued)

be used, either stabilized on the teeth with modeling compound or held in position by a baseplate.

A self-curing resin baseplate is adapted to the diagnostic cast so that it covers all the occlusal surfaces of the posterior teeth and leaves uncovered the lingual surfaces of the teeth to be prepared. With the cast still mounted on the surveyor, the paralleling instrument is slipped onto a special analyzing rod (made from a bur to exactly fit the bur guiding sleeve) and is mounted on the baseplate with self-curing resin so that the sleeve is parallel to the predetermined path of insertion.

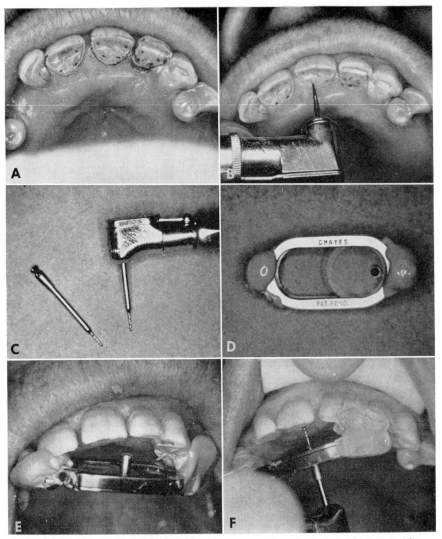

FIGURE 100.   *A*, Lingual surfaces of three maxillary incisors with preparations outlined and finishing lines prepared. Locations of pinholes marked.

B, Countersinking points of entry for pinholes.

C, Drills 0.023 inch in diameter.

D, Loma Linda Parallelometer with modeling compound on ends. Disk rotates and moves in frame. Sleeve guides bur to make all holes parallel.

E, Parallelometer secured to arch and aligned for preparation of left lateral incisor.

F, Parallelometer set for lingual path of insertion on right central incisor.

The baseplate is removed from the cast and taken to the mouth, where it can be held in position. The pinholes, when drilled, will be parallel to each other, regardless of the number.

In Figures 101 and 102 four teeth (both laterals and both cuspids) are involved. Before attempting to drill the pinholes, all other phases of the preparation were completed and a carbide bit was used to indent the enamel at the points on the ledges where the pinholes should start.

These pinholes were cut 2.0 to 2.25 mm. deep and were made parallel to the normal path of insertion. However, had there been reason for it, with the paralleling device the path of insertion could have been angled more to the lingual. Under some circumstances, particularly when using pinledges for splinting teeth, the holes may be made at right angles to the plane of the lingual surfaces, in which event ledges need not be cut on the lingual surfaces. There also may be some advantage to this linguo-labial path of insertion when abutment teeth have diverging or converging long axes and

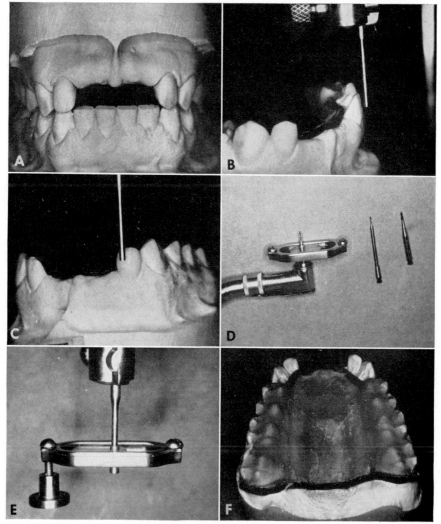

FIGURE 101.   *A,* Articulated diagnostic casts with altered mandibular incisal edges. (See case history in Chapter 36.)

B, C, Using surveyor to help determine path of insertion.

D, Loma Linda Parallelometer and 0.023 inch drill.

E, Parallelometer placed on analyzing rod of surveyor. Attachment for baseplate has been added.

F, Resin base free of abutments but covering all other occluding surfaces.

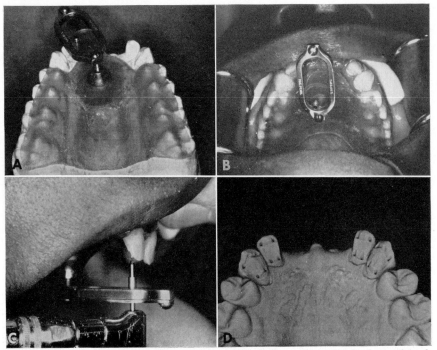

FIGURE 102. *A,* Parallelometer secured to acrylic resin palatal plate with sleeve parallel to predetermined path of insertion.

B, Device transferred to maxillary arch.

C, Four abutments have been prepared up to sinking pinholes. Points of entry have been indented with No. ½ round bur. The sixteen pinholes—four in each tooth—will be parallel.

D, Cast of prepared teeth.

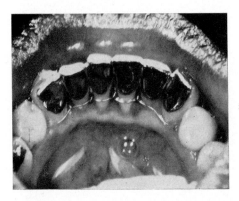

FIGURE 103. Mandibular anterior splint made by this technique.

incisal seating could endanger a pulp. When the lingual approach is being used on an individual tooth, the paralleler may be stabilized on supporting teeth with modeling compound.

On a very thin tooth the holes in the incisal one-third, suitable for pins of bent wire (24-gauge PGP wire*), can be made with a No. ½ round

* The J. M. Ney Company, Hartford, Conn.

bur. With such pins, owing to the color of the wire, there possibly is less chance that a shadow will show through the labial enamel. However, cast posts or pins will serve the purpose in almost every case and under almost all conditions. For example, in mandibular incisors, regardless of bulk, the closer-fitting, even though shorter (1.3 to 1.5 mm.), cast pins give a snug fit that is impossible on these teeth with bent wire pins. On a maxillary lateral or central, when the cingulum is deeply indented, a pin 1.25 mm. long and the size of a No. 702 or 703 bur may be used. With the Pinwaxer these can be waxed directly or indirectly, without flaws.

The Finishing Line and Incisal Bevel. The finishing line for a pinledge is in three sections. The lingual surface segment is a chamfer and is accentuated by using a small round stone from the incisal edge to the point where the proximal cut and cingulum reduction join. The proximal cut has produced a chisel-edge margin on that surface admirably suited for a finishing line. The incisal edge and angle must be beveled, although not drastically. This phase of the finishing line is the final step in this preparation.

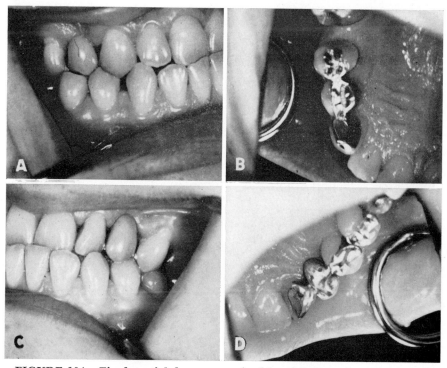

FIGURE 104. Fixed partial dentures retained by pinledges.

A, B, First bicuspid pontic retained by pinledge on cuspid and inlay in second bicuspid.

C, D, Replacing upper cuspid. Pinledge on lateral incisor abutment; inlay in first bicuspid.

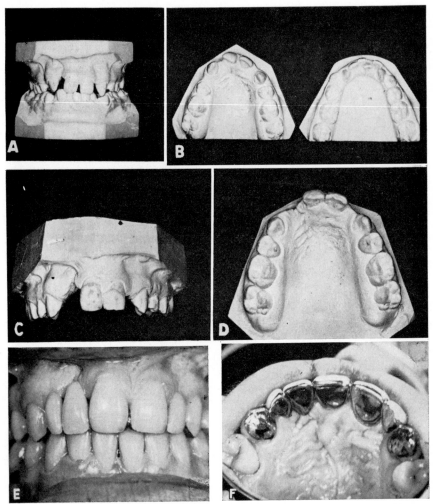

FIGURE 105. Replacing maxillary lateral incisors; repaired cleft between right cuspid and central incisor.

A, B, Casts of mouth before orthodontic treatment.

C, D, Upper arch after orthodontics. The left lateral space is normal in width; on the right it is approximately two-thirds wider than the left. The cuspids have no proximal surfaces. The left central is normal; the right is ultraconcave on the lingual. The right ridge is abnormal, owing to closed cleft.

E, Fixed partial denture retained by four pinledges, each with two incisal wire pins and two cast pins in the cingulum.

F, Three lateral incisor pontics.

DIRECT WAXING

If the operator prefers a direct waxing technique, the pinholes can be made with No. 700 or 701 taper fissure burs, with drills, or with No. ½ round burs. The pins can be waxed in holes made with taper burs by using a Pinwaxer or a No. 23 explorer. Wax is pressed against the preparation and partly carved. The Pinwaxer or explorer is heated, seated in the pinhole, and slowly withdrawn. Molten wax will flow in behind it. Tapered plastic pins, 1.0 mm. longer than the depth of the hole, can be fitted into the pinholes. The wax pattern is readily adapted around that portion which extends beyond the surface of the tooth. Nylon bristles of appropriate size or 24-gauge PGP wire should be used when the pinholes have been made with a drill or a No. ½ round bur.

When using tapered plastic pins or nylon bristles, soft wax is pressed against the prepared lingual and proximal surfaces. It is held in position while being carved to approximate form and dimensions. The wax is

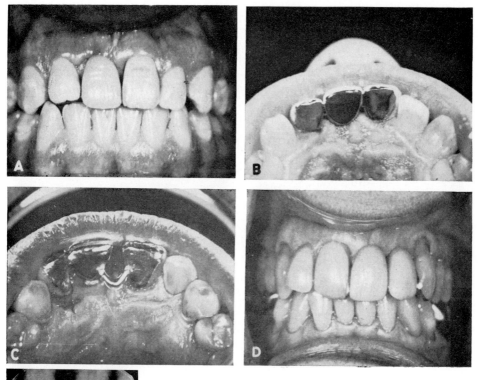

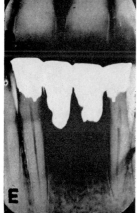

FIGURE 106. *A, B,* Labial and lingual views of central incisor supported by two pinledges.

C, Perpetuating diastema.

D, Replacing upper left central and lateral incisors. Pinledge on right central.

E, Replacing lower central incisors. Pinledges on laterals.

pooled over the pins and pressed lightly with a finger in order to fill all indentations or voids. Carving is completed. A small nodule of wax is placed in the center of the lingual surface, and with a No. 5 explorer point engaging the excess wax the pattern is removed.

Direct Waxing with Wire Pins

Each wire pin (24-gauge PGP wire) must be cut long enough to protrude 0.5 mm. from the orifice of the hole. The PGP wire must also have a horizontal extension of not less than 1.0 mm. It is imperative that this arm be bent sharply; otherwise the pins may not be held securely in the wax pattern on withdrawal, and the casting will not seat (Fig. 107).

After the preparation has been moistened with saliva, the wire pins, grasped by cotton pliers with the arm pointed into the mouth, can be placed in the holes without difficulty. They will be held there by the saliva and friction.

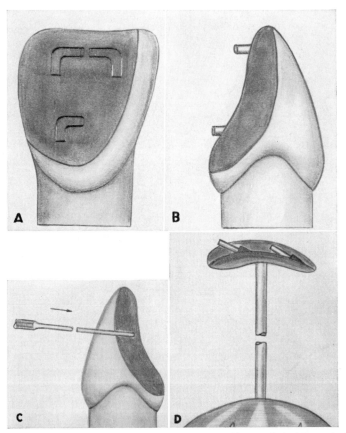

FIGURE 107.   *A,* Direct wax pattern showing outline and position of pins.
B, Setting pins in wax.
C, Disengaging pattern.
D, Spruing pattern.

The Wax Pattern

With the pins flat against the tooth surface, a softened piece of inlay wax is pressed to place against both the lingual and the proximal surfaces. It must be held against the tooth from the lingual while the incisal and proximal are being carved. The lingual wax is then pared almost to tooth form. The wax is pooled over each pin with a heated canal plugger, and the pins are turned perpendicular to the lingual surface. The wax is resoftened and the arms are rotated into their original positions against the tooth, thus assuring that wax completely surrounds the wire pins.

Just before the carving is completed, the pattern must be disengaged. If it cannot be removed with a No. 5 explorer point thrust into the lingual surface, the instrument is placed on the proximal and gentle pressure is applied toward the lingual. Minute movement will break the adhesion. It is then reseated, margins are readapted, carving is finished, and the wax is polished, leaving a little excess on the incisal only. A small bead of wax is placed and secured in the center of the lingual surface to facilitate the attachment of the sprue pin. The pattern is removed and sprued as described (see Fig. 107D).

(See Chapter 10, The Working Cast, for polysulfide rubber impressions of pinledge preparations. See Chapter 13 for Spruing, Investing, and Casting.)

REFERENCES

1. Grubb, H. D.: Fixed bridgework. J. Pros. Den., *3*:121, Jan. 1953.
2. Vedder, F. B.: Paper read before Crown and Bridge Symposium, Indiana Univ. School Den., April 1956.
3. Pruden, K. C.: A hydrocolloid technique for pinledge bridge abutments. J. Pros. Den., *6*:65, Jan. 1956.
4. Baum, L.: Progress report on intraoral precision drilling techniques. J. South. California D. A., 27:134, April 1959.
5. Baum, L.: Technics for utilizing intraoral aligning devices for achieving parallelism in cavity preparations. J. D. Res., *39*:768, July–Aug. 1960 (Abstract).
6. Baum, L.: New cast gold restorations for anterior teeth. J.A.D.A., *61*:1, July 1960.
7. Curtis, G. H., and Baum, L.: New concepts in splinting the mandibular anterior teeth. J. Periodont., *31*:393, Oct. 1960.
8. Johnston, J. F.: The application and construction of the pinledge retainer. J. Pros. Den., *3*:559, July 1953.
9. Alpert, C. C.: Anterior pinledge abutment. J. Dist. Columbia D. Soc., *34*:11, Feb. 1959.

Pinkerton, R. G.: Anterior fixed bridge prosthesis. J.A.D.A., *44*:393, April 1952.
Pruden, K. C.: Abutments and attachments in fixed partial dentures. J. Pros. Den., 7:502, July 1957.

8

THE INLAY RETAINER

The inlay is a retainer that should be employed only under the most favorable conditions and when workmanship is of the highest order.[1] When an inlay-retained bridge is constructed by one who understands its limitations and does not exceed its potentialities, the prosthesis will have a surprisingly long life. When its use can be justified, minimal tooth surface is covered by metal.

INDICATIONS

For the inlay to be used successfully as a bridge retainer, the span must be short, preferably no wider than one tooth; the mouth must be relatively caries-free or must have entered into a caries-free period; and the clinical crown must be of average length and in functional occlusion cannot be subjected to undue leverage. The tooth should be vital, with dentin lining all cavity walls. Theoretically only one joint should be soldered, and it should approximate the stronger of the two abutment teeth. With rugged teeth, there can be frequent exceptions to this rule. An inlay may be used to support the free end of a broken-stress bridge, since little or no stress will be transferred from the bridge.[2]

Inlays are being used in increasing numbers in the mouths of the young-age group because of the mounting evidence that crowns for adolescents cause considerable gingival irritation on the buccal and lingual surfaces, especially the lingual. While pulp size and crown length may make it necessary that the cavity preparations be shallow, pins can add to retention. In these cases, both joints are soldered.

144

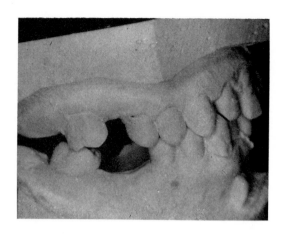

FIGURE 108. Mandibular molar has mesial tilt. Tooth should not be built up to occlusion on mesial with inlay retainer. Maxillary space suitable for inlay retainers.

CONTRAINDICATIONS

An inlay retainer is contraindicated for a tooth that is rotated, extensively carious, short (except in the very young), extruded, or pulpless, or that has a large cervical restoration. A cavity prepared in a rotated tooth will give substantial retention only when supplemented by two or more pinholes; even then the inlay may not offer an area receptive to the solder joint. Usually an inlay cavity in a broken-down or short tooth is not retentive. When one abutment is extruded beyond the occlusal plane, the load will be unorthodox and excessive for the surrounding tooth walls. A pulpless tooth is brittle and often the retainer must be supported by cement. When there is cervical caries or a cervical restoration, the walls may be incapable of resisting the force transmitted through the inlay.

An inlay should not be used to build up one section of the occlusal surface of a tipped tooth, because leverage from the protruding casting may overcome stability (Fig. 108). It is contraindicated in an older patient, whose teeth may be severely abraded, because the lateral walls probably will be checked or cracked and unequal to the strain induced by mastication. Thus, in order to cover the occlusal surface, the tooth must be shortened so much that the proximal surfaces cannot control displacement.

The inlay retainer should be either an MO or DO restoration. If the abutment is a first molar, it may have steps into the buccal and lingual surfaces.[3] An MOD inlay is contraindicated as the major support for a bridge, because the cavity walls will be unduly weakened by the preparation without there being an increase in holding power. A partial veneer or full veneer gold crown should be substituted.

CAVITY PREPARATION

When compared with a single-unit preparation, the cavity walls for

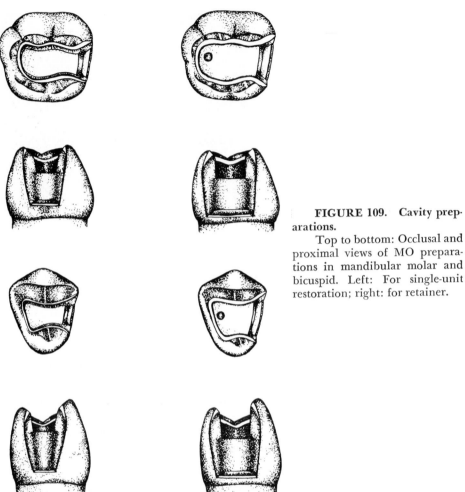

FIGURE 109. Cavity preparations.

Top to bottom: Occlusal and proximal views of MO preparations in mandibular molar and bicuspid. Left: For single-unit restoration; right: for retainer.

an inlay retainer must be more nearly parallel, there must be added depth and width, and the cavity outline should be extended into the auxiliary grooves (Fig. 109).[4] In width, the proximal step should include the buccal and lingual line angles, or go beyond one of them if the tooth is rotated. The occlusal margin should have a wider and heavier bevel so that the walls will have more protection during lateral excursions.

In a molar preparation a pinhole should be placed in the occlusal floor,[5] 1.0 to 2.0 mm. from the remaining marginal ridge. In a bicuspid it should be adjacent to the marginal ridge. Occlusal pinholes should be 1.5 mm. deep and should be made with a No. 701 or 702 taper fissure bur. Larger sizes are desirable occasionally. Location and depth are dictated by pulp position, form, and size. In the cervical seat of the cavity, pinholes should be made 1.0 mm. deep with a No. 700 bur and should be a continuation of grooved axial line angles. Pinholes must be in dentin, *not* in cement.

When an MO inlay is to be used in a maxillary first molar, the occlusal seat of the cavity need not cross the transverse ridge unless there is under-mining caries in the distal pit or on the distal surface. It should be deeper than the conventional preparation, and the pinhole, to be made with a No. 702 taper fissure bur, should be against the ridge and 1.5 mm. deep. The axial angles should be grooved with a No. 56 bur, and two pinholes should be made in the cervical seat (Fig. 110).

Retention in all inlay retainer cavities is effected not only through the parallel walls and width of the cavity floor but also by the parallel relation-ship of the pin in the occlusal pinhole with the casting fitting against the axial walls. An accurately fitting occlusal pin will limit forces against the buccal and lingual walls of the tooth, while pins in the cervical seat of the cavity will transmit any stress to the entire tooth rather than one specific area (Figs. 111 and 112). In an indirect technique, pinholes should be a little larger in diameter and more shallow.

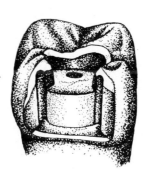
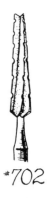

FIGURE 110. MO preparation for maxillary first molar.

#702

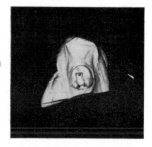

FIGURE 111. Preparation with three pinholes in mandibular molar.

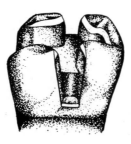
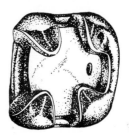

FIGURE 112. Preparation advocated by Markley for either maxillary or mandibular molars.

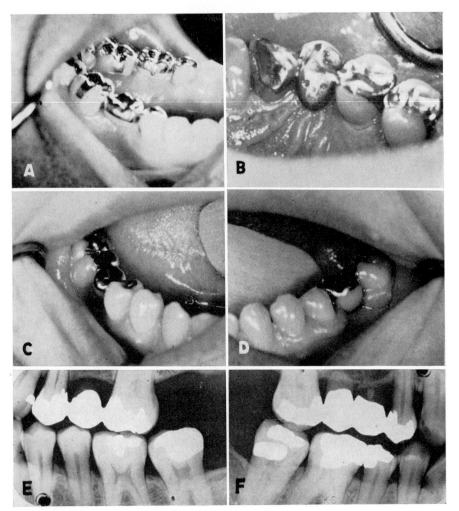

FIGURE 113.   Inlay-retained bridges.

A, Replacing mandibular right first molar. Markley-type inlay retainer in second molar; DO inlay in second bicuspid; distal joint soldered; mesial connector a subocclusal rest.

B, Inlay-pinledge bridge supplying maxillary cuspid.

C, D, Inlay-retained bridges in same arch. MO inlays in second molars; DO inlays in second bicuspids; anterior connectors are subocclusal rests.

E, Replacing upper second bicuspid. DO inlay in first molar (note pins) and MOD inlay in second bicuspid (note pin); two solder joints.

F, Four-unit bridge retained by two two-surface inlays. This technique (and also *E*) is recommended only for an operator who has exceptional skill and judgment.

The instruments and instrumentation are the same as for any inlay preparation.

THE WAX PATTERN

When carving an inlay pattern direct, a circular matrix band is fitted loosely around the tooth, the band being trimmed both occlusally and cervically to accommodate the opposing cusps and to avoid cutting the soft tissue. The inner surface of the band is coated with Microfilm and filled with softened inlay wax; then the surface to be applied to the cavity is warmed until the wax is quite soft, after which the band and wax are forced to place on the prepared tooth. (See Chapter 6, The Partial Veneer Crown.) The patient is asked to close and hold this position with no lateral movement until the wax has solidified.

The excess wax is trimmed from the occlusal and cervical of the band, using a suitable wax carver or a warm No. 23 explorer point. The band is loosened and removed from the tooth, with the wax being held in position in the tooth either by the finger or a pellet of damp cotton held by pliers.

At no time during direct carving should the carving stroke be in a direction that will remove the pattern from the tooth, unless it is maintained in its contact position under pressure.

Gross carving can be done with a Wagner or an Ash instrument, a No. 12 Crenshaw scaler, or any instrument most conveniently handled by the operator.

Final proximal carving is best done with the No. 23 explorer, or the tapered end of the Wagner, finishing at the cervical with the Tarno No. 1 and No. 2 wax burnishers. The No. 2 can be used with a lateral "push" or "pull" stroke.

The occlusal surface can be carved with the instrument of choice. Either the flat end of the Wagner instrument or the No. 5 explorer is most efficient. If a margin is uncovered, small amounts of wax may be added to the pattern, making sure that no saliva is incorporated and that a union between the added wax and the pattern is consummated.

Form must be produced that is compatible with the tooth being restored and with the occlusal pattern. If the tooth has abraded surfaces on the proximal or occlusal, such surfaces must be copied. If the patient is young, with normal convexities and grooves, then such form must appear in the carving.

There can be no overextended margins, occlusally, proximally, or cervically. Checking the wax pattern *before it is removed from the tooth* will disclose any such discrepancy. After the occlusal is polished with wet cotton and the proximal surface with smooth-edged seam binding tape, the pattern can be removed from the tooth, using an explorer on the proximal, or two explorers if the pattern is an MOD.

Spruing

The pattern should be attached to the sprue pin at once, letting the pattern rest in the palm of the hand and applying the heated pin to the contact area in a direction that bisects the angle on the cavity surface. It must be invested immediately.

REFERENCES

1. Pruden, K. C.: Abutments and attachments in fixed partial dentures. J. Pros. Den., 7:502, July 1957.
2. Markley, M. R.: The practical application of sound principles to the field of restorative dentistry. J. Pros. Den., 3:96, Jan. 1953.
3. Markley, M. R.: Broken-stress principle and design in fixed bridge prosthesis. J. Pros. Den., 1:416, July 1951.
4. Thom, L. W.: Principles of cavity preparation in crown and bridge prosthesis. III. The inlay abutment. J.A.D.A., 41:541, Nov. 1950.
5. Ante, I. H.: Abutments. J. Canad. D. A., 2:249, 1936.

9

THE MACBOYLE RETAINER

The MacBoyle retainer, like the inlay, will be a serviceable retainer if meticulously designed and constructed. Its application is limited, but in a few instances it supersedes all other retainers.

INDICATIONS

The MacBoyle retainer may be used on mandibular central and lateral and maxillary lateral incisors, even though these teeth have proximal caries or large pulps. It is akin to the partial veneer crown, but the preparation is not as deep and the retention is derived from grooves at the labial line angles instead of on the proximal surfaces. It is indicated particularly for adolescents, but it will be satisfactory for any patient who does not object to a display of metal. It should be considered primarily as a retainer for temporary bridges.

PREPARATION

The steps in the preparation are as follows:
(1) reduction of the mesial and distal surfaces,
(2) reduction of the lingual surface from the crest of the cingulum to the incisal edge, and
(3) reduction of the incisal edge;
(4) beveling the mesio- and disto-labial line angles;
(5) grooving the mesio- and disto-labial bevels;

151

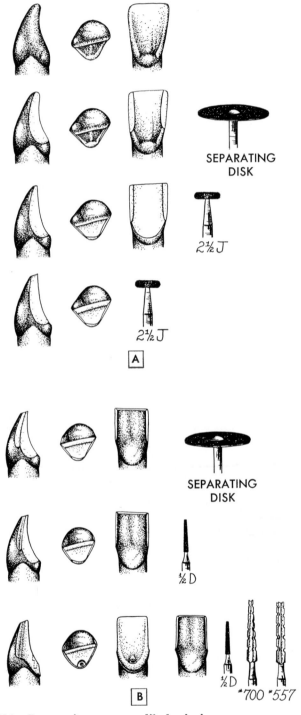

FIGURE 114.   Preparation on a mandibular incisor.

A, Top to bottom: Uncut tooth; proximal slices; lingual reduction; incisal bevel.

B, Top to bottom: Labial line angles beveled; labial chamfer; finishing line, lingual pinhole, and rounded angles at labio-incisal.

(6) reduction of the cingulum and establishing the cervical finishing line; and

(7) placing a pinhole in the cingulum.

The mesial and distal cuts, made with a disk in a straight handpiece, should be parallel to the path of insertion. Labially they can extend beyond the line angles but should converge lingually less than the proximal cuts for the anterior partial veneer crown (Fig. 114*A*).

The lingual surface may be prepared 0.5 mm. deep, with a round-edge wheel stone of appropriate size. This cut, starting on the cingulum, must include the incisal edge. Here the reduction is made at an angle similar to the abrasion, or indicated abrasion, on this surface. Using a disk or stone, the labial line angles can be beveled from 0.3 to 0.5 mm. onto the labial surface and as far cervically as the contour of the tooth will permit, which usually is three-fifths or two-thirds of the length of the surface (Fig. 114*B*). A small cylindrical or tapered stone is used to make the bevels concave but not so deep that their axial margins are at right angles to the labial enamel surface.

The cingulum is shaped the same as for a partial veneer crown. The cervical finishing line is continued onto the proximal surface and may go into the gingival crevice, although this is not a requisite.

A No. 700 or 701 taper fissure bur is used to make a pinhole in the cingulum, 1.0 mm. deep and parallel to the path of insertion. The labial

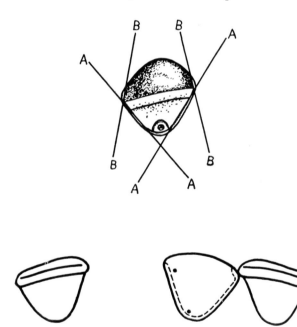

FIGURE 115. Schematic explanation of MacBoyle preparation, showing retentive grasp on labial. MacBoyle preparation combined with pinledge on rotated tooth. Lines A-A designate the direction of the proximal cuts; lines B-B show the labial convergence of the labial bevels, which provides resistance to lingual displacement.

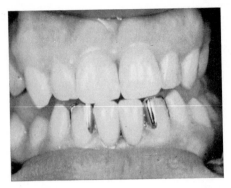

FIGURE 116. Lower anterior bridge constructed for adolescent. Pulps large, deep proximal caries. New bridge, with veneered crown retainers, will be built when pulps have receded sufficiently to permit adequate preparations.

margin at the incisal edge is beveled only enough to protect the enamel rods.

When accelerated speeds are used for this preparation, the proximal surfaces should be reduced with a disk to avoid an exaggerated display of metal at the labial line angles. Otherwise, instrumentation closely follows the initial steps for a partial veneer crown.

Direct wax patterns may be carved using the same technique advocated for the maxillary anterior partial veneer crown.

The sprue should be attached outside the mouth and in the same manner as for a pinledge retainer.

10

THE WORKING CAST

Many types and combinations of impression materials have been used for the fabrication of the fixed partial prosthesis, each having advantages and disadvantages. The rubber base impression materials have become increasingly popular since their introduction, displacing hydrocolloid in many areas. Their merit lies in reduced armamentarium and simplicity of use, not in greater intrinsic accuracy.

RUBBER BASE IMPRESSION MATERIALS

The rubber base materials fall into two broad classifications, the polysulfide rubbers and the silicones, of which there are many brands now on the market. Among their advantages over hydrocolloid may be listed: (1) the ability to pour two stone casts in one impression; (2) the possibility of seating metalized dies in a full arch impression and producing a working cast with removable units; (3) the ability to withdraw plastic pins and nylon bristles and thus reproduce all sizes and lengths of pinholes in the stone cast; (4) slightly extended working time; and (5) a more varied application in many offices.

Selection of a material probably will be based on office routine, mastery of the material, and objective handling characteristics. Discussion of the manipulation of some of these materials follows in this chapter.

POLYSULFIDE RUBBER IMPRESSIONS

The polysulfide rubber is prepared by combining two pastes. One tube contains a mercaptan, a compound having extremely reactive –SH terminals

155

on the molecule.[1,2] The other tube usually holds lead peroxide and small amounts of sulfur, and such agents as zinc oxide, stearic acid, and calcium sulfate are added to regulate certain properties. Polymerization, and thus curing of the paste in the mouth to an elastic impression, is accomplished by mixing the second paste with the first. The basic compositions of these synthetic rubbers have now been well established and shelf life and quality fluctuations among batches are no longer problems.

The polysulfide rubber materials generally are brown in color and have a rather pungent odor (although less noticeable to the patient than to the operator), are sticky, and for the inept can be somewhat messy to use. Clothing must be protected.

As with hydrocolloid, the manipulation of each of these materials must be carefully standardized. The variables that influence precision and sharpness of detail are common to both.

Construction of the Tray

In contrast to hydrocolloid, a lesser bulk of material is desirable in making rubber base impressions. Accurate dies and casts cannot be produced routinely when ordinary stock impression trays are used. Since research has shown that the accuracy of the rubber base impression is in part dependent on a thin, uniform layer of material, with an optimal thickness of 1.0 to 2.0 mm., a tray must be built to assure an even, minimal thickness of impression material around the preparations and working area in order to construct well-fitting, complicated restorations such as bridges.[3] It must be emphasized that a stiff tray, adherence of the rubber to the tray, and proper control of bulk are all essential to accuracy.

Several satisfactory self-curing resin tray materials are available and the techniques for their use are basically the same. One layer of baseplate wax is adapted over a diagnostic cast to create the space needed for the rubber (Fig. 117). This space is maintained in the oral cavity by stops that make contact with teeth or ridge tissue and preclude further seating of the tray. They are made by removing wax from the occlusal surfaces or incisal edges of three or more teeth that will not be used as abutments. These supporting teeth should be as widely separated as possible, to form a tripod that will allow the tray to be held without movement during setting of the impression material. If the remaining teeth are insufficient to stabilize the tray, then one or two of the stops should be in contact with the ridge tissue, although definitely not in areas associated with the prosthesis.

Tin foil is burnished over the wax to keep it from contaminating the inside of the tray, and thus prevents the impression material from pulling away and being permanently deformed when removed from the mouth. The tray resin is mixed in accordance with the manufacturer's directions and pressed over the prepared cast. It should fill the spaces

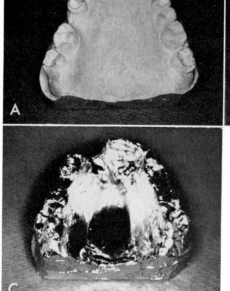

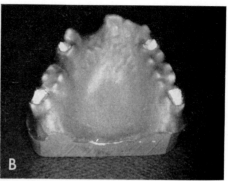

FIGURE 117. *A,* Diagnostic cast with tray stops outlined on four teeth.

B, Wax over diagnostic cast to provide space for impression material. Stop areas cut through wax.

C, Wax tin-foiled to prevent contamination of tray resin.

cut out for the stops. The tray should include enough of the soft tissue area so that pontics can be aligned, but should not extend so far apically that deep tissue undercuts are involved needlessly. To do so would make removal from the mouth difficult and might cause deformation of the impression material. If an extensive undercut must be included, it should be blocked out with wax before covering the cast with the single sheet of baseplate wax (Fig. 118).

After the material has set, the tray is removed from the cast, the tin foil and wax are stripped from its inner surface, and the borders are trimmed with an acrylic bur or stone.

Preparation of the Tray or Band

The tray, or the band for an impression of a single tooth, must be rigid. A pliable matrix will invariably distort when taken from the mouth. Likewise, the material must be held tenaciously by the tray or band. The rubber cement, as a rule supplied by the manufacturer, works very well if the surface of the vehicle is clean, sparingly coated, and then set aside for at least 6 or 7 minutes before it is filled.

The Gingival Crevice

Before preparing the abutment teeth the gingival crevice should be

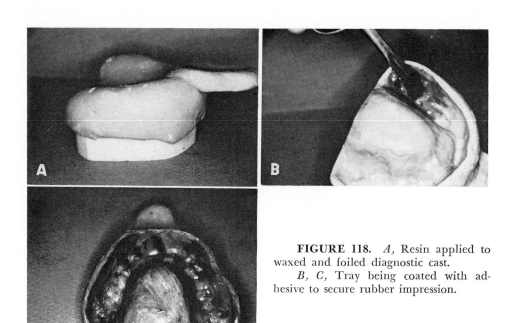

FIGURE 118. *A,* Resin applied to waxed and foiled diagnostic cast.

B, C, Tray being coated with adhesive to secure rubber impression.

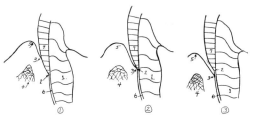

1 DENTIN
2 CEMENTO-ENAMEL JUNCTION
3 GINGIVAL ATTACHMENT
4 ALVEOLAR PROCESS
5 GINGIVAL CREST
6 CEMENTUM
7 ENAMEL
8 3-5 = DEPTH OF CREVICE

FIGURE 119. Types of gingival crevices. Left to right: adolescent; adult; slight recession. (Courtesy of J. F. Jelenko & Co., Inc.)

explored (Fig. 119). In the young patient it will be shallow and the gum will be more troublesome to retract. In the adult patient the depth is customarily more than 1.0 mm., giving room not only to place the cervical margin where, theoretically, it will be protected against both recurrent caries and recession, but also to displace the tissue for an elastic impression. If extension of the preparation into this crevice is impracticable, the type of cervical finishing line and its outline must be determined by the preference and judgment of the operator.

Mouth Preparation

Elastic impression materials will not significantly displace tissue, saliva, blood, mucus, or debris, and contact with any one of these, excepting tissue, will ruin an impression. Therefore the most urgent aspects of mouth preparation are lateral movement of the gingival tissue to uncover the cervical margin, and cleaning and drying of the total area to be included in the impression.

Methods of Tissue Displacement

Displacement of tissue, or exposing the margin of the preparation, may be done by mechanical pressure alone, which is slow and occasionally uncomfortable, or by mechanical pressure and drugs that will relax the soft tissue and inhibit the seepage of blood or serum (Fig. 120).[4] Surgical removal of gingival tissue requires a perfected technique and demonstration, and will not be discussed here.

Mechanical Displacement.   The mechanical method is applied most often to full veneer gold crown preparations or when surgical intervention is not warranted to correct an irregular or high gingival outline. An aid to, rather than a means of, marginal exposure, it is done with an aluminum shell that has been trimmed to conform to the gingival contour and *to rest on the occlusal surface* of the prepared tooth **without impinging** at any point on the tissue. The patient should be asked to close and contour the occlusal surface of the shell, then occlusal irregularities must be smoothed and the cervical margin–gingival tissue relationship rechecked. This shell, coated at the cervical margin or partially filled with a soft

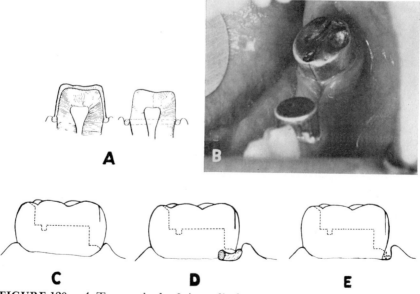

FIGURE 120.   *A,* Two methods of tissue displacement.
B, Mechanical displacement of tissue.
C, D, Displacing gingival tissue with cord and astringent liquids.
E, Correct type of displacement.

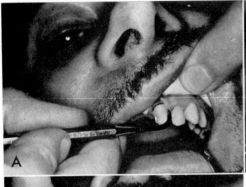
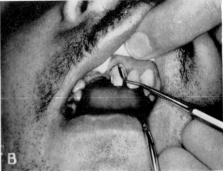
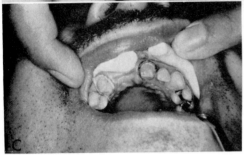

FIGURE 121. *A, B,* Packing gingival crevice with cotton fibers saturated with an alum solution.

C, Packing in position around each tooth. Alum was activated by an application of Hemodent. Displacement was lateral.

temporary stopping that has been heated until flexible, is replaced in its predetermined position on the tooth. The stopping will be extruded, displacing the gingiva.

Outside the mouth, the cervical of the temporary stopping must be trimmed so that the tissue will be displaced laterally without blanching. A drop of cavity varnish or of zinc oxide and eugenol paste is placed inside the temporary crown, which is returned to the dried tooth for at least 12 hours. The stopping in the gingival crevice should be smoothed with a warm instrument.

If preparations and impressions cannot be made at the same sitting, this mode of coverage and displacement is acceptable. It is also suitable on posterior teeth prepared for partial veneer crowns.

WARNING: Displacement of tissue, if sustained for the entire construction period, may cause prolonged or even permanent recession. The resultant uncovered neck of the abutment may be sensitive and susceptible to caries.

Cotton Fibers, Alum, and Hemodent or Orostat for Tissue Displacement. Gingival tissue can be displaced safely with alum-saturated cotton fibers* and Hemodent† or Orostat‡ (8:100 racemic epinephrine). While the elapsed time is longer than needed for zinc chloride, the tissue damage

---

* Westwood Dental Mfg. Co., Inc., Los Angeles, Calif.
† Premier Dental Products Co., Philadelphia, Penna.
‡ Surgident Ltd., Los Angeles, Calif.

is negligible, and packing may be repeated at once if desirable. The area should be dried and *kept dry* throughout the procedure, and the impregnated fibers should be packed into the crevice in all areas where the preparation is below or at the gingival crest. If the crevice is deep, more than one layer of cotton may be needed. Hemodent or Orostat, carried between the beaks of cotton pliers, may be used to dampen, but not flood, the string (Figs. 121 and 122).

After 10 minutes, the crevice should be examined for displacement of tissue. If too little has been effected, or if hemorrhage or tissue seepage continues, the area must be repacked with fresh material for an additional 5 minutes.

Cord in various sizes may be soaked in a saturated solution of alum, dried, stored, and cut off as needed, but a kit now on the market is convenient and sufficiently well stocked.*

The packing should push the gingival tissue laterally and expose the tooth surface 0.35 to 0.5 mm. past the cervical margin. If the impression material is hydrocolloid, after the mouth is rinsed, a clean, unimpregnated No. 8 thread may be tamped into the crevice to continue displacement in order that two impressions may be taken.

There are cogent reasons for using Hemodent rather than Orostat. It has none of the side effects of epinephrine, while Orostat is several times

---

* Westwood Dental Mfg. Co., Inc., Los Angeles, Calif.

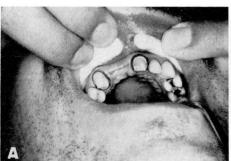
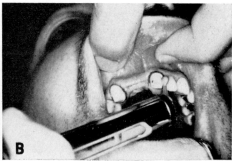
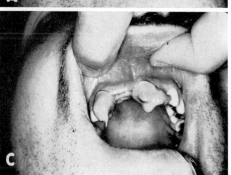

FIGURE 122. *A,* Tissue displaced laterally and to a depth well beyond margins of preparations. Area is isolated so that field may be kept dry during injection and seating of tray.

B, Starting the injection in interproximal area has a tendency to help force rubber into crevice. Syringe may be moved either to labial or lingual, but crevice and cervical margin must be covered first; then, with a circular motion, crown is covered, finishing at incisal.

C, Abutments and adjacent teeth covered with syringe material.

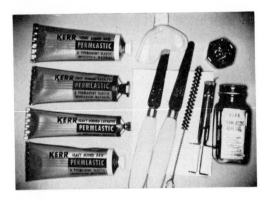

FIGURE 123. Material and equipment needed for the impression.

stronger than the maximal dosage recommended by many authorities. Hemodent does cause a granular residue in the presence of blood, but this can be removed.

Cord and Zinc Chloride in Tissue Displacement. The use of zinc chloride in the displacement of tissue has been replaced, to a great degree, by cotton fibers saturated with alum and Hemodent. Harrison[5] has shown conclusively that zinc chloride drastically affects the soft tissue and that healing following its use takes up to 60 days. However, some operators who are still using hydrocolloid continue to advocate its use.

While zinc chloride will effectively displace tissue, lasting damage can be inflicted if it is mishandled. Protective equipment, such as cotton rolls and holder, and the saliva ejector should be adjusted meticulously and kept under observation, because the quadrant must be isolated and dry or the tissue of the approximating cheek and tongue as well as that surrounding the tooth can be severely burned. The residual moisture in the crevice will activate the drug, which will relax the tissue.

After approximately 4 minutes, the impregnated string must be removed and the tissue rinsed, dried, and examined. If the cervical margin has not been exposed, it will be necessary to resort to other means. It is seldom wise to make a second application of zinc chloride, because the cervical gingiva may be cauterized beyond the point of normal repair.

Preparation of Polysulfide Rubber

A stiff yet slightly flexible spatula should be employed (Fig. 123). The manufacturer's directions for proportions must be methodically followed, as even seemingly trivial digressions may cause erratic setting.[6] Increased room temperature or high humidity definitely hastens the setting. In some climates, an air-conditioned operating room is essential to establish atmospheric conditions that will ensure sufficient working time.

Most of the materials are furnished in at least two consistencies, which are very similar to the syringe and tray hydrocolloids. One is thin, to be used for injecting into the cavity preparation, and the other is heavy-bodied, for filling the tray. A double-mix technique will minimize trapping of bubbles. Better adaptation and increased accuracy will result from careful injection followed by pressure from the less resilient rubber in the tray.

The syringe material is mixed until all streaks are gone, and is then transferred to a Dappen dish. The open end of the syringe barrel is placed into the mixture, a sufficient quantity is drawn into the barrel, the excess is wiped off the outside, and the nozzle assembly is screwed on. (Wiping off the excess should be done with care, or the syringe may be difficult to disassemble and clean.) The heavy-bodied material is mixed and the tray loaded.

Injecting and Seating the Tray

The use of a syringe for injecting polysulfide rubber impression material is highly advantageous and will facilitate flow into the intricacies

FIGURE 124. Cross section of two polysulfide rubber impressions. One at left was single mix and shows more and larger internal bubbles than one at right, which was taken with a double-mix procedure. These bubbles are dangerous, since their collapse results in distortion.

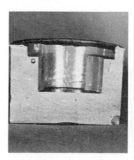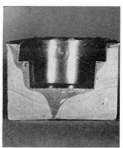

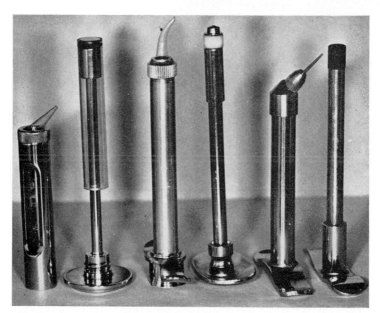

FIGURE 125. Three different syringes available for polysulfide rubbers.

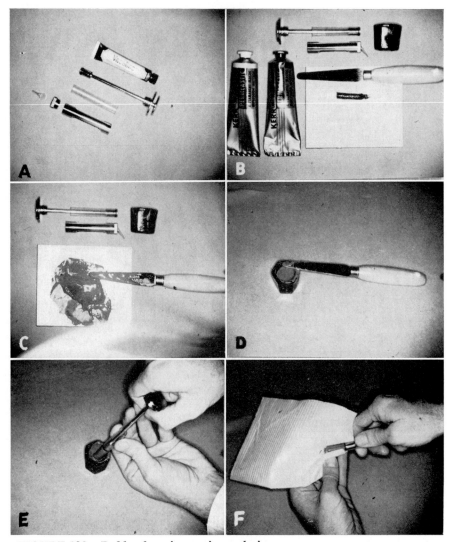

FIGURE 126.   Rubber base impression technique.
A, Syringe.
B, Armamentarium assembled.
C, Rubber mixed.
D, Transferred to dish.
E, Filling syringe.
F, Cleaning syringe.

of the preparation and lessen the possibility of trapping bubbles (Fig. 124).[7, 8] Several types are available (Fig. 125). One that can be loaded easily by drawing the material into the barrel seems to be preferable (Fig. 126).

The syringe tip is placed in one of the cervical angles of the preparation, very near the tooth surface. These are the areas to be filled first, the syringe being manipulated so that the gingival crevice is filled under light

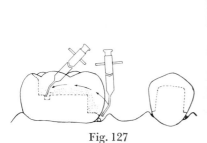

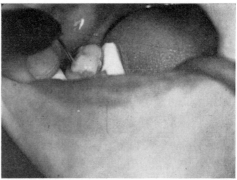

Fig. 127   Fig. 128

FIGURE 127. Syringe should be placed first at cervical margin and moved toward occlusal extremity of the preparation. (Courtesy of J. F. Jelenko & Co., Inc.)
FIGURE 128. Covering all surfaces of abutment tooth with rubber base injected from syringe.

but positive pressure (Fig. 127). The syringe tip is moved up to and across the occlusal. If the tooth has an MOD or PV preparation, the syringe is placed in the other cervical area, again very close to the tooth surface, and this area is filled as the syringe is moved toward the occlusal (Fig. 128). The occlusal surfaces of the approximating teeth and all surfaces of the abutments are covered. For a full crown, the gingival crevice is filled first; then with the syringe tip against the tooth and working with a circular motion around the tooth toward the occlusal, this surface is covered last. (See Fig. 122.)

When pinholes have been made with taper fissure burs, they will accept the small size syringe tip and may be injected and reproduced with polysulfide or silicone rubber. Immediately following injection with the syringe, the tray is filled with heavier material, is seated in the mouth, and held immobile.

Clinical Manipulation

One of the most common causes for failure is premature removal of the impression. Curing continues for some time, and adequate polymerization must take place before it is taken from the mouth. The shortest possible length of time from the start of the first mix until the impression is removed is 10 minutes, during which time the tray is seated in the mouth approximately 7 or 8 minutes.

One of the publicized arguments for the use of the rubbers is their excellent dimensional stability, which supposedly will permit safe storage of the impression indefinitely. These claims are *not* based on fact.[9] There is no doubt that some dimensional change does occur with time and that these changes are due to continued polymerization and to release of internal

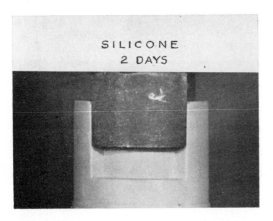

FIGURE 129. Gross distortion resulting in a silicone impression poured at 2 days. Casting was made on original die and will fit stone cast if impression is poured at once.

stress. Distortion, particularly on preparations involving long and parallel walls, can be detected readily in a matter of hours (Fig. 129). Although in regard to storage there probably is somewhat greater leeway than with hydrocolloid, it is advisable to pour the rubber base impression within the first 2 hours, especially if the first cast poured is to be removed after 1 hour and sectioned for dies (Fig. 130). The second, or working, cast would then be poured not more than 3 hours after removal from the mouth. The safety range beyond this interval is questionable.

The Die

The cast to be sectioned for dies should be trimmed and a fine jeweler's saw used to cut it from the ridge through to within 3.0 mm. of the base. Pressure at either end will fracture the sections. If those sections which contain the reproductions of the abutments are trimmed so that the cervical margin of the preparation will have the greatest circumference on the die, there will be room for carving, and any tooth contour cervical to the margin of the preparation will be visible.

Using another method for die construction, one impression may be poured to 2.5 mm. above the cervical margins of the teeth (Fig. 131).[10] Just after the stone is poured, dowel pins, flat on one side, should be set into the abutments approximately parallel to the long axes of those teeth. Wire loops are placed to engage the second pouring of stone. Centering and paralleling the dowel pins in the impression can also be done mechanically.[10]

After the stone has set in a humidifier, the stone surface is dried and lubricated with either petrolatum or shellac, and the ends of the dowel pins are covered with small balls of wax. The remainder of the impression is then filled, covering the wax on the ends of the dowel pins. As a guide to sectioning, the added stone should differ in color from the original.

Using a jeweler's saw, the abutment teeth are sectioned through the initial pouring of stone. The die can be detached by cutting out the wax

THE WORKING CAST **167**

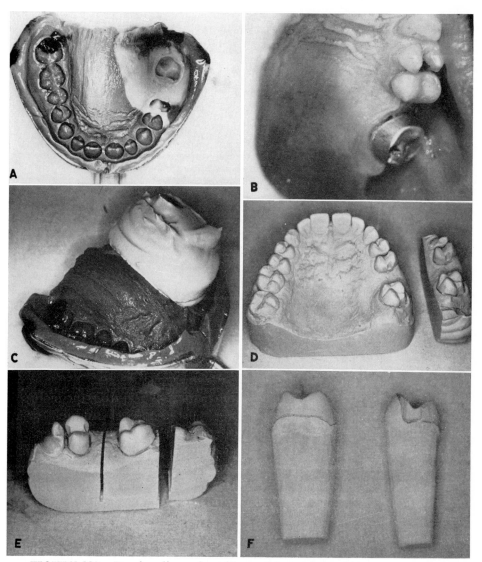

FIGURE 130. Pouring dies and working cast in one impression.

A, The impression.

B, Prepared teeth covered with aluminum shell filled with temporary stopping, and resin PV crown.

C, Prepared teeth poured for dies.

D, Casts trimmed for mounting and sectioning.

E, Sectioned die cast.

F, Dies trimmed.

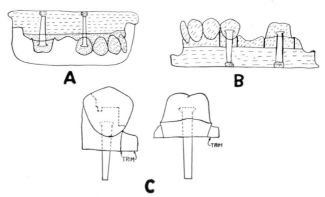

FIGURE 131.   Method for pouring impression in sections to produce removable dies.
A, Two mixes of contrasting colored stone are used.
B, Dies are sectioned through first pouring.
C, Dies trimmed.
(Courtesy of J. F. Jelenko & Co., Inc.)

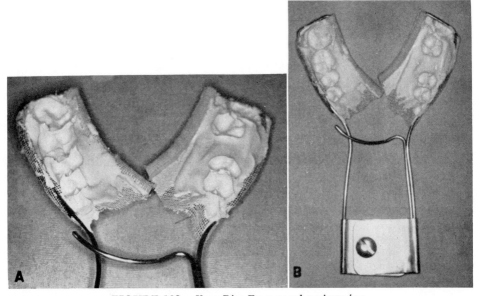

FIGURE 132.   Kerr Bite Frame and registration.

at the end of the dowel pins and tapping the pins with a metal instrument. The stone must be trimmed from the cervical margin to give access for carving the wax pattern.

The Opposing Cast

The impression for the opposing cast may be made with polysulfide rubber or alginate and poured with stone. If the operator chooses to work against a metal cast, a plaster of Paris or rubber impression may be taken.

The occluding cast must be made from an impression just as accurate as that taken for the working cast and should be poured soon enough to avoid distortion. The casts must be articulated and mounted with the maximal degree of accuracy that the available equipment will allow.

The Registration

The registration is made, using a Kerr Bite Frame (Fig. 132) with a zinc oxide and eugenol impression paste which sets hard. The impression material is applied to both sides of the gauze bib on the Bite Frame, which is then placed over the prepared teeth and two or more posterior teeth in the adjoining quadrant. The patient is instructed to close in centric occlusion and to maintain this position. After the paste has hardened, the registration is put aside along with the locked face-bow for safekeeping.

MOUNTING THE CAST

After being trimmed, the maxillary cast must be mounted on an articulator capable of simulating the movements dictated by the occluding surfaces of the opposing teeth. The mandibular can be related to it, using the registration procured with the Kerr Bite Frame, and secured to the instrument.

Casts should be mounted using a face-bow (Fig. 133). The technique to be described accepts the existing orientation even though it be an

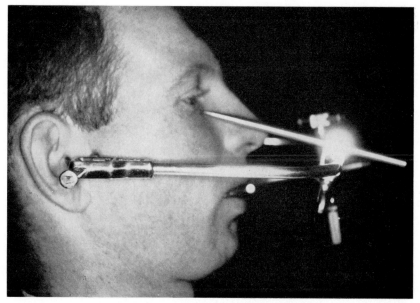

FIGURE 133.   Making face-bow registration.

eccentric jaw relation. Hundreds of thousands of bridges and other restorations that have given many years of comfortable, efficient, nondestructive service have been built in this way. The authors are not opposed to reconstructing mouths using the hinge axis mounting, but are presenting a plea for sanity in the approach to the making of the small, badly needed fixed partial prosthesis.

Many prosthodontists believe that it is not necessary to mount casts with a face-bow registration. This may be true for the construction of complete dentures. However, bridges, constructed over casts that have been mounted on an adjustable articulator with the assistance of a face-bow, have better alignment and require less equilibration when placed in the mouth.

The condyle should be located on each side of the face. The fork, covered above and below with two thicknesses of medium-soft baseplate wax, should be placed in the mouth and the patient instructed to close with enough force to indent the wax approximately 2.0 mm. The face-bow is adjusted and locked and the assembly is transferred to the articulator (Fig. 134). The maxillary cast, whether it be the opposing or working cast, is secured to the fork and then attached to the articulator with plaster of Paris. Using the Kerr Bite Frame registration for position, the opposing cast should be luted to the upper cast and fixed on the articulator.

The plaster of Paris must be trimmed and smoothed so that no crumbs will break off and interfere with carving the wax patterns. The condyle slots of the articulator should be set to accommodate the lateral and protrusive movements of the articulating surfaces. (See Fig. 135.)

Any articulator used in constructing a bridge should be capable of reproducing, in a general way, the centric, lateral, and protrusive positions of the mandible. The dictatorial introduction of extremely complex mechanical armamentarium into the offices of all dentists who should be making bridges replacing one or two teeth will result only in bridges not being built. Prosthodontics need not be so spectacular. Small crown and bridge articulators possibly may be adequate when short posterior replacements are being constructed by the direct technique, but larger, more versatile instruments and full arch casts, needed for either direct or indirect construction of longer or anterior prostheses, will serve much better.

Dies Separate from the Working Cast

When a pattern for a casting is made by an indirect technique, certain preliminary requirements must be met. The die must be constructed so that it can be removed from the articulated working cast, or it may be separate entirely if produced from the same impression or from the same type of elastic impression. The accuracy of the die or the method for making the die must be proved. If the die was made by metalizing a copper band-modeling compound impression, a cast transfer can be made. If this casting fits the die, seats on the tooth, and fits the preparation, the die can be used. If a synthetic rubber or hydrocolloid impression was used to pour the die, accuracy may be taken for granted, provided that the fundamentals of impression-taking have not been violated.

The pattern can be carved, polished, and invested with the expectation

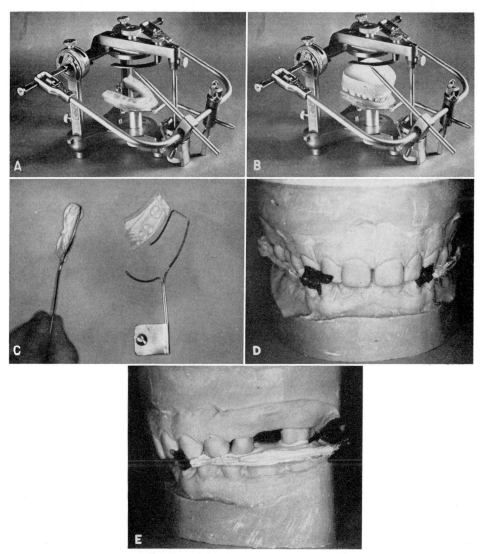

FIGURE 134. *A,* Face-bow registration transferred to articulator.
B, Upper cast oriented for mounting.
C, Kerr Bite Frame and registration; left section removed from frame.
D, E, Lower cast articulated with and luted to upper cast, which has been attached to articulator.

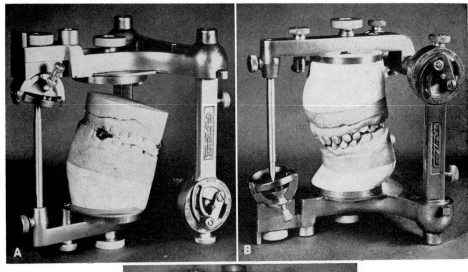

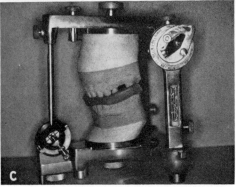

FIGURE 135. *A,* Articulator in position for mounting lower cast.
B, Mounted working cast.
C, Wax registration for setting protrusive or lateral position.

that the casting will fit the prepared tooth exactly as the pattern fitted the die and that adjustments in occlusion will be minimal.

It is certainly advantageous to be able to pour two accurate casts from a single rubber base impression. Separate dies and working casts may be secured in this way without the expenditure of additional time and materials. The first cast, poured in the washed and dried impression, should include only the prepared teeth, and the die stone should be mixed sufficiently stiff so that its flow can be controlled. After the stone has set (1 hour), the dies are removed easily. By this procedure the possibility of distortion of the impression is also minimized. The working cast is poured in the same material, this time pouring the complete arch.

Metalized dies may be seated and secured in rubber impressions (Fig. 136). The working cast constructed here will have detached dies. Their stone roots should be lubricated with petrolatum to facilitate removal.

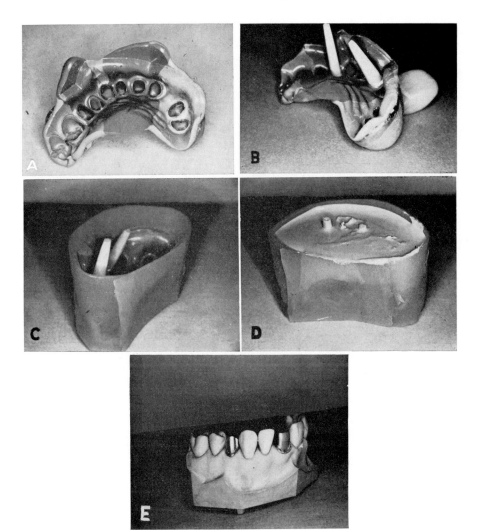

FIGURE 136. Constructing working cast from polysulfide or silicone rubber impression and metalized dies.

A, Impression.

B, Dies seated and waxed to impression at gingival line. Stone roots have been lubricated with petrolatum.

C, Impression boxed.

D, Cast poured.

E, Cast separated.

RUBBER IMPRESSIONS OF PINLEDGE PREPARATIONS

With the use of the small orifice syringe tips now available, accurate and complete polysulfide or silicone rubber impressions may be obtained of pinholes made with No. 700 or 701 burs. This probably is the method of choice.

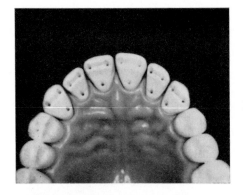

FIGURE 137. Model, with six pinledge preparations, which was used for both hydrocolloid and rubber impressions.

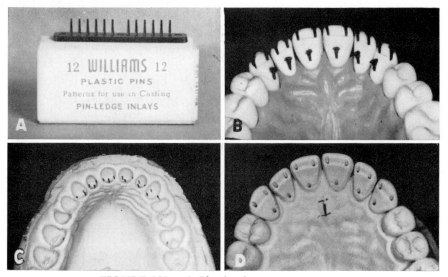

FIGURE 138. *A,* Plastic pins.
B, Plastic pins in position.
C, Rubber base impression showing pins removed.
D, Cast with impression and pins removed.

Another very good indirect technique for use with tapered pinholes made with a No. 700 or 701 bur combines polysulfide or silicone rubber impressions with tapered plastic pins* inserted in the pinholes (Fig. 137). If the holes are too long for the pins, sections of the base may be included and the ends given a cylindrical form. For shorter holes the pins are broken off the plastic base. Retentive tack-type heads are made on each by pressing the ends of the pins vertically with a warm spatula until the plastic flows. The heads should be wide and must extend laterally in all directions from the pins to prevent their breaking out of the rubber. The head of the pin should extend 1.0 mm. beyond the tooth surface to allow bulk of impression material. The pins should be lightly coated with

---

* Williams Gold Refining Co., Inc., Buffalo, N. Y.

petrolatum before being placed in the tooth. This will hold them in position and also make removal easy (Figs. 138 and 139).

When applying impression material with a syringe, it must be ejected in line with the pins; otherwise, they must be held in place so that the flow will not displace them.

With polysulfide rubber, as with silicone, the tray must be removed following the long axis of the pins. This makes it necessary to build an individual tray, so constructed that the undercuts will be blocked out and the labial flange of the tray shortened even with the gingival line.

When bridges retained by tapered pins are constructed by indirect

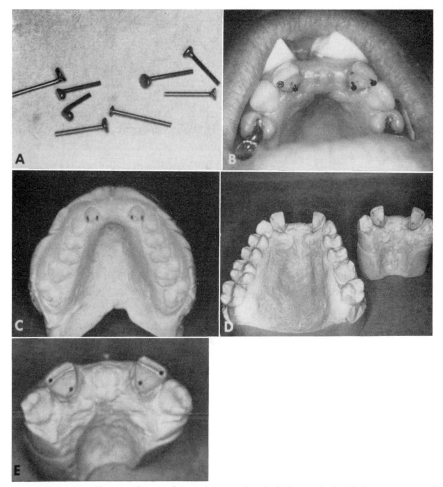

FIGURE 139. Impression and cast from nylon bristles and elastic impression.
A, Nylon bristles cut and headed.
B, Bristles in preparation pinholes.
C, Full arch rubber or silicone impression.
D, Two casts poured in same impression.
E, Cast to be sectioned for dies.

methods, hydrocolloid impressions can be recommended also, provided that the material can be forced to the bottoms of the pinholes.

When the pinholes have been made with drills, they will be too small for injecting. Usually only 0.023 inch in size, nylon bristles of 0.022 inch in diameter, with tack-type heads, are cut to protrude 2.0 mm. from the pinholes when fully seated. A special pair of cotton tweezers, which has been grooved to hold the pins firmly, is used to place them in the holes. No lubrication is necessary.

A rubber base or silicone impression is taken and is removed on a line parallel to the path of insertion. The area of the prepared teeth is poured in stone and allowed to set for approximately 1 hour. This block of stone is removed to be sectioned for dies. The full arch impression is then poured and this cast will be used for an intact working cast.

SILICONE RUBBER IMPRESSIONS

The silicones, first used in Germany, are cleaner than polysulfide rubber, have no offensive odor, and can be colored easily. Their formula contains the element silicon, and polymerization occurs through the connecting hydroxyl groups. The curing is effected by the addition of a catalyst, the exact nature of which is not publicized. Compared with the polysulfide rubber, the major advantage of the silicones lies in their esthetic qualities. However, their shelf life, while much improved, is limited, and deviations in normal setting time are more prevalent.

A custom-built tray is used, and the mixing technique for silicone duplicates that for polysulfide rubber. Thorough mixing is easier than with polysulfide rubber because one ingredient is a liquid. Elapsed time from beginning the mix until removal from the mouth should be at least 10 minutes.

A special adhesive is provided for silicone rubber and it must be used in the tray. Silicone rubber flows somewhat more readily than polysulfide rubber, and for this reason it is a preferred material for duplicating small pinholes.

REVERSIBLE HYDROCOLLOID IMPRESSIONS

Since it was presented to the profession, reversible hydrocolloid, because of its inherent desirable properties, has been widely used. Its accuracy and ease of handling have made possible exact duplication of the cavity or abutment preparations and their relationship, with reduced effort and time for both the dentist and the patient.

As with all dental materials, ultimate success with the hydrocolloid technique is dependent on a working knowledge and careful control of all variables. If suitable equipment is available, if office or clinic routine is organized, and if strict attention is given to all steps, true reproduction of the involved areas can be expected. The technique is unexcelled for the indirect construction of restorations for individual teeth and partially edentulous mouths.

To appreciate fully the importance of certain manipulative variables, the composition and mechanics of gelation must be understood. Hydrocolloids may be classified as reversible or irreversible.[11] They are suspensions of aggregates of molecules in a dispersing medium of water.

The base of reversible hydrocolloid is agar (a seaweed), which at elevated temperatures forms a colloidal fluid sol and may be safely injected into the prepared cavity. By means of water-cooled trays, the sol material is converted into a firm yet elastic gel. Agar forms a complete gel at a temperature of approximately 102° F. This process of gelation is essentially a physical change only and is thermally reversible. In dentistry these materials generally are referred to merely as hydrocolloids. The hydrocolloid is usually supplied in tubes for filling the tray, and in jars of small cartridges for syringe injection into the cavity preparation. These slender sticks have a higher water content and thus increased fluidity, and they spread readily into all areas.

Preparation of the Hydrocolloid

The first step is the proper liquefying of the gelled material furnished by the manufacturer. The gel latticework must be broken down into a fluid sol that will precisely reproduce the cavity preparations. This is fundamental, since all succeeding phases of the technique rely on correct preparation of the hydrocolloid.

The tubes and loaded syringes are placed in the boiling compartment of the conditioner, which is basic apparatus (Fig. 140). Most agars will go into a complete sol at temperatures above 206° F. if the temperature is held sufficiently long. Boiling water is a convenient medium for liquefying the material, giving assurance that the minimal temperature has been attained. No less than 10 minutes of boiling time is imperative in order to obtain a smoothly flowing and nongrainy substance. The real danger in preparing the hydrocolloid, and a frequent cause of disappointment and failure, is inadequate heating. There are no serious consequences from prolonged boiling. If it is allowed to re-gel, approximately 3 minutes should be added *each* time the material is reboiled in order to bring the gel into a sol condition.

The hydrocolloid, when thoroughly liquefied, can be stored until needed (Fig. 141). With good equipment it may be boiled at the beginning of the day and maintained in a workable state for at least 8 hours. This

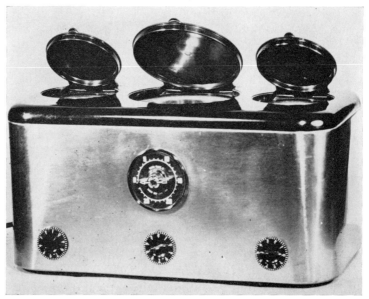

FIGURE 140. Example of one type of commercial hydrocolloid conditioner. Bath at left is for boiling, middle compartment for storage, while tempering of tray material is carried out in bath on right. Equipment of this type is essential to the technique.

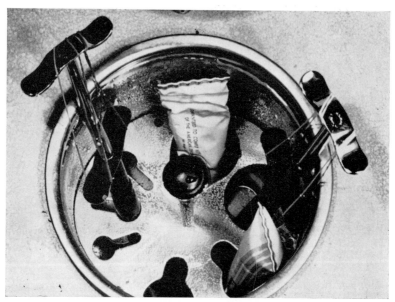

FIGURE 141. Tubes of hydrocolloid and syringes in storage compartment (145 to 155° F.). Material may be kept fluid all day at this temperature.

fluid material must be stored at a temperature that will prevent any appreciable gelation, because as gelation proceeds fluidity decreases and the material will not flow into all fine lines of the cavity.

Since gelation of hydrocolloid is a function of both time and temperature, it will progress at any temperature if the material is held long enough. However, at 150° F. the gelation is retarded, and storage at that temperature will give the operator a usable material throughout the working day. Storage at temperatures below 150° F. may produce a stiff, granular mass that will be incapable of injection into the less accessible areas of the preparation. There is no risk of injury to the pulp by injection of the material at 150° F., or even 155° F., because as the hydrocolloid passes through the needle and onto the relatively cool tooth surface the temperature drops quickly.[12] Checking the temperature control indicators of the conditioning unit for erroneous readings should become a routine phase of this procedure.

Although the hydrocolloid in the syringe is now ready to be injected into the cavity preparation directly from the storage bath, the material in the tube, which will be used to fill the tray, must be cooled to below 150° F. "Tempering" is necessary to induce some gelation and to diminish the temperature so that the large bulk of hydrocolloid will be neither uncomfortable to the patient nor difficult to contain in the tray. Likewise, the thermal contraction will be lessened, with better reproduction of cavity detail as a consequence.

The degree of gelation of the agar and the speed of its formation

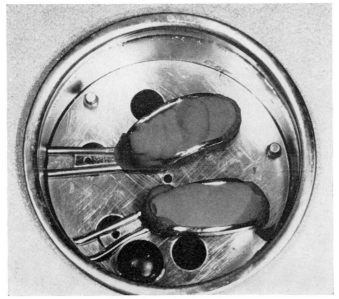

FIGURE 142. Filled trays being tempered to reduce temperature and produce some gelation.

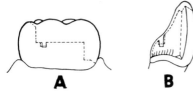

A   **B**

FIGURE 143.   Pinholes should be changed in size for hydrocolloid technique.

will be governed by the temperature of the tempering bath and the length of time it remains in the bath at that temperature (Fig. 142). Various combinations have been suggested. Naturally, the cooler the tempering bath, the more rapid will be the drop of the temperature of the impression material in the tray, with an accompanying decrease in the time required to secure adequate gelation for insertion into the oral cavity. If the tempering temperature is low, then the period that the tray is stored in the tempering bath is quite critical. A few extra minutes at a low temperature, say 103° F., will lead to excessive gelation and unusable hydrocolloid. Accordingly, a slower gelation achieved at a somewhat higher tempering temperature is more conducive to a favorable outcome.

While the time-temperature ratio may hinge on the consistency most suited to the operator's needs, the recommended method is to temper at 115° F. for approximately 10 minutes.[13] Other procedures are applicable but more demanding (Table 16). Different materials, and even different batches of the same brand of hydrocolloid, may necessitate a slight alteration in the proposed tempering time. The tray material can be tempered during the final moments of tissue displacement and while the teeth are being prepared for injection of the syringe material.

Abutment Preparations for Hydrocolloid Bridges

With an indirect impression technique, standard preparations should be made on the abutment teeth. However, if pinholes are to be placed in the abutment, it is helpful if they have greater diameter and less depth. For example, a pinhole in the occlusal of an inlay preparation, in the cusp tip of a partial veneer preparation, or in the cingulum area of a partial veneer preparation ordinarily would be made with a No. 701 bur, 2.0 mm. deep (Fig. 143). To reproduce easily with hydrocolloid, the pin-

Table 16.   Time-Temperature Combinations for Tempering Hydrocolloid

TEMPERATURE	TIME
115° F.*	10 minutes
110° F.	5–10 minutes
105° F.	5 minutes
102° F.	2 minutes

* Recommended method.

hole should be made with a No. 701 or 702 bur and reduced in depth to 1.5 mm. With the use of extra pressure and a special needle on the syringe, a pinhole made with a No. 700 bur may be reproduced. The cervical finishing line must be distinct.

For *Gingival Displacement,* see page 159.

Selection of Trays

In an indirect technique, full arch impressions are indispensable for working *and* opposing casts. There are no articulated retainers to assist in relating the casts or to pilot their movements; hence occlusion of the unprepared teeth is essential.

The tray must be selected with this in mind. It should extend distally past all teeth, be fitted with tubes for cooling (Fig. 144), and have room for 3.0 mm. of material around the teeth occlusally and laterally. Black tray compound is the best material for the "stops" that will guide the tray into position over the teeth. (Red and green compound and wax become too pliable in the tempering bath.) A black compound dam (Fig. 145) is built in the metal tray beyond the most distal abutment tooth, even though it may be supported by soft tissue, and trimmed so it will not contact an abutment during gelation. A second stop should be located mesially to the most anterior prepared tooth, and a third one in the approximating

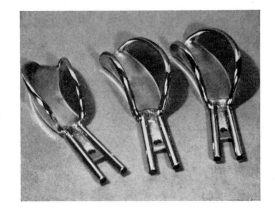

FIGURE 144. Trays fitted with flanges and tubes for retention and cooling of impression material. A complete arch impression should be made for the working cast.

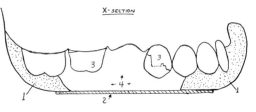

FIGURE 145. Cross section of compound stops for seating tray. (Courtesy of J. F. Jelenko & Co., Inc.)

1. Compound
2. Tray
3. Preparations
4. Space for Hydrocolloid

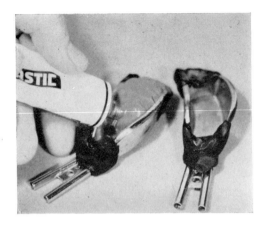

FIGURE 146. Filling tray.

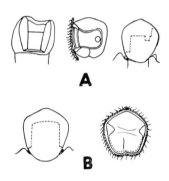

FIGURE 147. Gingival crevice packed with No. 8 thread. This will prolong displacement of tissue in order that two impressions may be made. (Courtesy of J. F. Jelenko & Co., Inc.)

quadrant. They will form a tripod for positioning the tray. The compound in the tray is molded by pressure over the occlusal surfaces of the teeth or over the retromolar pad. Trays should be prepared before tissue displacement is begun, but filling the trays with liquefied impression material and tempering should be done during displacement (Fig. 146). If the trays are without perforations or rim locks, compound must be added to the inner borders to stabilize the impression material during removal.

The hollow point, or needle, on the syringe should be no larger than is needed to permit a free flow of hydrocolloid. The smaller the stream of impression material, the less likely will be the trapping of air. On the other hand, if there is resistance to pushing the hydrocolloid through the needle, there may be some uncontrolled movement of the needle point, with a chance of bubbles, or abrasion of the tissue, and hemorrhage.

Preimpression Steps

After the gingival crevice has been examined, it is washed and dried and may be repacked with a single strand of No. 8 thread (Fig. 147), which will not attach to the impression.[4] The field must be isolated by placing cotton rolls to the buccal and the lingual of the teeth. Warm air should be used cautiously to rid the surface of moisture or debris; otherwise the gingival tissue may hemorrhage. The surface now should produce no discrepancies in the impression.

Use of the Syringe

The syringe is taken from the storage bath and ½ inch or more of the material is ejected as waste inasmuch as the hydrocolloid in the syringe tip may have been contaminated by water or air during conditioning. Air pockets must be avoided, because even the smallest nodule on a critical margin or in the angle of the cavity will render the die useless. The tip of the syringe must be confined to or actually dragged along the tooth surface.

Taking the Impression

During the period of injection the assistant will have removed the tray from the conditioning bath and attached the hose for circulation of water. Some operators merely blot the surface of hydrocolloid with a towel, but a much better practice is to scrape off the layer that has been in contact with the water in the conditioning bath (Fig. 148). Neglecting to remove this outer surface may hinder union between the tray material and the hydrocolloid that has been injected around the prepared tooth. The tray is now forced over the teeth until the compound stops are in position. Although haste is unnecessary, if too much time elapses between injection and seating the tray, there will be a poor bonding between the syringe and tray materials.

The tray is held passively for at least 5 minutes (Fig. 149). This will produce a gel strong enough to resist deformation or fracture. If the tray is withdrawn before 5 minutes have passed, the gel that has formed will

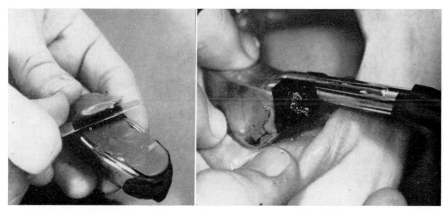

Fig. 148   Fig. 149

FIGURE 148. Surface of conditioned hydrocolloid should be scraped.
FIGURE 149. Seated tray must be motionless for at least 5 minutes.

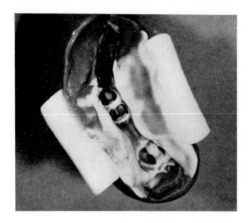

FIGURE 150.   Impression removed. Cotton should be left, as its removal could tear impression.

not have strength to withstand the applied stresses. Premature removal is a habitual basis for inaccuracy.

The temperature of the circulating water should be approximately 60 to 70° F. Ice water should not be used, since it is annoying to some patients and may cause undue stress to be in the impression.[14] Cold water for the last 2 minutes probably has no deleterious effect but must be avoided during the first 3 minutes. If the water in the unit is too cool during the winter months, the temperature of the tray can be regulated by turning the water on at short intervals only, instead of using an uninterrupted stream.

The tray is removed with a quick thrust, parallel, if possible, to the long axis of the tooth or preparation (Fig. 150). It must not be teased or rocked from the cavity preparation. Contrary to prevalent opinion, this type of material will deform or rupture much less readily when subjected to a sudden movement than a constant pressure.

Treating the Impression

The impression should be gently washed free of blood, saliva, and debris with approximately room-temperature water and immersed in a solution of 2 per cent potassium sulfate (Fig. 151) for 5 minutes while the stone is being weighed and mixed (Fig. 152). This will impregnate the surface of the hydrocolloid with the sulfate ion, accelerate the set of the adjacent stone, and yield a harder and denser surface (Fig. 153).[15, 16] Moreover, should the cast not be separated from the impression within a few hours, it will prevent deterioration of the surface. The surface of the hydrocolloid is always covered with a watery film, and unless the stone sets rapidly, this exudate will dilute the stone and produce an inferior surface.

The final impression is essentially a suspension of water held in the micelles of the agar and it constitutes approximately 75 to 85 per cent of the composition. These materials will tend to lose water (syneresis) or

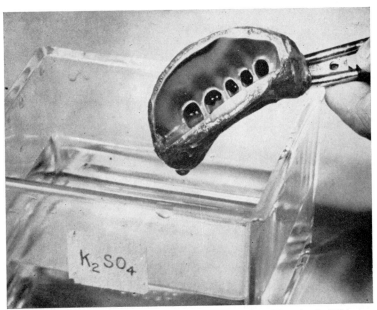

FIGURE 151. Placing clean impression in potassium sulfate bath. This step, carried on while mix of stone is prepared, improves surface of stone cast.

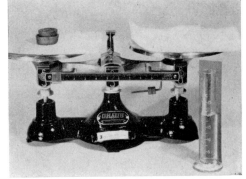

FIGURE 152. Balance for weighing stone.

gain water (imbibition), processes that result in dimensional change and distortion within the impression.[14, 17, 18] Also there is a residual stress pattern in the impression, which will be relieved upon storage and cause distortion.

Pouring the Cast

Unfortunately, no chemical solution or storage environment that will maintain an equilibrium within the impression has yet been developed for use in the dental office. One of the recognized limitations of the hydrocolloid technique is the absolute necessity for pouring the cast without delay. This is true with most impression materials, but particularly with the hydrocolloids. Nevertheless, many operators still indulge in the bad

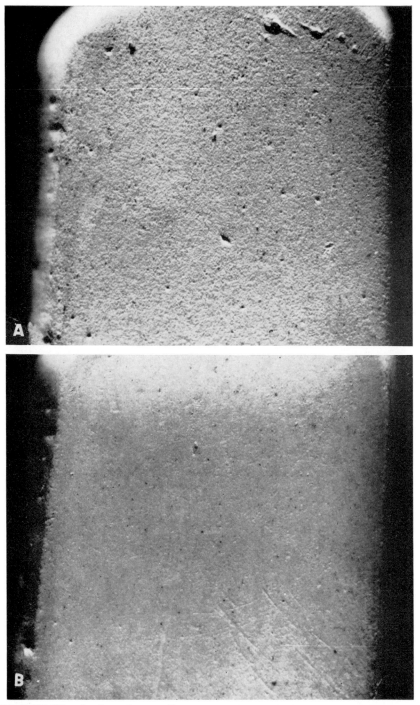

FIGURE 153.   Surface of stone die (*A*) may often be chalky if potassium sulfate treatment of impression is omitted. Superior surface (*B*) results if solution is used.

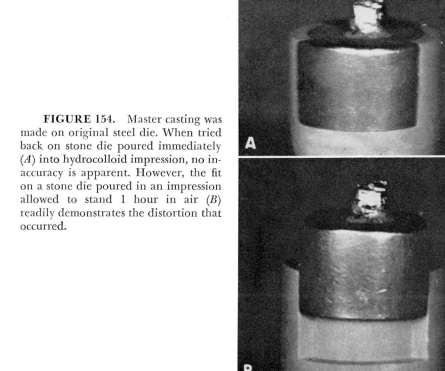

FIGURE 154. Master casting was made on original steel die. When tried back on stone die poured immediately (*A*) into hydrocolloid impression, no inaccuracy is apparent. However, the fit on a stone die poured in an impression allowed to stand 1 hour in air (*B*) readily demonstrates the distortion that occurred.

habit of permitting the impression to stand for varying periods of time before pouring the cast. Undoubtedly, this is one of the most frequent reasons for distortion and inaccuracy. It has been shown that, on some types of preparations, distortion is evidenced within 30 minutes after removal from the mouth (Fig. 154). It bears repeating that a cardinal rule, which must be followed if the exactness of the impression is to be preserved, is to pour the cast within 15 minutes after the impression is taken from the mouth.

Construction of the Die

To guarantee a continuous correct relationship between the abutment teeth, bridges should be constructed and assembled on solid, complete arch casts from which no portion may be removed. Therefore two impressions of the prepared area must be taken. The cast that appears to have the better reproduction of the abutments will be partitioned for the dies. The other may be articulated and used as the working cast. After the impressions have been taken for the dies and the working and opposing casts, a registration should be made with the Kerr Bite Frame.[19]

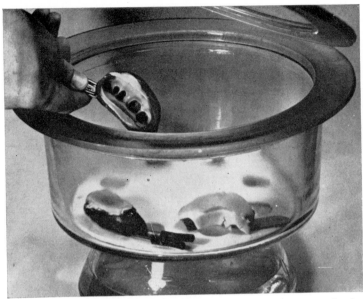

FIGURE 155.   If storage is necessary, the best storage environment for hydrocolloid is an arrangement such as that shown. Water in bottom and tightly fitting lid provide atmosphere of approximately 100 per cent humidity.

If, in an emergency, this policy of pouring the cast at once cannot be followed, what is the most reliable storage environment? This will change with the brand of material. The safest medium, one more dependable than either air or water, is an atmosphere of 100 per cent humidity—that is, a humidifier (Fig. 155). However, in view of the questionable behavior in any environment, storage is an unpredictable variable that can be—and certainly should be—eliminated from the technique.

Excess droplets of the potassium sulfate solution should be gently blown from the impression, being mindful not to dehydrate and subsequently distort the hydrocolloid. The surface of the impression should have a moist appearance.

Several stones for constructing the dies are on the market, e.g., Vel-Mix and Duroc.* These newer materials are harder and have a low (approximately 0.06 per cent) setting expansion as compared with the older stones.[11] Little difference exists in the physical properties of the brands, and selection may be governed by color and contrast to the wax pattern.[20]

The cast must be poured with care, since a chalklike surface, nodules, or other imperfections may require another appointment and impression. The manufacturer's directions should be followed in regard to the water-powder ratio for each stone, because variation influences surface smoothness as well as strength and setting expansion. Mechanical spatulation,

---

* The Ransom & Randolph Co., Toledo, Ohio.

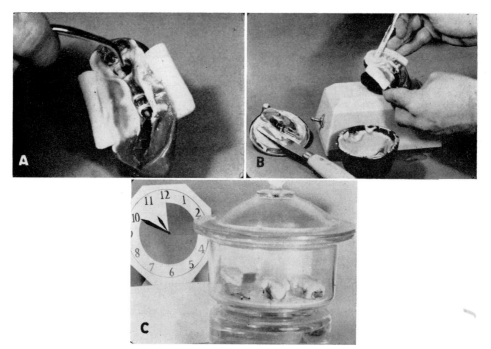

FIGURE 156. *A,* Removing excess potassium sulfate solution before pouring cast.
B, Pouring cast.
C, Setting stone is stored in humidifier.

preferably under vacuum, is valuable in assuring a compact, smooth surface. The stone is added in small increments and is mechanically vibrated into the mold, using *mild* agitation. The tendency is to use too much vibration, which results in holes in the die.[15] While the stone is setting, the poured impression is placed back in the humidifier in an atmosphere of 100 per cent humidity. The stone gains its strength slowly; therefore the die should not be removed from the impression in less than 30 minutes, and preferably an hour (Fig. 156). Premature separation will cause a rough surface. Although it is desirable to separate the die within 2 or 3 hours, generally no harm will be done by waiting longer (for example, overnight) if the impression was treated in the potassium sulfate solution. No attempt should be made to fabricate the wax pattern until the stone has fully hardened, approximately 24 hours later.

IRREVERSIBLE HYDROCOLLOID (ALGINATE) IMPRESSIONS

The irreversible hydrocolloids, commonly called alginates, gel by means of a specific chemical reaction. Alginates often are considered for indirect restorations or bridges because their use is somewhat less complicated. However, at present the reversible hydrocolloid still offers superior characteristics, such as greater accuracy on a long span, a better surface on the working die, and sharper detail.

Stock, perforated trays are used with alginate. These are available in many sizes, but for an extra large arch it may be necessary to add wax to the posterior border to furnish extra length. Wax may be needed in the center of an upper tray to push and hold the impression material against the palatal surface.

Alginate should be proportioned and mixed according to the directions furnished by the manufacturer. Setting time in the mouth is 2 minutes after it becomes obvious that gelation has begun. The impression should be washed and the cast poured immediately.

PLASTER OF PARIS IMPRESSIONS

The use of a plaster of Paris impression to produce a working cast minimizes variables, reduces armamentarium, and requires only that the plaster impression for the working cast be taken and reassembled precisely. However, many small pieces of the impression frequently are lost or cannot be reassembled. As a consequence, details inherent in a cast made from an elastic impression are missing, and the setting and removal of the impression material are quite distasteful to many patients.

In the construction of the small bridge, the jaws, hinged as they are at the temporomandibular joint, make an accurate and satisfactory preliminary articulator for establishing the exact relationship of the retainers to opposing teeth. However, there is the disadvantage of extra appointments for the patient. For a long bridge, the working cast must duplicate the entire arch.

After the castings have been polished, washed, adjusted for occlusion and contact, and reseated on the abutment teeth, a registration is made, using the Kerr Bite Frame.

Selection of the Tray

The tray should always extend distally beyond the most posterior abutment and across the median line to include at least the bicuspids on the opposite side (Fig. 157). There may be an exception for a bridge supplying only one tooth. A shorter working cast will suffice if the occlusion is well defined, since during pontic construction lateral movements will be guided by the previously equilibrated occlusal surfaces of the retainers and the uncut teeth in that segment.

The tray must clear the teeth buccally, lingually, and occlusally by 3.0 mm. and must not impinge on the lingual gingival tissue. The tray

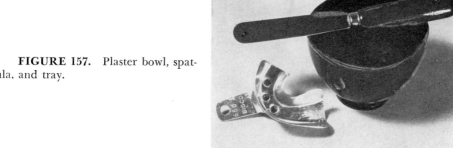

FIGURE 157. Plaster bowl, spatula, and tray.

need not be oiled or greased before taking a plaster of Paris impression, but it *must* be clean.

The Impression

Impression plasters differ from model plasters primarily in setting time and greatly reduced strength. Mixing plaster of Paris for taking impressions calls for more understanding and intuition than technical skill. Snowwhite No. 2* is an impression plaster that will harden quickly and break cleanly. Enough cool water to fill the impression tray one and one-half times is placed in a bowl. The plaster is gently sifted into the water, using a sieve or a spatula, and the liquid is stirred after each addition of plaster until the mix is creamy but thin. Spatulation is continued until just before setting begins, a point the operator will learn to recognize only by experience. The plaster is transferred to the impression tray and the tray is positioned in the mouth so that there is an equal thickness of plaster over the buccal, lingual, and occlusal surfaces. It is held until the plaster has set. Setting can be gauged by testing small pieces of the plaster left in the mixing bowl. When it cannot be crushed between the thumb and finger, begins to feel warm, and breaks sharply, the impression is ready for removal. This should be accomplished speedily before the plaster becomes excessively hard and hot.

Removal of the Impression

The tray is removed and laid to one side. Beginning at either end, a finger is placed under the buccal edge of the impression and pressure is exerted with some force labially and occlusally. As a rule, this will induce fracture and a section can be lifted out and placed in its relative position on a tray or napkin. This procedure is repeated until the outside wall of the impression has been disengaged (Fig. 158).

If the occlusal and lingual portion cannot be lifted out intact, a

---

* Kerr Mfg. Company, Detroit, Mich.

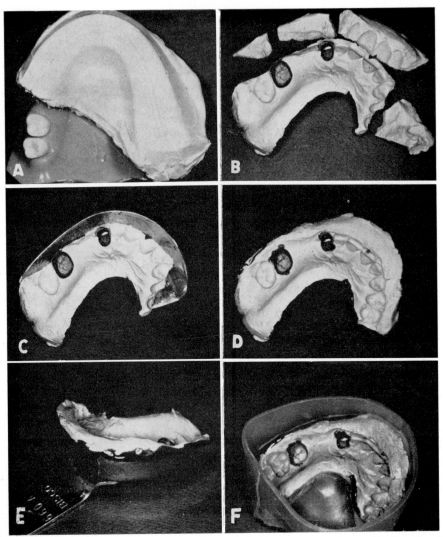

FIGURE 158. *A,* Tray removed and impression scored to provide guide lines for fracturing.

B, Sections of impression arranged on removal from mouth.

C, Largest piece cleaned and seated in tray. It may be necessary to lift or remove this segment in order to adapt buccal parts to area of fracture.

D, Retainers seated in the assembled impression and secured with wax.

E, Impression luted to tray.

F, Impression coated with separating medium and boxed for pouring.

groove must be cut at the most advantageous point, generally at the lingual of a cuspid, so that pressure on the ends of the impression and toward the center of the mouth will split the remaining section. A knife or chisel may be helpful, but their indiscriminate use may induce so much fragmentation that reassembly of the impression will be impossible.

When all parts of the impression have been collected, the patient should be permitted to rinse with a flavored wash. (See Fig. 158.)

Reassembly of the Impression

Only after all minute chips have been brushed from each surface of the impression, the retainers, and the tray, is it possible to reassemble and stabilize the impression and the retainers in the tray. Irregularities and inaccuracies are inevitable if the sections are joined outside the tray.

The retainers, if movable, are fixed to the impression with beeswax. The plaster should be coated with a separating medium, of which many are available. After this has dried, the impression is placed in water for a few minutes and then poured.

Pouring the Cast

Hydrocal, commonly called stone, is used because of its strength. The alginate impression for the opposing cast can be poured at the same time and with the same mix. It is never a good policy to pour a working cast with soldering investment, inasmuch as it breaks and abrades readily.

After the stone has hardened for a minimum of 1 hour, the alginate impression is removed and discarded. The plaster of Paris impression must be taken off one piece at a time, being careful in the application of force not to break an abutment tooth. No working cast, fractured in an area directly connected with the construction of the bridge, can be mended so that the parts will be correctly joined. A new cast must be made. If instructions have been followed strictly, any plaster of Paris impression should separate without difficulty (Fig. 159).

Technique for Constructing a Cast Transfer

A transfer is a nonanatomic cover for a tooth, which may be removed in an impression and used as a receptacle for dies to assure their correct relationship in the poured working cast (Fig. 160). It may be made of resin, low-fusing metal, or cast gold alloy, which is preferable. A cast

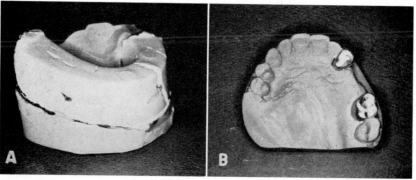

FIGURE 159. *A*, Cast poured and tray removed. *B*, Cast.

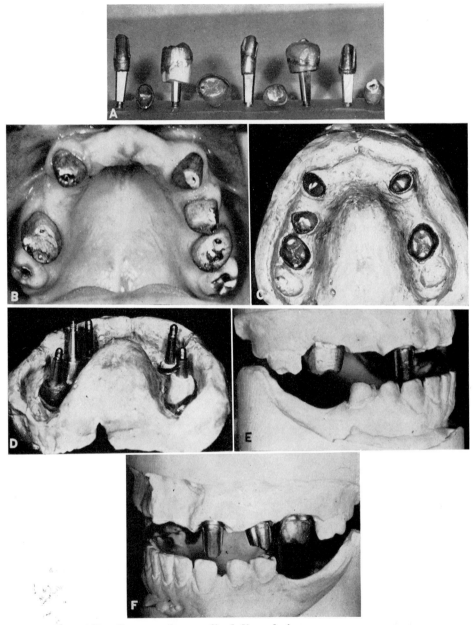

FIGURE 160. Cast transfer-metalized die technique.

A, Dies and cast transfers for the five abutments of a twelve-unit upper bridge.

B, The transfers on the abutments. The windows make it possible to check seating.

C, The transfers removed in a plaster impression.

D, The dies seated in the transfers. Threaded and tapped dowel pins were used for greater accuracy in replacing the dies in the cast.

E, F, The working cast.

transfer may be used as a coping, to become an integral part of the finished restoration. If it fits both the die and the tooth, accuracy of the die may be accepted. Fit of the retainer castings may be judged in advance, owing to the hardness of the gold.[21]

When the pattern is waxed on the die, it must contact all surfaces and be carved to marginal fit. The wax need be only thick enough to ensure a complete casting. Anatomic form is not essential except at the cervical periphery. The final step in producing the pattern is the removal of several square millimeters of wax down to the surface of the die, from a buccal cusp or incisal edge, without disturbing the adaptation of the wax. This opening will make it possible to check the seating of the casting.

The pattern is sprued at the same angle and invested with the same ratio of cristobalite to control powder that would be needed for a permanent restoration. The casting may be made with any dental gold, or if the coping technique is being followed, with the alloy to be used for the second casting. The sprue is cut off, leaving a stump of 1.0 to 2.0 mm. This stump and the window will orient the casting in the plaster of Paris impression. Cervical fit and occlusal or incisal adaptation should be checked on the die before the transfer is taken to the mouth.

The Working Cast. With the transfers on the teeth, a full arch plaster of Paris impression is made and reassembled with the castings seated in the impression. The plaster is luted to the tray, and the dies are placed in the transfers and supported in position by wax or rods. After separating medium has been applied and allowed to dry, the impression is soaked for a short time and poured in stone.

A mechanical vibrator should not be used unless the hand is placed between the impression tray and the instrument to reduce the agitation to a minimum. Otherwise the dies will loosen and the cast will be worthless. Model stone will flow into all recesses of the impression if the impression tray is tapped lightly against a rubber block or bench top. The casts are trimmed and mounted on an adjustable articulator with a facebow.

Cast transfers may also be seated in rubber or alginate impressions, especially if a plaster core was placed over the occlusal surfaces of the teeth before the elastic impression was taken.

REFERENCES

1. Roydhouse, R. H.: Elastic impression materials. New Zealand D. J., *52*:187, Oct. 1956.
2. Fettes, E. M., and Jorezak, J. S.: Polysulfide polymers. Indust. & Engin. Chem., *42*:2217, Nov. 1950.
3. Bailey, L. R.: Acrylic resin tray for rubber base impression materials. J. Pros. Den., *5*:658, Sept. 1955.

4. Jelenko, J. F. & Co., Inc.: Crown and Bridge Construction Using Hydrocolloid Impressions. 2nd ed. The company, 1956.
5. Harrison, J. D.: Effect of retraction materials on the gingival sulcus epithelium. J. Pros. Den., *11*:514, May–June 1961.
6. Skinner, E. W.: The properties and manipulation of mercaptan base and silicone base impression materials. D. Clin. North America, Nov. 1958, p. 685.
7. Sturdevant, C. M.: Mercaptan rubber impression technique for single and multiple restorations. D. Clin. North America, Nov. 1958, p. 699.
8. Myers, G. E.: Rubber base impression technics for operative dentistry. J. Michigan D. A., *39*:251, Oct. 1957.
9. Schnell, R. J., and Phillips, R. W.: Dimensional stability of rubber base impressions and certain other factors affecting accuracy. J.A.D.A., *57*:39, July 1958.
10. Jelenko, J. F. & Co., Inc.: Crown and Bridge Construction. A Handbook of Dental Laboratory Procedures. 5th ed. The company, 1964.
11. Skinner, E. W., and Phillips, R. W.: The Science of Dental Materials. 5th ed. Philadelphia, W. B. Saunders Company, 1960.
12. Phillips, R. W.: Physical properties and manipulation of reversible and irreversible hydrocolloid. J.A.D.A., *51*:566, Nov. 1955.
13. Thompson, M. J.: Standardized indirect technic for reversible hydrocolloid. J.A.D.A., *46*:1, Jan. 1953.
14. Phillips, R. W., and Ito, B. Y.: Factors influencing the accuracy of reversible hydrocolloid impressions. J.A.D.A., *43*:1, July 1951.
15. Phillips, R. W., and Ito, B. Y.: Factors affecting the surface of stone dies poured in hydrocolloid impressions. J. Pros. Den., *2*:390, May 1952.
16. Skinner, E. W., and Gordon, C. C.: Some experiments on the surface hardness of dental stones. J. Pros. Den., *6*:94, Jan. 1956.
17. James, A. G.: Maintenance of equilibrium in reversible hydrocolloid impressions. J. D. Res., *28*:108, 119, 447, April and Oct. 1949.
18. Skinner, E. W., Cooper, E. N., and Beck, F. W.: Reversible and irreversible hydrocolloid impression materials. J.A.D.A., *40*:196, Feb. 1950.
19. Emmert, J. H.: A method for registering occlusion in semiedentulous mouths. J. Pros. Den., *8*:94, Jan. 1958.
20. Peyton, F. A., Liebold, J. P., and Ridgley, G. V.: Surface hardness, compressive strength, and abrasion resistance of indirect die stones. J. Pros. Den., *2*:381, May 1952.
21. Schweitzer, J. M.: Oral Rehabilitation. St. Louis, The C. V. Mosby Company, 1951, p. 946.

11

INDIVIDUAL DIES CONSTRUCTED FROM TUBE IMPRESSIONS

This chapter will discuss making a die, or reproduction of a single prepared tooth, to be placed in an impression to become a removable part of a working cast or as a detached unit for freehand carving. It must be done precisely.

Polysulfide rubber base and modeling compound impression materials have specific advantages and disadvantages. Silver-plated or copper-plated surfaces, stone, and amalgam for producing the die have their proponents. (Impressions of polysulfide and silicone rubber and hydrocolloid for quadrant and complete arch casts and dies are discussed in Chapter 10.)

FITTING THE BAND

A copper band, stiff or annealed, depending on the impression material being used, should be selected as soon as the peripheral dimension of the preparation has been established, because when judging it for size and marking it for contour, manipulation on the tooth is far easier if one does not have to contend with a shoulder or prominent finishing line. For elastic materials a *stiff* band must be used and have at least 0.35 mm. clearance at all points. For modeling compound the *annealed* band should fit the cervical margin snugly. For either material the band should be about twice the length of the prepared clinical crown.

The band should conform to the silhouette of the preparation as seen from the occlusal. Its cervical outline must follow the configuration of the gingival tissue surrounding the tooth. If the preparation has been extended 0.5 mm. into the gingival crevice, then the band must be trimmed and

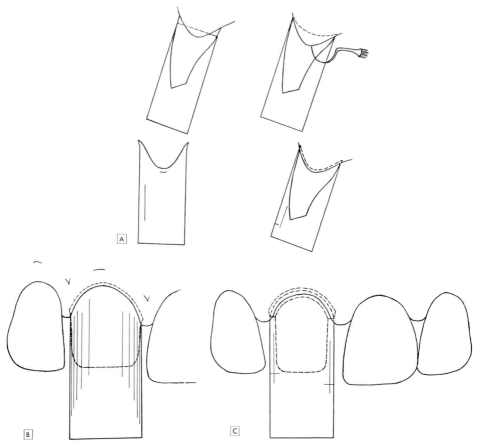

FIGURE 161.   Fitting the band.
A, Marking and contouring the band. Guide lines marked.
B, Band on partially prepared tooth.
C, Band on prepared tooth showing how guide lines help in positioning band.

contoured to extend evenly 0.3 mm. beyond the cervical margin of the preparation. While still uncut on the end, it can be placed over the tooth until it touches the gingiva, and these points of contact marked with a sharp instrument. Other marks should be made to indicate the distance of the labial and lingual edges from the tissue.

The band is removed and trimmed with shears or a stone to duplicate the cervical contour of the preparation, the edge is smoothed with a fine stone, the labial surface identified, and it is put aside until the preparation is completed (Fig. 161).

Guide Lines

Before filling the band, it should be placed on the tooth in the position it must occupy in order to secure a satisfactory impression. If there are approximating teeth, perpendicular guide lines can be placed on both the mesial and distal. A horizontal line to show cervical positioning can be made at any point where it will have a related object. If there are no adjacent teeth, seating the band will offer no problem.

TAKING THE IMPRESSION

Polysulfide Rubber Technique

When polysulfide rubber is used in taking a tube impression, the incisal end of the ordinary copper band must be plugged with modeling compound (Fig. 162). It should come within 2.0 to 3.0 mm. of the incisal of the prepared tooth, in order further to reinforce the band against deformation upon removal of the impression and to control the thickness of the material. This will force all of the excess to flow out at the cervical, presumably carrying away any bubbles of air that may have been trapped on the tooth surface as the band was seated. A selection of closed-end copper bands, which do not require the use of modeling compound, is available.*

The inner surface of the band and compound is painted with a thin coat of the tray adhesive that accompanies the impression material. This is allowed to dry for at least 6 or 7 minutes. The band is filled completely with heavy base or regular tray polysulfide rubber, seated over the prepared tooth, and held without movement for 10 minutes (Fig. 163).

This technique seems to be somewhat less exacting than that needed to obtain an accurate modeling compound impression. Also, the elastic material can be withdrawn from cervical undercuts without deformation or fracture of the impression.

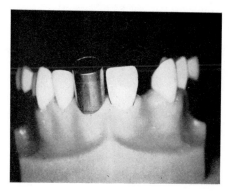

FIGURE 162. Copper band plugged with modeling compound to confine and limit the amount of polysulfide rubber.

---

* Blue Island Specialty Co., Inc., Blue Island, Ill.

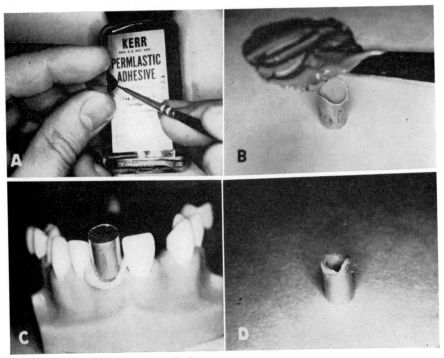

FIGURE 163. Impression technique.
A, Painting band.
B, Band filled.
C, Band seated.
D, Impression.

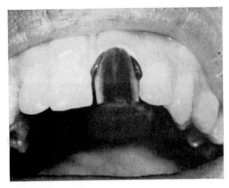

FIGURE 164. Modeling compound impression.

Modeling Compound Technique

The compound should be softened, preferably in boiling water; if dry heat is used, the surface that will contact the tooth must be tempered in hot water. The opening of the band must not be closed with the finger tip while trying to seat the band and compound; instead, a little compound should be forced out at the cervical, and the band should be guided into position before putting pressure on the impression material (Fig. 164).

The impression should be chilled with cold water and pulled incisally from the tooth with a steady vertical pressure. It must *not* be rocked or rotated during removal. Grasping the band with a dry napkin, a fine sandpaper strip, or a pointed clamp will give traction.

Every effort must be made to avoid taking the same impression repeatedly, as this may cause excessive thermal shock to the tooth, or it can traumatize the soft tissue, cut the periodontal membrane attachment, and stimulate gingival recession.

DIES

The Silver-Plated Die

One of the virtues of the polysulfide rubber impression is the ease with which it can be plated with silver. Hydrocolloid, alginate, or silicone impressions cannot be electroplated satisfactorily without some change in form.[1, 2]

After the impression has been washed with tap water and dried, a fine silver powder* is burnished into all areas with a soft brush. The powder should contact the copper band, the excess being blown out. The copper band is wrapped with masking tape or wax, extending 2.0 to 5.0 mm. (the same distance at all points) beyond the open end of the impression. The band is waxed onto the cathode holder and all conducting surfaces not to be plated are covered with wax. Other metalizing agents, such as bronze or graphite, may be employed, but silver powder produces a superior surface (Fig. 165).

A silver cyanide bath,* which must not be polluted with acid or other chemicals, is used for plating. To avoid trapping air bubbles, the metalized impression is meticulously filled with the solution and is then lowered into the electrolyte. The upper end of the cathode is attached to the negative D. C. source. The silver anode is placed about 4 inches away and is attached to the positive D. C. terminal. Plating is carried out for approximately 12 hours at 10 milliamperes for each square centimeter of surface. If, on examination during the first half hour, some areas are not plating, the impression should be washed, dried, and remetalized with silver powder.

Forming the Root. Stone, low-fusing metal, or self-curing resin may be used to form the root, which should be tapered and without irregularities. Stone will expand very slightly when setting, whereas metal and resin contract. For this reason and because of its uncomplicated working properties, stone is recommended for the support and root section of a metalized die.

---

* Kerr Mfg. Company, Detroit, Mich.

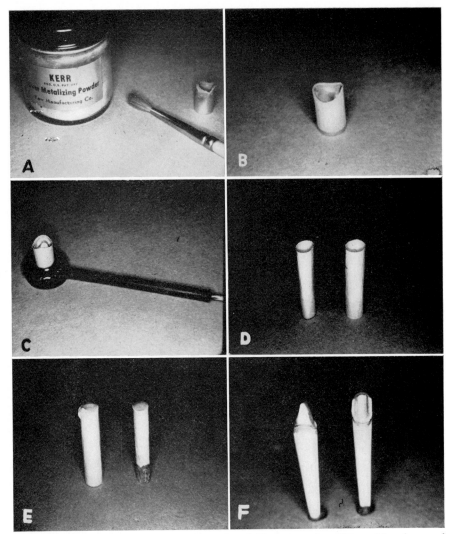

FIGURE 165. Construction of silver-plated die from polysulfide rubber impression.
A, Impression and metalizing powder.
B, Impression metalized.
C, Impression protected by tape and waxed to cathode holder.
D, Plated dies wrapped for pouring roots.
E, Roots poured.
F, Completed dies with roots tapered.

The Copper-Plated Die

For a copper band–modeling compound impression to be plated with copper, the inside, or preparation surface, must be metalized. The most accurate reproduction of the surface and the sharpest marginal detail will result when metalizing is accomplished through the chemical reduction of silver nitrate. From this reaction, a film of pure silver 2 millionths of

an inch thick is deposited on the surface of the impression.[3] Dietrich's*
compound or wax impressions may be metalized by the same method.

Solutions. Three solutions are needed. All must be handled carefully because they produce dark stains on almost all substances, including the skin and porcelain lavatories.

The sensitizing solution is made from

Stannous chloride	1.0 gm.
Hydrochloric acid	1.5 cc.
Distilled water	100.0 cc.

After the stannous chloride has dissolved, the clear liquid is poured off and bottled. The remains are discarded.

The silver nitrate solution requires

Silver nitrate	2.1 gm.
Distilled water	45.0 cc.

The reducing solution is made of

Pyrogallic acid	0.5 gm.
Citric acid	0.1 gm.
Distilled water	15.0 cc.

The sensitizing solution may be prepared in quantity and stored for a time in a brown glass bottle. The chemicals for the other solutions should be weighed and the designated amounts kept in capsules, to be emptied individually as needed.

Metalizing. The impression must be placed in the sensitizing solution for 3 to 5 minutes, with all surfaces in contact with the liquid. During this period the silver nitrate and reducing solutions may be mixed separately. The impression must be rinsed, placed in a cup, and the silver nitrate solution poured over the impression, moving the cup to assure complete wetting. After the liquid reducing reagent is added to the silver nitrate, the solution in the cup should be agitated, then allowed to set for 5 or more minutes. The impression is removed, rinsed, dried, and examined. If there are voids in the silver film, the process must be repeated. Paper drinking cups make suitable receptacles for the metalizing chemicals.

Plating. After metalizing, the bottom of the impression band must be scraped clean in order to make good contact with the cathode holder. It is then waxed to the holder, covering all surfaces not to be plated. A collar of 32-gauge wax or masking tape is placed around the impression band to extend evenly from 2.0 to 3.0 mm. beyond the open end. If an eye dropper is used to fill the impression with the copper solution before attaching it to the plating apparatus, there will be less chance of trapping an air bubble and having an area unplated. The impression is attached to the negative pole, the copper anode to the positive pole. The distance between the anode and cathode is not critical, but a maximal distance

---

* The Hygienic Dental Mfg. Co., Akron, Ohio. See p. 188.

up to 8 inches is desirable. The current required will depend on the number of impressions being plated, roughly 20 milliamperes per average impression.

After approximately 20 minutes, the cathode should be removed, rinsed, and examined. If coverage is complete, plating may be continued. If there is an unplated area with a definitely circumscribed border, a bubble of air was trapped. Again completely filling the impression with solution, plating is continued for at least 5 hours. When the impression has been plated to the desired thickness, it should be removed and rinsed with water and a sodium bicarbonate bath to eliminate all traces of acid. After plating, the impression is filled with a core of stone or resin and a root is formed.

The Stone Die

If the die is to be poured in stone, the band must be wrapped with a wax collar or masking tape extending about 10.0 mm. beyond the cervical margin. The stone mix, using the recommended water-powder ratio, should be vacuumed. Vibration, if used very sparingly, will cause the stone to flow into the impression without forming voids at the incisal angles. Excessive vibration must be avoided. Also, introducing very small increments of stone along one side of the impression and tapping the band vigorously on the bench will condense the material and give a good surface.

A die poured of stone will be as accurate as the impression and may be used for waxing a pattern for the indirect-direct technique or for a cast transfer. If carefully handled, a platinum matrix may be swaged over such a die; however, owing to abrasion and chipping, the end result is unpredictable.

The Amalgam Die

For an amalgam die the modeling compound impression is fitted with a wax collar and is boxed in an inlay ring. Standard* inlay investment is a satisfactory boxing material, because it liberates little heat during setting and, being granular, is easy to cut away when removing the die. Any standard die alloy may be used. A pointed or beveled orangewood stick is used for the crown portion, but the root should be compressed with regular amalgam condensers so that excess mercury is eliminated. Condensing must be followed by the maximal setting time (approximately 6 hours) before the die is removed from the impression and the root portion trimmed (Fig. 166).

The greatest circumference of the die must be at the cervical margin,

---

* The Ransom & Randolph Co., Toledo, Ohio.

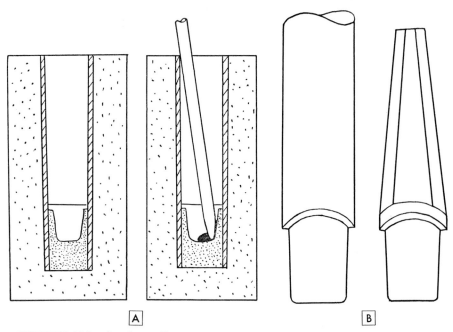

FIGURE 166. Amalgam die.
A, Packing amalgam die.
B, Untrimmed and finished die.

to provide access for carving and observation. The root portion must be tapered without irregularities, and if the die is to be seated in a working cast, one side should be flattened and grooved to act as a key for seating. The root can be shaped with coarse disks and then smoothed.

The amalgam die frequently has dimensions greater than those of the tooth, owing either to setting expansion or, more likely, to the pressure of condensing. The increased circumference may be advantageous in jacket crown construction. While it is stronger in the swage than an all-stone die, amalgam is inferior to dies with silver- or copper-plated surfaces. The grindings from the tapered root can contaminate casting alloys.

Quadrant Plating

A wax collar is not necessary when a quadrant or full mouth impression is to be plated. The cathode holder can be an insulated silver or copper wire, contacting the impression at some noncritical spot. Only the areas which are to be plated should be metalized, with silver-powdered wax strips leading to the wire cathode. When the impression is examined after 30 minutes, if the deposits are found to be satisfactory, these "leads" can be waxed over so that plating will not be continued in those areas.

REFERENCES

1. Phillips, R. W., and Schnell, R. J.: Electroformed dies from Thiokol and silicone impressions. J. Pros. Den., *8:*992, Nov.–Dec. 1958.
2. Hudson, W. C.: Clinical uses of rubber impression materials and electroforming of casts and dies in pure silver. J. Pros. Den., *8:*107, Jan. 1958.
3. Phillips, R. W., and Dettman, F. J.: A study of some variables associated with copperplating of dental impressions. J. Pros. Den , *6:*101, Jan. 1956.

Eastman, R. F.: Individual copper band rubber base impressions for inlays and crowns. J.A.D.A., *59:*966, Nov. 1959.
Hoffman, J. M.: Common problems in the construction of the full cast crown. J.A.D.A., *48:*272, March 1954.
Schnell, R. J., and Phillips, R. W.: Dimensional stability of rubber base impressions and certain other factors affecting accuracy. J.A.D.A.. *57:*39, July 1958.

12

WAX PATTERNS

Wax patterns for individual restorations or cast retainers may be fabricated in three ways: (1) by carving the pattern on a die expected to be devoid of dimensional imperfections (indirect), then making the casting; (2) by carving the pattern to completion on the prepared tooth (direct), then making the casting; or (3) by carving the pattern on a die suspected of having some imperfections, transferring the pattern to the prepared tooth for the correction of marginal defects (indirect-direct), and investing and casting without returning the pattern to the die.

The *indirect* technique is suggested whenever reproductions of the preparations can be made, because much of the procedure can be delegated to a technician, time will be saved, and usually the restoration will be superior in contour, adaptation, and marginal fit.

The *direct* method for carving wax patterns (forming them in the mouth on the prepared teeth) should be restricted to anterior partial veneer crowns, pinledge retainers, and inlays. (This has been discussed in detail in Chapters 6, 7, and 8.) Wax must be applied to the tooth in such a way that all fine lines of the preparation are copied, so that there is ample material to permit carving to form, rather than building to form by the addition of wax, and so that the closed relationship of the teeth may be registered while the wax is confined to the tooth surface. While the ability to produce patterns by this method is rapidly becoming a lost art, some of the more conservative partial veneer and inlay preparations demand that it be used. Also, total construction time can be lessened in many cases.

The *indirect-direct* procedure is not recommended, but it may be used when carving patterns for full veneer gold crowns and for partial veneer crowns.

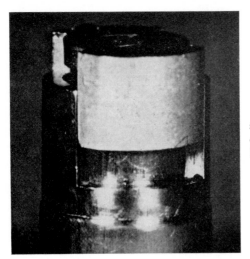

FIGURE 167. Wax pattern was stored off of the die for 24 hours and then casting was made. Distortion is result of release of internal stress.

Stress and Distortion in Wax Patterns

Any wax pattern contains a certain amount of internal stress due to carving, molding of the wax, spot heating, or the natural tendency of wax to contract on cooling. The stress can be reduced in any pattern by avoiding undue patching and pooling of the wax and by forming the pattern at as high a temperature as possible.[1] While it is true that a pattern fabricated by flowing wax on the die, as in the indirect method, has minimal stress, some exists in any pattern.[2] This stress probably is insignificant if the pattern is invested immediately after it has been removed from the cavity preparation or die.

The two factors exerting the greatest influence on the degree of distortion in the wax pattern before investing are the length of time between removal of the pattern and investing, and the temperature at which the pattern is stored. The stress will be relieved over a period of time even though the storage temperature remains constant. Some types of patterns will distort enough in only 30 minutes to prevent critical fitting of the casting (Fig. 167). The degree of distortion will increase as the storage temperature is raised, because the lowered yield point and increased flow allow the internal stress to be liberated more easily.

The direct pattern should be placed in a refrigerator if it must be stored overnight, since any change in form is minimized at lower temperatures. Storage in a cup of water does *not* prevent warpage. The bad habit of leaving patterns off the preparations, as in a direct technique, to accumulate throughout the day, is a common cause for distortion and failure. Also, investing multiple patterns on a single sprue former is contraindicated because of the danger of distortion through uneven expansion.

Patterns should be free of inner surface defects or creases. Outer surfaces should be smooth, polished, and without pits or blemishes. Grooves and sulci should not be scratched or retain small, almost-detached crumbs of wax. Margins should be definite, regular, minutely excessive in bulk, and have substance to resist deformation.

An overwhelming majority of castings are made from patterns carved on dies that reproduce teeth prepared so that the surfaces are covered with minute ridges and grooves. If the cut surfaces have been smoothed with fine carborundum stones or paper disks, or if the walls converge occlusally, removal of the carved pattern can be easy. If the tooth or die shows bur or stone marks, the inner surface of the pattern may be made of a thin layer of softer wax, and removal must be established before it takes final form.

With the indirect technique, it is imperative that all margins be checked just before investing. Even on a stone die, the wax may distort slightly during the interval between fabrication and investing. Once the pattern has been surrounded by set investment, it may be cast when convenient.

Indirect Wax Patterns

While the expert can carve near-perfect direct wax patterns for anterior partial veneer crowns, pinledge retainers, and inlays, routinely the best patterns are made in the laboratory on dies produced from elastic impressions. This is because of freedom from interferences found in the oral cavity, lack of tension associated with a "helpful" and uncomfortable patient, better access, and the use of auxiliary personnel unconcerned with other problems.

The die and working cast must be lubricated before the die is dipped into molten wax to assure a thin, contracting film next to all the prepared surfaces (Fig. 168). In this way there will be no creases in the internal surface. Regular inlay or Kerr's* blue sprue wax may be used. The latter makes the built-up wax easier to remove from some dies, but before the cervical margin is perfected, this wax should be cut away 0.5 mm. short of the finishing line and a more rigid wax added. Marginal contour can be developed more readily with harder wax.

Using a No. 39 or 40 inverted cone bur, a circumferential groove may be cut around the die about 0.3 mm. below the margin of the preparation to act "as a guide in carving the wax pattern, in checking the seating of the crown on the die and in finishing the crown to the margin."[3] This is an excellent method for finishing crowns constructed by an indirect technique (Fig. 169). (See Chapter 10, The Working Cast.)

When waxing patterns on stone dies made from elastic impressions, a warm, blunt instrument, rather than one that is sharp, should be used

---

* Kerr Mfg. Company, Detroit, Mich.

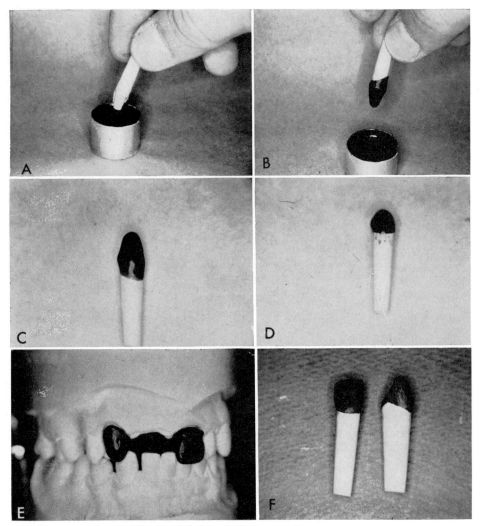

FIGURE 168.   *A,* Dipping lubricated die into molten wax.

B, C, First application of wax at the beginning of formation of wax pattern for retainer casting.

D, Wax trimmed to margin of preparation.

E, Patterns, roughly contoured, transferred to working cast to establish occlusion, length, contacts, and width, and to help in forming labial contour.

F, Wax patterns returned to dies for refinement of margins and completion of veneering areas.

to carve the margins. Otherwise, scarring the stone may lead to a discrepancy in the casting. The pattern can be tried on the working cast to position and gauge the strength of the contacts and to study occlusal carving and alignment (Figs. 170 and 171). It is then returned to the die, the margins are corrected, and the pattern is polished. It may be wise to examine all margins with a magnifying glass or loupe so that patterns will be more carefully waxed (Fig. 172).

FIGURE 169.

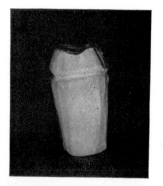

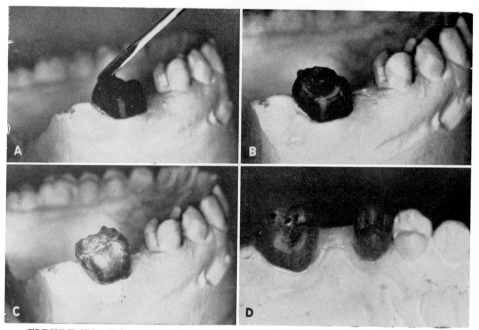

FIGURE 170. The wax pattern.

A, Wax being applied to lubricated working cast.

B, C, Occlusal height and pattern registered by closing articulated casts.

D, Patterns checked for occlusion in lateral and given final form. High spots were carved to a form which contacted but did not interfere with opposing tooth.

The full veneer gold crown, partial veneer crown, pinledge, and inlay will be included here, but the veneered gold crown will be discussed later.

The Full Veneer Gold Crown

The diagnostic cast, taken before preparation of the tooth, will show the form to be given to the carving. Close attention should be paid to the exact location of the contact areas, the height of contour on both buccal and lingual, the area between the cusp tips, the relation of the cusp tips to the anatomic center of the tooth as determined from the height of contour

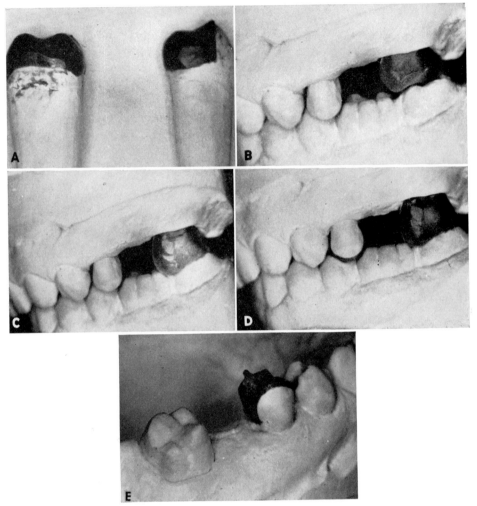

FIGURE 171.   Forming the wax pattern.

A, Wax is flowed on the lubricated die, or the die may be dipped in molten wax if all surfaces of the tooth have been included in the preparation.

B, C, Crudely formed pattern is transferred to the lubricated working cast to establish occlusal pattern.

D, Giving occlusal form to second wax pattern.

E, Occlusal pattern formed on bicuspid.

viewed from the occlusal, the relative size of the cusps, and the relation of the cusps to the marginal ridges. The wax pattern should represent exactly the form of the finished restoration that will be placed in the mouth.

The beginning student or the less apt technician must make some allowances at the cervical margin of a full veneer gold crown pattern. While the pattern must not extend beyond the cervical margin of the preparation, it should have just a little extra bulk in that area, possibly an added thickness of 0.3 mm., so that the casting can be polished without producing a margin that is short of the finishing line of the preparation,

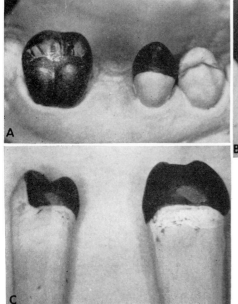
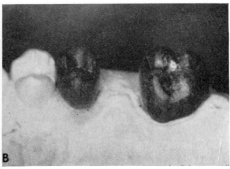

FIGURE 172. Forming the wax pattern (continued).
A, B, Patterns carved and refined.
C, Patterns returned to dies for refinement of cervical margins.

a common failing. Marginal fit requires adaptation to the prepared surface, with the pattern extending just to the finishing line, and in respect to convexities and concavities, a reproduction or continuation of the tooth form at the junction line. The pattern can be polished with wet cotton.

The Partial Veneer Crown and MacBoyle Retainer

The pattern for a partial veneer crown or for a MacBoyle retainer may be produced by dipping, adding wax, and carving, or by fitting a band, filling it with softened wax, pressing it on the tooth, and carving.

The Pinledge Retainer

The pattern for a pinledge retainer may be all wax or may utilize plastic pins or nylon bristles in the pinholes with wax flowed around and securely holding them.

Pruden[4] says: "The wax pattern is made by melting inlay wax over the well-lubricated stone cast, and driving it into the pinholes with a very hot pointed instrument, such as an old explorer point. The trapped air will bubble through the melted wax, and a dense smooth wax pattern can be removed from the stone cast with surprisingly little difficulty."

This technique is good when the pinholes have been prepared with taper fissure burs and the impression made using tapered plastic pins. However, even here plastic pins are very helpful in pattern construction.

When the holes in this preparation were made with drills, nylon

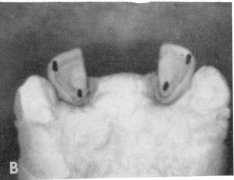

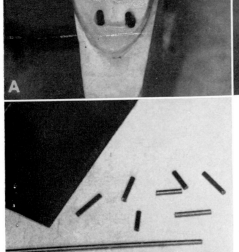

FIGURE 173.   *A,* Die showing preparation on maxillary cuspid. Surface has been lubricated. Bristles are in place.

B, Die of maxillary lateral incisors ready for application of wax.

C, Cut bristles.

bristles, slightly smaller in diameter, are cut, headed, and placed in the lubricated die. Wax is flowed onto the cut surface and held in position with a finger until cool (Fig. 173). This prevents curling and pulling pins out of position (Fig. 174).

After the pattern has been carved and polished and the margins checked, a very small semicircular mound of wax is placed in the center of the lingual surface to provide an attachment for the 18-gauge sprue pin. Spruing is done best off the die, and the pin should be at right angles to the lingual surface. If the pattern is sprued on the die, the added wax must be closer to the incisal and the pin *must* be in line with the path of removal.

The pinledge pattern is the only one attached to the sprue pin so that molten metal enters the mold and strikes a flat or concave surface at a 90 degree angle. The 18-gauge pin is also the smallest used.

The Inlay Retainer

When making a pattern for an inlay, wax may be flowed into the lubricated die or be confined and forced to place with an adjusted matrix band. Carving and removal may be done readily. The sprue pin is attached to the contact area and pointed so that the molten gold will divide and flow in at least two directions.

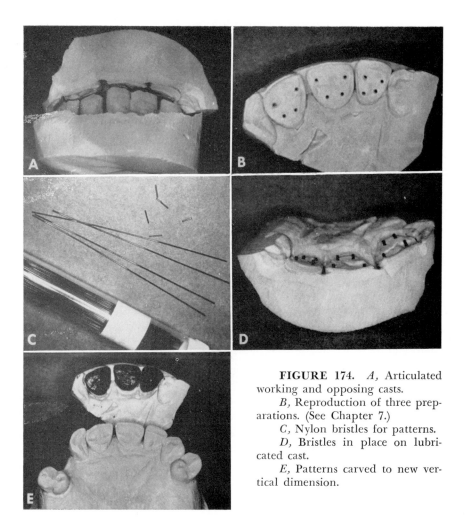

FIGURE 174. *A,* Articulated working and opposing casts.

B, Reproduction of three preparations. (See Chapter 7.)

C, Nylon bristles for patterns.

D, Bristles in place on lubricated cast.

E, Patterns carved to new vertical dimension.

Indirect-Direct Patterns

Full veneer and partial veneer patterns may be carved on a disassociated die without benefit of a full arch working cast and then checked in the mouth for position and strength of contact areas and occlusion. For this technique, it is well to make a single tooth occlusion registration before putting a temporary covering on the prepared tooth.

Softened inlay wax is placed on the occlusal and forced onto the mesial, distal, and lingual prepared surfaces. The patient is asked to close in centric and to open immediately. The wax is readapted to the tooth and the patient is again asked to close and to hold this position until the wax has become rigid. It is removed and stored until the die is available.

To keep the wax from sticking, the die must be lubricated with

Microfilm, Slikdie,* or Die-Sep.† The wax registration is adapted to the die and inspected for conformation to all surfaces. All areas not contacted by the opposing or approximating teeth are cut away. Discrepancies in adaptation can be filled by flowing melted inlay wax into the crevices.

The purpose of the registration is to help establish proximal contacts and to guide occlusal and peripheral carving. To some extent this is achieved. However, the inner surfaces of such a pattern usually show creases and irregularities, which tend to weaken the casting and lessen resistance to deformation through loss of dimension by wear or equilibration.

Testing the Wax Pattern in the Mouth

The indirect-direct pattern must be checked on the tooth. The prepared tooth stump must be cleaned, leaving the surface moist but with no vestige of gutta percha or other foreign matter when the wax pattern is seated. Very light pressure should be used, at the same time watching the contact area with a mirror. If the contact has been overbuilt and is binding, the wax should be touched at the point of interference with a hot instrument, and the pattern gently seated. The approximating tooth will pare the wax to the proper thickness. The pattern must be replaced on the die and the proximal surface and cervical recontoured.

After the thickness and position of the contact area have been revised, the harmony of the pattern with the arch and the cervical convexities and embrasures of the remaining teeth must be observed. The occlusion can be tested by having the patient close until some obstacle is met and then move the mandible to burnish the wax pattern. It is then placed on the die and the scored spots are recarved. The occlusion of the wax pattern should be left high, rather than out of contact.

The cervical margin must be checked. The curved shank of a No. 5 S. S. White explorer or a No. 12 Crenshaw scaler or burnisher can be used to plane off any excess wax. Uncovered margins of the preparation can be discovered by rubbing the curved angle of the explorer occluso-cervically over the junction. The point of the explorer must not be used.

Wax should never be added to the cervical portion of the pattern while it is on the tooth, as moisture would be incorporated and an imperfect pattern would result. The pattern must be removed, dried thoroughly, placed on the die, and the wax added *outside* the mouth. Then the pattern can be returned to the tooth and carved to form. It is polished on the tooth, using moist cotton, and it should not be returned to the die after it has been polished.

---

* Slaycris Laboratories, Portland, Ore.
† J. F. Jelenko & Co., Inc., New Rochelle, N. Y.

REFERENCES

1. Lasater, R. L.: Control of wax distortion by manipulation. J.A.D.A., *27*:518, April 1940.
2. Phillips, R. W., and Biggs, D. H.: Distortion of wax patterns as influenced by storage time, storage temperature, and temperature of wax manipulation. J.A.D.A., *41*:28, July 1950.
3. Smith, G. P.: The marginal fit of the full cast shoulderless crown. J. Pros. Den., *7*:231, March 1957.
4. Pruden, K. C.: A hydrocolloid technique for pinledge bridge abutments. J. Pros. Den., *6*:65, Jan. 1956.

Hollenback, G. M.: Brief history of the cast restoration. J. South. California D. A., *30*:8, Jan. 1962.
Kasloff, Z.: Recent advances in casting techniques and their evaluation. Internat. D. J., *13*:331, June 1963.

13

SPRUING, INVESTING,
AND CASTING*

The objective in any casting technique is to produce from a wax pattern a casting that will fit snugly on the preparation and be free of porosity. Success of the inlay or crown depends on minute accuracy and maintenance of the high physical properties of the alloy necessary to resist deformation and corrosion. Probably the most difficult problem facing the dentist or technician is to obtain the vital over-all adaptation of metal to tooth surface and to margins.

While it is true that the perfect casting has never been made, dental casting procedures have progressed to a point today where failure, which has become the exception, usually can be traced to a lack of respect for the basic principles associated with a sound technique. The process of fabricating an accurate and dense small casting cannot be a haphazard one and short cuts inevitably lead to failure. Each operator must adjust his own technique to the fundamentals, inasmuch as the fundamentals cannot be altered to accommodate every empirical method of investing or casting.

Zinc phosphate cement, the common luting medium, is soluble in oral fluids,[1] particularly the weak organic acids,[2] which may be present for limited periods at the critical marginal areas. The less exact the fit of the gold restoration, the greater the margin of cement that will be exposed and the sooner this margin will deteriorate, owing to dissolution of cement. A magnifying lens will show quickly that even the best inlay or crown attainable fits none too well. Unquestionably, slight marginal seepage of fluids occurs with any gold restoration, as well as other restorative materials.[3, 4]

---

* Investing and casting for *bonded porcelain veneers* is discussed in Chapter 22.

Longevity of the crown or bridge rests to a notable extent on minimizing such leakage. If the casting conforms with precision, disintegration of the thin layer of cement is of secondary importance.

Likewise a smooth surface and density are requisites in the gold casting. Any porosity will result in pits or voids that drastically lower the physical properties and thus increase the possibility of distortion or fracture during mastication. Corrosion and discoloration will occur also, although surface roughness or contamination of the alloy are the usual causes for corrosion.

The finished casting can be no better than the original wax pattern; therefore it follows that extreme care must be taken to assure maximal reproduction of the cavity preparation for the sake of stability, anatomical contour for function, and freedom from distortion to enhance seating.

SPRUING

Too much weight cannot be placed on the necessity for cleanliness in the investing process. Any separating medium, saliva, blood, or crumbs of wax must be removed from the pattern by gently brushing it with a soft brush, soap, and room-temperature water. The sprue base, also, must be free of any particles of old investment, which will leave a frayed or rough surface after separation.

The sprue pin should be made of a rustproof metal so that no oxide will form and remain on the investment to contaminate the gold as it enters the mold. When joining the pin to the pattern, the pin must not be overheated or it will melt or distort the adjacent area on the pattern, and as the wax resolidifies it will contract and perhaps draw away from

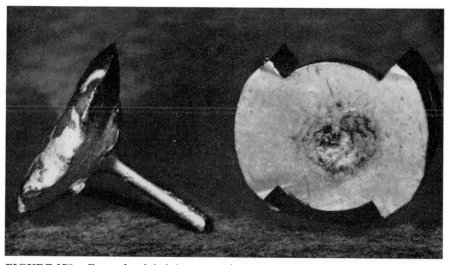

FIGURE 175. Example of shrinkage porosity due to use of a sprue that was too small.

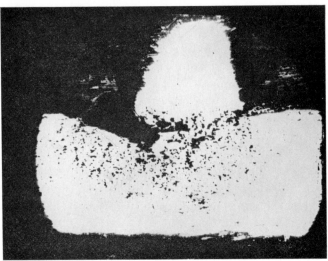

FIGURE 176.   Shrinkage porosity as shown by metallographic picture. Porosity extends deeply into casting.

the margins. A drop of wax may be added where the pin is to be attached and the pin can be inserted without disturbing the body of the pattern.

The size of the sprue will influence the density of the casting.[5] If it is too small, the gold will freeze in the sprue first, and as it contracts will pull metal from the casting itself. (See Fig. 175.) The ensuing porosity is termed "shrinkage porosity" and usually is located at the point of sprue pin attachment (Fig. 176). For the average size or large pattern, the sprue pin must be not less than 14-gauge, preferably 12-gauge. When the pattern is very small or thin, an 18-gauge sprue pin should be used to avoid distortion of the wax. Reservoirs are often recommended as an aid in eliminating any inclination toward shrinkage porosity, but they are unnecessary if the sprue is of appropriate size.

The sprue pin should be placed at the bulkiest part of the pattern, but not where it will mutilate carving designed to promote function in lateral excursions or in centric closing, with the inside or open area of the pattern toward the top of the ring. Fixing the pin at an angle, rather than vertically to a flat area, will lessen considerably the chance of gold "turbulence" and consequent porosity.[6] (See Fig. 177.)

A mandibular full veneer gold crown pattern, in most instances, can be sprued on the lingual surface of a lingual cusp or on the surface approximating an edentulous area. A maxillary crown pattern will not be damaged if the sprue pin is placed on the buccal surface of a buccal cusp. A partial veneer pattern can have a reduced contact restored by spruing to such an area, but if the contact has been carved and adjusted, the pin should be placed either on the opposite proximal surface or lingually to the cusp tip (Fig. 178). An inlay pattern seldom can be sprued advantageously other than at the contact point. A pinledge or a MacBoyle pattern must be joined to the sprue pin in the center of the lingual surface, perpendicular to the plane of that surface (see Fig. 179). Pins should be attached to pontics to allow the molten metal to flow along, rather than directly against, metal backings.

Generally double sprues are not essential for the crown and bridge casting, but when an occlusal or a surface to be veneered is shallow in comparison with the proximal walls, a double sprue or vent must be

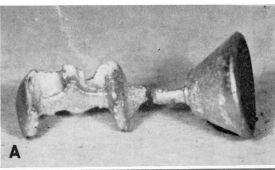
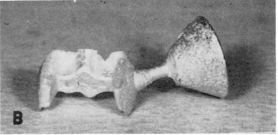

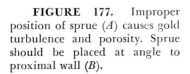

FIGURE 177. Improper position of sprue (*A*) causes gold turbulence and porosity. Sprue should be placed at angle to proximal wall (*B*).

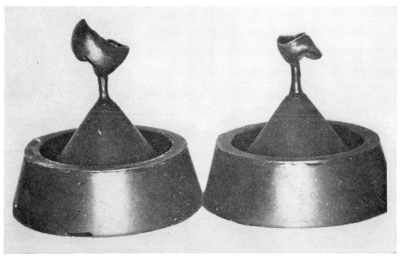

FIGURE 178. Points and angles of attachment for attaching sprue pins to upper posterior patterns.

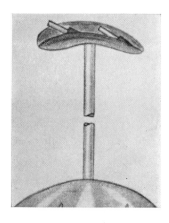

FIGURE 179. Spruing pinledge pattern.

employed or the metal will tend to freeze first in the thinner area and lead to porosity or an incomplete casting.[7] (See Chapter 19, The Veneered Gold Crown.)

Location of Pattern in Ring

The location of the pattern in the ring is another variable that markedly affects the density of the final casting. After the wax has been burned out, gases remain in the evacuated mold, and as the gold is forced into this space these gases must filter through the investment and out the end of the ring. If they are not eliminated, the gold cannot fill the pattern area, and, owing to the backward thrust of the gases that are still present, "back pressure" porosity results.[8] Often wrongly ascribed to other causes, this is one of the most frequent types of porosity seen in dental castings. It is prevalent especially in the full cast crown, in which the large inner core of investment slows the gas escape from the occlusal area. (See Fig. 180.) The porosity pattern is inconstant and may

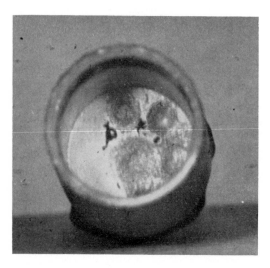

FIGURE 180. Example of back-pressure porosity caused by gases not being completely forced out of the mold. This type of porosity can be evidenced in many other ways.

be evidenced in various ways, such as rounded margins, general porosity, or a hole in the casting. The sprue pin should be long enough to place the end of the pattern within ¼ inch of the end of the ring (Figs. 181 and 182). In this position the gases can be readily expelled through the investment. If the diameter of the sprue pin is adequate, the length may be safely increased in order to locate the pattern close to the end of the ring.

Another factor in this phenomenon of back pressure is the casting pressure. It must be sufficient to force the gases out. Within reasonable limits, little danger exists from too much pressure. At least four turns of

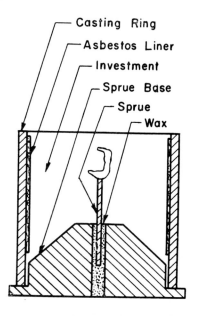

— Casting Ring
— Asbestos Liner
— Investment
— Sprue Base
— Sprue
— Wax

FIGURE 181. Schematic drawing to show proper location of pattern in ring and the various components which are used in making a dental casting.

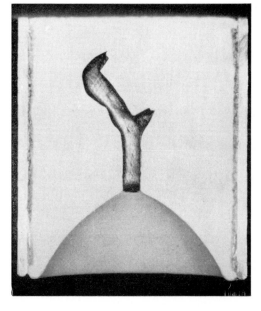

FIGURE 182. Section cut through an invested pattern to show the location in ring.

the casting arm will be needed with a centrifugal machine; a minimum of 15 pounds should be used if air pressure casting is employed. Some of the newer casting machines make use of vacuum, either wholly or in conjunction with centrifugal force or air pressure. Properly used, all these devices produce comparable results.

THE ASBESTOS LINER

In order that the investment not fall out, the asbestos liner should be positioned so that it is approximately 1.5 mm. short of the ends of the ring. (See Fig. 181.) Likewise, placing the liner somewhat short of the end of the ring will tend to minimize any distortion of the pattern or in the mold. The expansion of the investment is always greater in the direction toward the open, unconfined ends of the ring than toward the sides of the ring. Thus, if the liner is slightly short, the contact of the investment with the ring helps to restrict the expansion of the investment in that direction and equalize the dimensional changes that occur during setting, hygroscopic, and thermal expansion. (See Fig. 182.)

The purpose of the asbestos is to permit free expansion of the investment, which would otherwise be hampered and restrained by the metal ring. Before mixing the investment, the liner must be soaked with water. There is no doubt that the liner does affect the expansion and the size of the mold because of greater freedom for thermal and setting expansion, some hygroscopic expansion from the water in the liner, and the compressibility of the liner, which offsets the contraction of the more rapidly cooling ring during the time the gold is being melted and the casting made. Use of additional layers of asbestos can provide a noticeable additional expansion on certain preparations.

INVESTMENTS

Many investments, and techniques for their use, are advocated for making the small dental casting. All are concerned basically with the problem of expanding the mold to compensate for the contraction of the gold as it solidifies. This contraction has been measured at approximately 1.25 per cent,[9] although some recent studies indicate that it may fluctuate with the alloy composition.[10] Inasmuch as 1.25 per cent is a mean and accepted value for the alloys generally used for small castings, it is used for the technique to be described in this book.

To counterbalance contraction of the alloy and to make certain the casting has as nearly as possible the same dimensions as the wax pattern, the investment must enlarge in some manner to form an oversize mold.

A dental investment has three potential types of expansion: thermal, setting, and hygroscopic. In fact, all three appear to some extent with every technique. However, two basic procedures are favored. One relies chiefly on the thermal expansion of the investment to compensate for the contraction of the gold, while the other utilizes hygroscopic expansion plus a certain amount of thermal expansion. In the latter technique, the hygroscopic expansion is secured in diverse ways, such as by the use of a water bath for immersion of the invested pattern,[11] or by the addition of a controlled quantity of water to the top of the setting investment.[12]

Both the thermal and the hygroscopic methods have discernible advantages, as well as limitations, with the human equation playing a vital role. As with most dental materials, ease of mastering a technique and the behavior of a given material will vary for each individual. All the techniques mentioned can be used to produce habitually sound and accurate gold castings. Regardless of technique, the fundamentals remain the same, and emphasis in this chapter is on these fundamentals. However, only the thermal expansion process will be stressed and covered in detail here, its selection having been based upon several factors.

1. Provided that the thermal expansion technique is standardized and customary caution is exercised, it has not been demonstrated that superior results can be attained with any other method.

2. All the variables are so well defined that the reason for a failure can be recognized promptly and proper steps can be taken to prevent a recurrence.

3. It has proved to be a simple method with uniformly accurate and consistent results in the hands of both the beginner and the expert. Discouragement with the thermal expansion technique invariably stems from lack of attention to a few easily observed fundamentals, such as burnout temperature and time.

With any one of the investments or the investing techniques, varying percentages of expansion will be required for the diversified classifications of cavities. Restorations that fit cannot be made for all forms of cavity preparation with one range of expansion. Even though the original pattern be most intimately and routinely reproduced with a given validated technique, both the ease of seating the casting onto the cavity preparation and the fit will be regulated not only by the size of the casting itself but also by the frictional resistance between the gold and the tooth structure. Wherever the cavity walls are long and parallel, the casting will contact them immediately, the friction will increase, and the casting will be more difficult to seat; hence the casting must be of such size that it will seat in spite of this frictional resistance. Conversely, when the preparation is conical or walls are short, they will not touch the casting until it is practically seated; therefore, a smaller casting will be desirable in order that it may fit snugly. The longer the preparation occluso-cervically and mesio-distally, the greater the expansion required. The "effective" setting or hygroscopic expansion will also vary with the type of preparation and the exact location in the inlay ring.[13] Thus the configuration of the preparation must be considered in order to achieve ideal results.

Etching or altering the inside surface of the casting in any way, or changing the cavity preparation in an attempt to "engineer" a better fit, will decrease the considerable mechanical retention needed in a bridge retainer. The fit of the casting may be properly attained by control of the investing fundamentals, not by reliance on alteration of the final restoration or preparation.

Stability in a casting means that it has the form and adaptation that will make it resist all forces tending to cause motion and, to a lesser degree, movement directed opposite to the path of insertion. The casting should fit closely on the preparation, but it should slip to place with finger pressure or light tapping with a mallet and an orangewood stick or metal instrument, which can be accomplished only by modifying the size of the casting within certain limits.

Expansion of Investment

The latitude in expansion needed to accommodate the numerous types of cavity preparation used in the field of crown and bridge can be managed by altering the degree of thermal expansion. The setting expansion is quite uniform (0.3 per cent, approximately), and the small amount of hygroscopic expansion from the wet asbestos liner, although not definitely known, is constant; however, the thermal expansion can be varied in a number of ways to secure the shifting values required to control the size of the casting. A simple device is to alter the composition of the investment.

Silica, in some form, is the constituent in the investment that induces the thermal expansion.[1] Two physical forms of silica are used principally in dental investments. One of these is the cristobalite form, which expands thermally approximately 1.3 per cent when heated to 1200° F. If the quartz form of silica is used, maximal thermal expansions between 0.75 per cent and 1.1 per cent may be expected (Figs. 183 and 184). By mixing together different proportions of a cristobalite* and a quartz investment* (referred to as the "control powder"), thermal expansion ranging from approximately 0.75 per cent up to 1.3 per cent may be insured, thereby obtaining castings slightly smaller or larger than the original pattern.[14]

It must be emphasized that the trade name of "control powder" is not to be construed to mean an ingredient that solves all casting problems. It is simply a quartz investment which, in conjunction with the cristobalite

---

* Kerr Mfg. Company, Detroit, Mich.

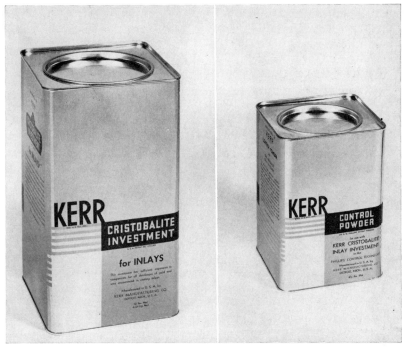

Fig. 183   Fig. 184

FIGURE 183. Cristobalite investment.
FIGURE 184. Control powder.

investment, may be used to provide a wide range of thermal expansion in the investment.

Weighing and Proportioning Investments

The Phillips[15] control technique, advocated by the manufacturer of one of the cristobalite investments, was originally designed to compensate not only for the shrinkage of cooling metal but also for the shrinkage of a direct wax pattern on its removal from the oral cavity into a cooler temperature in the room. A chart and automatic scale (Figs. 185 and 186) are used to determine and weigh the proportions of cristobalite and control powder indicated for patterns of various types, sizes, and shapes. The system is predicated on room temperature and on the theory that the wax pattern will change in dimension if subjected to temperature fluctuation.

It is necessary to have a thermometer reading when patterns are taken from the mouth to the laboratory. When the chart suggests a below-room-temperature investing, it will call for less control powder to be included, with greater expansion occurring. If an above-room-temperature mixture is used, more control powder will be added, thus retarding expansion.

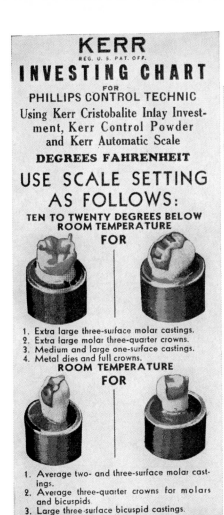

KERR
REG. U. S. PAT. OFF.

INVESTING CHART
FOR
PHILLIPS CONTROL TECHNIC

Using Kerr Cristobalite Inlay Investment, Kerr Control Powder and Kerr Automatic Scale

DEGREES FAHRENHEIT

USE SCALE SETTING AS FOLLOWS:

TEN TO TWENTY DEGREES BELOW ROOM TEMPERATURE
FOR

1. Extra large three-surface molar castings.
2. Extra large molar three-quarter crowns.
3. Medium and large one-surface castings.
4. Metal dies and full crowns.

ROOM TEMPERATURE
FOR

1. Average two- and three-surface molar castings.
2. Average three-quarter crowns for molars and bicuspids.
3. Large three-surface bicuspid castings.
4. Small one-surface castings.

FIVE TO TEN DEGREES ABOVE ROOM TEMPERATURE
FOR

1. Average two- or three-surface bicuspid castings.
2. Large three-quarter crowns for anterior teeth.

TEN TO TWENTY DEGREES ABOVE ROOM TEMPERATURE
FOR

1. Most anterior three-quarter crowns.

IMPORTANT—The amount of expansion is easily and exactly controlled. If more expansion is desired, balance the scale below the prevailing room temperature, and if less is desired balance above the prevailing room temperature.

Where weighing temperature is 60° or less use straight Cristobalite.

KERR MANUFACTURING CO.
DETROIT, 8, MICHIGAN, U. S. A.

PRINTED IN U.S.A.   1215-12

FIGURE 185. The Kerr Investing Chart. These values were developed for patterns taken directly from the mouth and invested in a different temperature environment. With indirect techniques, where patterns are not subjected to mouth temperatures, a constant room temperature of 80° F. makes a suitable basis for calculating ratios of Cristobalite investment and Control powder.

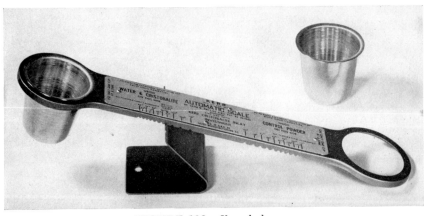

FIGURE 186. Kerr balance.

A decision as to the amount of control powder to use must be based on judgment derived from a combination of chart study and an observation of results. A tabulation of investing percentages used and the quality of fit obtained can become of great help in establishing an investing routine. A rule of thumb that all patterns of a given type should be invested without using control powder would produce many castings too loose for any practical purpose (e.g., a full cast crown on a long parallel wall preparation as compared with a crown on a short tapered preparation).

The technique of investing a wax pattern does not demand haste; nevertheless, all materials and equipment needed should be at hand in order that attention can be focused entirely on investing the pattern, without delay or confusion.

In the more recently developed indirect techniques, shrinkage of wax due to thermal change is avoided by allowing the formed pattern to remain on the die until it has cooled to room temperature and by subsequent use of room-temperature water and investment. Therefore, the use of the automatic scale with the indirect technique necessitates some modification in the procedure of proportioning the investments.

The authors have found that by utilizing the ranges of figures on the Kerr balance shown in Table 17, accurately fitting castings can be made for the various preparations.

When employing the scale in this procedure, the numbers should no longer be thought of as degrees of temperature but rather as uniform increments of a range of expansion. The figure 80 is used for the "average" partial veneer crown. Restorations needing more expansion (less taper, longer walls, smaller diameter of preparation) will require the use of a lower number. Those needing a lower percentage of expansion (greater taper, shorter walls, greater diameter) require a higher number.

The necessity for expansion increases as the number and length of the parallel surfaces increase. When the walls are shorter and tapered, there is less reason for expansion.

Most full veneer crowns are invested at 70 and veneered crowns at 60 (straight cristobalite). Occasionally, with a small diameter veneered crown such as a mandibular incisor, a double asbestos liner must be used to take advantage of all available thermal expansion in order to get a satisfactory fit. Pinledges, as a general rule, have short walls and pins and need only minimal expansion.

Table 17

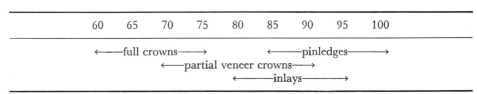

	60	65	70	75	80	85	90	95	100

In the techniques described here, the amount of water used is the same for all proportions of the two investments and is weighed at the figure 95 on the investment balance. The water-powder ratio is critical, variations causing quite noticeable changes in the amount of mold expansion. Some manufacturers of cristobalite investments take note of this characteristic and vary the expansion of the investment by altering the water-powder ratio rather than by the control powder method. The amount of expansion ensuing is in an inverse relationship to the amount of water used. In other words, the heavier the mix, the greater the setting expansion. However, thermal expansion is not significantly affected.

The special high-fusing gold alloys used in the construction of fused porcelain veneer crowns must have the greater expansion afforded by the phosphate bonded investments. This material and its properties will be discussed in Chapter 22.

Hand Investing

Wax patterns can be invested regularly by hand without resultant nodules or imperfections on the gold casting,[16] although care and experience are invaluable in overcoming the human variables.[17] Whether the pattern is to be invested by hand or by vacuum equipment, strict adherence to the powder-water ratio is a must. Deviations from the recommended ratio will influence not only the setting and thermal expansion but also, and of more consequence, the surface smoothness of the casting. If the mix is too thick, the investment will flow sluggishly onto the surface of the pattern and air bubbles may be formed. A thin mix will have a lower strength, increasing the possibility of fracture, particularly at the margins, during burnout or casting.

Nodules on the surface of a casting are due to air that was either incorporated in the investment itself or trapped during the investing process. If investment and water are blended with a mechanical spatulator, any large air bubbles will be broken up. A wetting agent, painted on the surface of the pattern before investing, will decrease the likelihood of enclosing air, but more than a very light coat will actually produce surface imperfections on the casting; therefore, any excess should be taken up with a dry camel's-hair brush. Vibration should *not* be employed when a wetting agent has been used, because the liquid tends to flow irregularly and to foam.

When the right powder-water ratio has been used, the consistency of the mix will be such that a small portion of the investment, placed on an inside edge of the pattern, will flow onto the floor of the pattern as it is gently pushed with a brush (Fig. 187). It should be applied from only one spot, because bubbles can be trapped wherever two separate portions of investment join. After the pattern has been covered, the

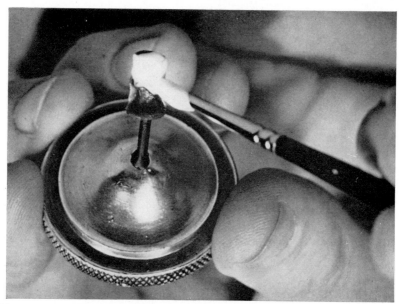

FIGURE 187.   Investment is gently flowed onto pattern with a small brush, applying from only one spot. Note clean surface on sprue base. If wetting agent is used, it must be a very thin coat.

investment may be blown off the surface, leaving a thin film and disengaging any large bubbles. The pattern should be repainted, the inlay ring filled, and the invested pattern cautiously seated in the ring with a vibrating motion; or the ring may be placed over the painted pattern and the investment flowed in on one side until the ring is filled (Figs. 188 and 189). A mechanical vibrator should not be used, because any air remaining in the investment seems to collect around the pattern.

Vacuum Investing

Castings free of nodules can be secured routinely by either hand or vacuum investing, but if it is astutely handled, vacuum investing is certainly more nearly foolproof.[17] With it, reproduction of minute marginal detail is sharper and the surface density of the gold is greater. This is due to the presence of a denser mass of investment adjacent to the pattern.

Many types of vacuum equipment are at the disposal of the profession (Fig. 190). Perhaps the most satisfactory is one in which both the mixing and the investing are done under vacuum. Directions for using two types follow.*

---

* Whip-Mix Corporation, Louisville, Ky.
  Kerr Mfg. Company, Detroit, Mich.

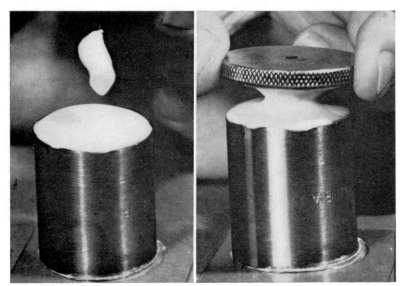

Fig. 188   Fig. 189

FIGURE 188.   Painted pattern is carefully vibrated into filled ring.
FIGURE 189.   Final step in seating pattern in ring. If proper powder-water ratio is used there is no danger in breaking off pattern.

Equipments and their Use

The mixing bowl, spatulator, and vacuum line must be free of investment. If the equipment has not been used recently, the pump should be operated (with the mixing bowl, spatulator, stainless steel casting ring, and rubber crucible former in place) to make certain that vacuum up to 26 to 28 pounds is available.

The ring designed for the investor being used is lined with one or more layers of asbestos of proper width. The wax pattern is sprued in the same manner as for hand investing. To resist pull from force of the vacuum, it is mandatory that the pattern be firmly attached to the sprue pin. The pattern is cleaned, and, if desired, painted with a very small quantity of wetting agent. Any excess should be removed with a dry brush.

The sprue pin is placed on the special rubber crucible former, which is fitted to the asbestos-lined casting ring. Room-temperature distilled water and investment powder (previously measured and weighed to meet specifications) are placed in the bowl and mixed with a plaster spatula.

The clean, dry spatulator is placed on the mixing bowl and the inlay ring inserted into the spatulator (Whip-Mix), or placed on the bottom of the rubber bowl (Kerr) after removing the plug. The motor operating the vacuum pump is turned on and the vacuum hose is connected to the spatulator. Atmospheric pressure will hold casting ring and crucible former in place.

The spatulator shaft is attached to the rotating motor shaft and the investment is mixed under vacuum (15 to 20 seconds on the Whip-Mix equipment; 30 to 60 seconds with the Kerr). The vacuum inlets must be turned upright to minimize the possibility of having them filled with investment. The mixing bowl must be tipped rather slowly from horizontal to vertical while vibrating the investment and causing it to flow from the mixing bowl into the ring. Vibration is transmitted from the vibrator of the investing unit through the rubber crucible former and casting ring to the mixing bowl. If the casting ring is carried to a vertical position too rapidly, bubbles may be formed on the surface of the wax pattern adjacent to the sprue pin.

When the ring is filled with investment, the vacuum tube should be removed from the spatulator. With the Kerr machine, it is advisable to remove the vacuum tube slowly and to continue mild vibration while doing so. Since the casting ring will drop away from the bowl upon removal of the vacuum, it must be held against the bowl during this operation. When the Whip-Mix machine is used, vacuum may be terminated suddenly.

The investment-filled casting ring should be set aside until the investment has hardened. The bowl, spatulator, and vacuum line must be cleansed thoroughly before the setting of any investment which they may have accumulated.

Vacuum investing equipment may be used also for vacuum mixing only, but the small-sized bowl will not handle enough investment for two casting rings. If the bowl is overloaded, investment will be forced into the vacuum line and must be cleaned out promptly. The vacuum line and vacuum pressure must always be inspected before use.

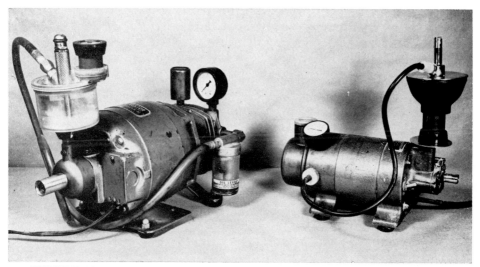

FIGURE 190. Various types of vacuum equipment for investing patterns are available.

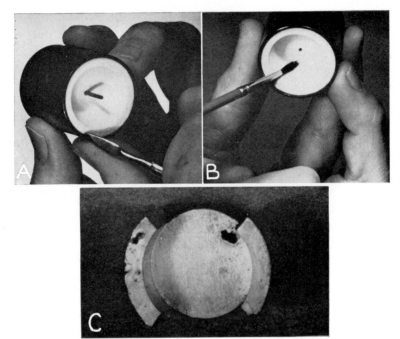

FIGURE 191.   *A,* Investment should be trimmed from edge of ring to prevent flakes from falling into sprue hole.

B, Dry brush may be used, holding ring inverted, to brush off investment chips after pulling sprue out.

C, Any bits of investment or charcoal from flux which get into mold will result in sharp, well-defined deficiencies as seen here.

Hygroscopic Technique

In the hygroscopic technique, after surrounding the wax pattern with a specially compounded investment, the casting ring is immediately immersed in a water bath at a temperature of approximately 100° F. The contact of the setting investment with the warm water produces an added expansion, referred to as hygroscopic expansion. The hygroscopic expansion is probably a prolongation of the normal setting expansion.

In most of the present hygroscopic expansion techniques, the degree of hygroscopic expansion desired is controlled by regulating the water-powder ratio. Generally, the thicker the investment mix the greater will be the hygroscopic expansion. Likewise, the longer the delay in time before the investment is immersed in the water bath the less will be the hygroscopic expansion. With some investments the expansion may be increased by using warmer water.

After the investment has hardened, the ring is removed from the water bath and the burnout completed as for the thermal expansion technique.

Controlled Water-Added Technique

In this technique, a soft flexible rubber ring is employed instead of the usual asbestos-lined metal ring. The pattern is invested normally. Immediately thereafter a specific amount of water is added on the top of the investment and the investment allowed to set, usually at room temperature. It is contended that the degree of hygroscopic expansion produced by the added water may be controlled by the amount of water used.

It should be emphasized that several investing techniques can produce comparable results. The dentist or technician should familiarize himself with different methods to find the one which will work best in his hands.[18] In any technique, however, the fundamentals described here will be applicable.

Removal of the Sprue Pin

The sprue pin and base should not be removed for approximately 30 minutes. The edge and outside of the ring should be cleaned of all flakes of investment that might accidentally fall into the sprue hole. The pin is heated over a burner and carefully pulled from the investment. It is advisable, too, to check the edge of the investment at the sprue hole and to detach any small irregular edges that might inadvertently enter the mold during burnout or casting. (See Fig. 191.)

BURNOUT

Elimination of the wax may be started as soon as the sprue pin has been removed (never before 30 minutes after investing), or it may be safely postponed indefinitely. While it is imperative to invest the pattern as soon as possible to avoid warpage, heating of the mold may be done at any convenient time. Once the burnout is started, the casting should be completed without allowing the mold to cool, as reheating a mold will cause a marked loss in strength, with the risk of frayed margins or an unacceptable casting.

The dental office or laboratory should contain an electric burnout furnace equipped with a pyrometer (Fig. 192). Calculated temperature control is essential in burning out the wax, and many failures may be traced to neglect of this precautionary measure. The pyrometer should be checked periodically, because it is not unusual to find these temperature-measuring devices to be inaccurate by as much as several hundred degrees. Dental gold manufacturers supply small cones of chemical compounds that melt at a specific temperature. These temperature indicators form a convenient method for checking the furnace temperature as registered on the pyrometer.

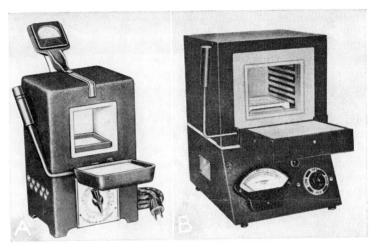

FIGURE 192.   Burnout furnaces. *A*, Jelenko, *B*, Huppert.

The temperature of the furnace should never be above 800° F. at the time the ring is inserted. Initial burnout temperatures above 800° F. cause too rapid heating, with danger of cracking the mold. The heating should be slow until the free water and the water of crystallization of the plaster have been evaporated. If the temperature is increased too quickly, steam may be formed and small pieces of investment will literally explode off the inside of the mold to produce a rough, defective casting. The furnace should be set on "Low" during the first 20 minutes.

Slow heating is especially important with a cristobalite-type investment since the inversion and thermal expansion occur quickly over a narrow temperature range. The ultimate temperature should not exceed 1250° F. As a matter of fact, with a cristobalite-type investment, provided that the burnout is complete, the casting may be made at a temperature as low as 1000° F. Thermal expansion will have reached its crest at that temperature. If lower temperatures are used during burnout (900 to 1000° F.), the ring should be held at that temperature long enough to assure complete wax elimination.

Extreme care must be exercised to avoid heating the investment to a temperature that will decompose the gypsum which is present as a binder. If any traces of carbon still remain in the mold, then the gypsum will break down at a temperature of only 1292° F. The sulfur that is liberated will then attack the gold alloy when it is forced into the mold. When gold is contaminated by sulfur, or by chlorine in some investments, it turns black, cleans up slowly on pickling, has low physical properties, and when cast is susceptible to corrosion and tarnish. If the temperature does not exceed 1250° F., there will be no danger of such contamination and the surface condition of the casting should be excellent. If the temperature of the mold is below 900° F., risk of subsurface porosity is increased.[19]

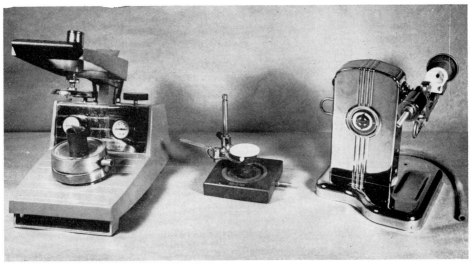

FIGURE 193. Various types of vacuum casting machines available.

CASTING

Gold alloys may be cast repeatedly with no impairment of physical properties if the metal has not been abused. Nevertheless, as a safety precaution, it is expedient to use approximately one-half new gold for each casting. The old sprue or button should be cleaned on a charcoal block to remove any occluded gases or small pieces of adhering investment. This can be conveniently done just before the ring is to be removed from the furnace, and the mass of metal may be carried to the crucible or inlay ring while still hot. In this way the time required to make the casting will be reduced. There is no reason for haste except that if the investment contains the quartz form of silica, as the investment cools it will contract and perhaps result in an undersize casting; therefore, the casting must be made within 2 minutes after removing the ring from the furnace. Sufficient metal should be used to fill the mold and produce a dense sprue and modest-sized button.

Centrifugal, air pressure, or well-designed vacuum equipment may be used to make the casting (Figs. 193 and 194). As yet no difference has been demonstrated in the marginal sharpness or the physical properties of metal cast in any of these machines.

Cleaning Metal

In cleaning an old button or sprue, the metal is placed on a charcoal block and melted (Fig. 195A). The molten metal should be sprinkled liberally with a reducing flux. A mistake frequently made at this point is to remove the flame from the metal and allow it to freeze. Exposed to

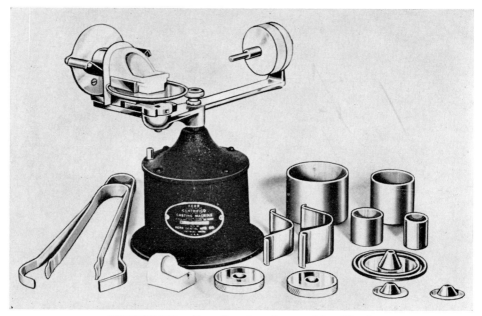

FIGURE 194. Centrifugal casting machine (Kerr).

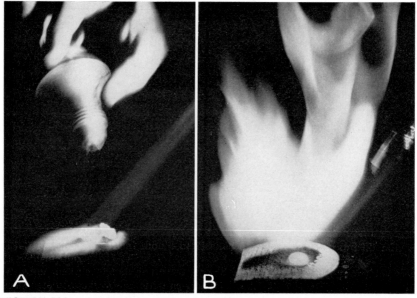

FIGURE 195. *A*, Metal should be cleaned on charcoal block and liberally covered with a reducing flux.

B, After melting, the air is turned off and metal freezes under protecting gas flame. When surface becomes frozen, torch may be removed.

air, the congealing metal will absorb gases, and the primary purpose of cleaning the metal is defeated. Instead, the air should be turned off and the gas flame played on the surface until the metal congeals (Fig. 195*B*). This flame is not hot enough to prevent the metal from solidifying, yet it will protect the alloy from occluded gases.

Fluxing

Flux should be added just after the metal has liquefied, and another small amount should be added just before casting. This thin film of flux on the surface aids in guarding the metal against accidental oxidation during melting. The most popular fluxes are mixtures of borax and powdered charcoal. The charcoal acts as a strong reducing agent by combining with any oxygen to form carbon monoxide or carbon dioxide, neither of which contaminates the alloy. Such a reducing flux must be kept from falling, or being blown, into the sprue hole, because any charcoal particles entering the mold will be entrapped in the metal, quite possibly on a critical marginal area.

A good flux for casting may be made by grinding together equal portions of fused powdered borax and powdered boric acid. The black reducing flux, which contains charcoal, is handily applied with a salt shaker but should be used only for cleaning old metal.

Melting Gold

Proper melting of the gold is of utmost importance. Naturally, the upper limit of the melting range must be exceeded to allow the metal to flow into the mold. This temperature may be reached by various types of torches. Gas and air are satisfactory if the peak of the melting range is not over 1950° F. and if the gas has sufficient B.T.U. The gas should be clean, as a high sulfur content may contaminate the alloy during melting. For higher melting ranges, oxygen and gas or acetylene must be used, but since they are exceedingly hot and a small mass of metal may be severely overheated, caution is necessary.

The paramount factor to be considered during this melting procedure, beyond liquefying all the metal, is the hazard of oxidation. Dental gold alloys, particularly the harder types, contain metals that are easily oxidized during melting. As the metal solidifies the dissolved oxygen is expelled, leaving voids throughout the casting. This is called "occluded gas" porosity and ordinarily is manifested in a general pitting of the surface (Fig. 196). Such porosity offers a choice harbor for oral fluids or debris, with discoloration resulting.

Hardness, strength, and ductility are lost rapidly in any porous area. If a gold alloy has been selected because of its applicable physical properties,

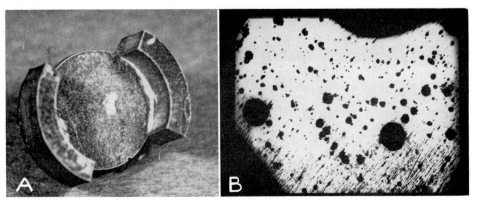

FIGURE 196.   Mistreatment of gold results in black castings that do not clean up on pickling. Similar effects may result if investment is overheated, breaking down; the liberated sulfur attacks the gold.

B, Section through casting shown in *A* shows typical example of severe internal "occluded gas" porosity. Surface of casting is usually pitted.

it must be dense in order to retain these properties. Porosity resulting from occluded gas can be controlled by governed use of the torch and by protection of the metal by fluxing. The reducing zone of the flame should be used; this is the hottest area and the only portion that will avert oxidation of the metal (Fig. 197*A*). The appearance of the gold reflects the part of the flame which is being used. That is, whenever the gold has a scum or film on the surface, the metal is being oxidized (Fig. 197*B*); when the surface is shiny and mirror-like (Fig. 197*C*), the metal is being reduced and the torch is in a suitable position. A brush-type flame is desirable since it is not quite as hot and will cover a larger area of the gold. Its position should be adjusted until this shiny surface appears.

The color of the molten gold, when it has reached its specific state for casting, cannot be described readily. Through experience this will become obvious instinctively. It will be noted that as it is heated the alloy first becomes somewhat spongy and small globules of melted metal appear. This stage is followed by a gradual change of the bulk of alloy to spheroidal form. The reason for this gradual change from solid to liquid is that gold alloys have a melting *range,* rather than a melting *point.* In the earlier phases of heating, the lower-fusing metals liquefy while the higher-fusing metals remain solid. All the alloy soon melts and a spheroidal mass is formed, having a dull red color at this point. Shortly thereafter the metal becomes almost transparent and begins to "spin." When the crucible of a centrifugal casting machine is shaken, the mass will roll around and will have assumed a light orange color. The gold is now ready to cast. Overheating the gold beyond this point does not burn out the base metal constituents, as was once believed, but it does heighten the danger of oxidation and will inevitably lead to frayed margins or a generally rough surface.

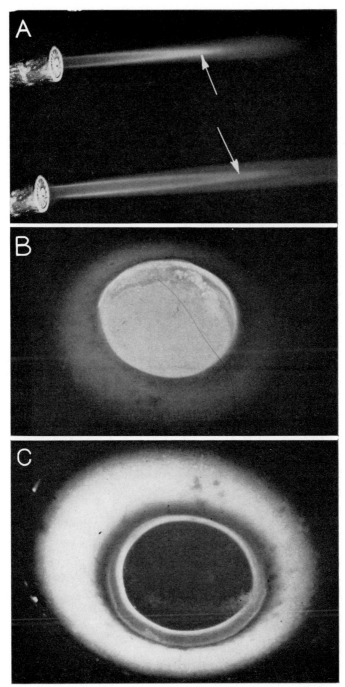

FIGURE 197. *A,* Two different adjustments of torch. Flame at bottom is preferable as it is not as hot and covers wider area of gold. The reducing areas to be used for melting alloy is shown by arrows.

B, Scum on surface denotes oxidation.

C, Shiny, mirrored surface indicates that metal is being treated kindly and not oxidized.

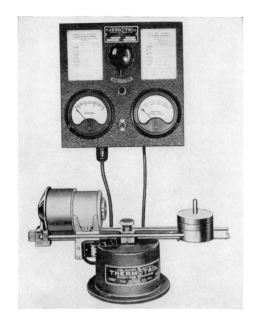

FIGURE 198. Thermotrol (Jelenko).

There is an ingenious instrument for melting the metal electrically, and for casting at a definite controlled temperature (Fig. 198).* While it does not turn out castings that surpass in physical properties those which may be obtained using a well-handled torch, it does minimize the human variables.

CLEANING AND HARDENING THE CASTING

The casting may be a little dark, owing to surface oxidation from the investment, but it can be cleaned readily by "pickling" in a 50 per cent solution of sulfuric acid or in solutions available from some dental gold manufacturers. If acid is used, the casting should be placed in a porcelain pickling dish or glass container, and the acid added and heated but not boiled. After the acid has been poured off, the casting must be thoroughly washed in tap water. Acid may be re-used, but it should be changed frequently to avoid possible contamination.

A casting should never be held with steel tongs, heated over a burner, and quenched in acid. Acid invariably contains traces of copper from previous pickling of gold castings, and insertion of the tongs into the acid will produce a galvanic current that will deposit a deep layer of copper on the casting, which will subsequently discolor in the mouth.

At this point the cavity surface of the casting should be examined with a magnifying glass. If any small nodules or irregularities are present, they must be removed with a bur or very small knife-edge stone before trying the casting on the die or tooth.

---

* Thermotrol, J. F. Jelenko & Co., Inc., New Rochelle, N. Y.

The conventional medium-hard crown and bridge golds are not usually receptive to a hardening heat treatment, and since a later soldering operation will rid the casting of all effects from such treatment, the ring may be plunged into water as soon as the button loses its red color. It should *not* be quenched while still red, because the sudden drop in temperature may distort a fine margin or thin area.

In the area of casting it is the good fortune of the dental profession to have access to results of research in materials and their handling, including rules to be obeyed, directions to be taken seriously, and precautions to be heeded. Acceptance of these findings will leave small room for contamination and failure. Ignoring them is only indulging in the foolhardy practice of asking for trouble.

POLISHING THE CASTING

If the wax pattern was smoothed and polished before investing, if the investment was treated properly during the burnout, and if the gold was not overheated, the casting will come from the pickling bath requiring minimal polishing.

The importance of a smooth, highly polished surface, or of a sound or dense casting, cannot be overemphasized, since saliva can wash across it freely, tending to keep it clean and bright. A rough, poorly polished casting will hold saliva and debris and greatly accelerate the formation of deposits or a film, which can become stained and unsightly. This discoloration may be mistaken for corrosion. Actually, chemical reaction of the metal is seldom involved, and as a rule cleaning with a toothbrush and dentifrice will remove the deposit and restore the original color and luster, provided that the surface is polished and the alloy has not been contaminated.

The polishing routine to be described embraces the systematic use of progressively finer abrasive instruments and materials.[20] There are no short cuts. The final appearance will be disappointing if a step is omitted.

A separating disk,[a] * moved back and forth with very little pressure

---

* The materials mentioned in the text that follows, indicated by superior letters, can be obtained from the following manufacturers:

[a, d] The S. S. White Dental Mfg. Co., 211 South Twelfth Street, Philadelphia 5, Penna.
[b] Mizzy, Inc., Clifton Forge, Va.
[e] Chayes Dental Instrument Corp., Miry Brook Road, Danbury, Conn.
[c, e, f] National Keystone Products Company, 2024 Market St., Philadelphia 36, Penna.
[d] The Ransom & Randolph Co., Post Office Box 905, Toledo 1, Ohio.
[f] Dental Development & Mfg. Corp., 653 Washington Avenue, Brooklyn 38, N. Y.
[g] J. F. Jelenko & Co., Inc., 170 Petersville Road, New Rochelle, N. Y.
[h] Buffalo Dental Mfg. Co., Inc., 2911 Atlantic Avenue, Brooklyn 7, N. Y.
[i, k] William Dixon, Inc., 32-42 East Kinney Street, Newark 1, N. J.
[j] Lever Bros., 390 Park Avenue, New York, N. Y.

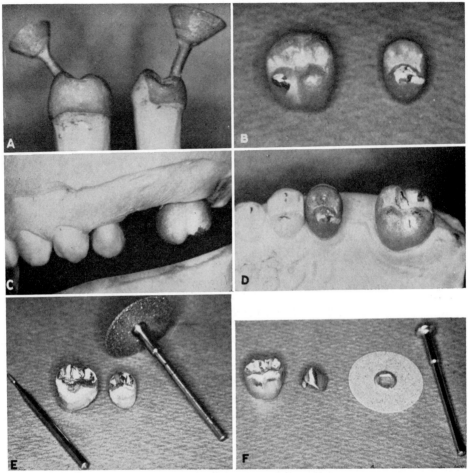

FIGURE 199. **Routine used to polish three-unit bridge.** This varies slightly from that described in the text but will produce excellent results.

    A, Castings pickled and seated on dies.

    B, Sprues cut off and areas contoured.

    C, Castings seated on working cast; occlusion being checked.

    D, Premature contacts registered.

    E, Occlusion adjusted and surfaces of castings stoned and burred.

    F, Surfaces smoothed.

and kept as close as possible to the casting, is used to cut off the sprue. It is followed by a heatless stone,[b] which blends the area of the cut-off sprue into the contour of the casting but leaves a coarse surface. A mounted green stone,[c] of a finer grit, is then used over the area previously ground.

    Because of the difficulty of polishing the sulci and maintaining the detail incorporated in the wax pattern, a dull No. ½ round bur[d] should be employed as a rotating burnisher, rather than a cutting instrument. A rubber point,[e] which can be kept sharp by rotating it against a heatless stone, will smooth the grooves of occlusal surfaces and other hard-to-reach areas which a round rubber wheel cannot touch.

A coarse 7/8-inch rubber wheel[f] is used with light pressure on larger surfaces. To preclude the formation of deep grooves, which might be made by rotating the rubber wheel in one direction only, the casting must be kept moving so that each successive cut is at right angles to the one previously made.

Next, a finer rubber wheel, the Green Burlew Disk,[g] will give a satin finish to all surfaces and prepare the casting for tripoli.

The occlusal and other finely carved surfaces may be polished with tripoli on a Robinson Bristle Disk, No. 11 Soft.[h] This brush is kept moving over the surfaces with enough pressure so that the bristles will spread out and reach all grooves and corners. It is followed by a 4-inch or larger lead center rag wheel,[i] adequately coated with tripoli. Medium pressure will produce the best surface.

The casting must be washed in a detergent[j] solution to remove all traces of tripoli before a reflecting surface is acquired from rouge applied with a rag wheel.[k] Every trace of rouge must be washed off. It is an antiflux, and if not removed will hinder the flow of solder.

It is much less complicated to polish individual units satisfactorily rather than the assembled bridge.

After the bridge has been soldered, it must be pickled. If the retainers and pontics were polished separately before soldering, only light polishing

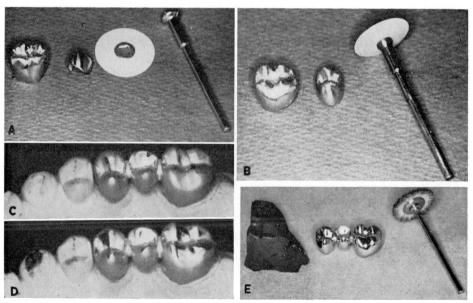

FIGURE 200. Polishing (continued).
A, Low polish produced by fine disk.
B, Smooth surface from rubber wheel.
C, Bridge soldered, pickled, and checked on cast for occlusion.
D, Occlusion corrected.
E, High polish produced by tripoli.

with tripoli, rouge, and No. 600 Carborundum powder* will be needed to prepare the bridge for cementation. After the bridge or crown is cemented, a higher luster can be obtained with a rubber cup and No. 600 Carborundum powder (Figs. 199 and 200).

CONTAMINATION AND FAILURE

A word should be said about the danger of contamination of the alloy. Certain contaminants, even though present in only minute amounts, have a profound effect on the physical properties. Usually the casting becomes brittle, the proportional limit is decreased, and the surface may be susceptible to corrosion. One of the possible contaminants, sulfur, was discussed earlier. A common hazard is mercury, and the consequence of its absorption by gold is dramatic. The casting metal must not come in contact with amalgam scrap and dies, contouring pliers, or base metal of any type, since the action of metals, such as lead or antimony, is extremely deleterious. Different types of golds should never be mixed. The resulting metal may form a eutectiferous alloy, which is often quite brittle and has low resistance to corrosion.

Casting failures should be most infrequent, but they do happen occasionally. As a rule, the cause for failure can be diagnosed readily. For example:

1. Rounded and shiny incomplete areas are indicative of incomplete burnout; the carbon left in the mold forms carbon monoxide, which acts as a strong reducing agent when the gold enters the mold.

2. Rounded margins that are dull instead of shiny may be attributed

---

* Silicon Carbide Grain No. 600, The Carborundum Company, Niagara Falls, N. Y.

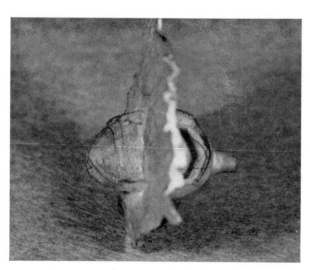

FIGURE 201. Casting failure due to investment fracture. This may be caused from burning out too rapidly, overheating gold, or too thin a mix of investment.

to inadequate casting pressure, to back pressure from improper orientation of the pattern in the ring, or to insufficient heating of the metal.

3. A sharp, well-defined deficiency, occurring usually at a margin, may be caused by the presence in the mold of some foreign object, such as a piece of investment or a bit of charcoal from the flux, or by the use of contaminated wax to form the pattern.

4. Frayed margins or a completely cracked mold are the result of burning out too rapidly, inaccurate water-powder ratio for the investment, or overheating the gold (Fig. 201).

5. Bubbles are associated with entrapment of air during investing or use of too much wetting agent.

CASTING ALLOYS

The choice of a casting alloy for a given bridge unit, when other requirements permit, should be harmonious in hardness with the alloys that may have been used for restorations made previously. Otherwise, wear, burnishing, and masticatory shock could be uneven; also, the rigidity needed to resist the transmitted forces, and flexing due to span length, must be inherent.

Rigidity is realized in part by using an alloy that is stiff after casting and soldering, and also by providing bulk in the casting. The thinner the occluding surface of a casting, the harder the alloy must be. Pinledges and many partial veneer crowns would be included in this group. Often partial denture alloys must be used, but conventional crown and bridge alloys should be considered first.

Whenever a variation in hardness exists in the alloys placed throughout an arch, more frequent examination and equilibration should follow.

REFERENCES

1. Skinner, E. W., and Phillips, R. W.: The Science of Dental Materials. 5th ed. Philadelphia, W. B. Saunders Company, 1960.
2. Norman, R. D., Swartz, M. L., and Phillips, R. W.: Studies on the solubility of certain dental materials. J. Den. Res., 36:977, Dec. 1957.
3. Sausen, R. E., Armstrong, W. D., and Simon, W. J.: Penetration of radiocalcium at margins of acrylic restorations made by compression and non-compression technics. J.A.D.A., 47:636, Dec. 1953.
4. Crawford, W. H., and Larson, J. H.: Dental restorative materials; amalgams, acrylics. J. D. Res., 33:414, June 1954.
5. Crawford, W. H.: Selection and use of investments, sprues, casting equipment and gold alloys in making small castings. J.A.D.A., 27:1459, Sept. 1940.
6. J. F. Jelenko & Co., Inc.: Dental Gold Structures. New York, The company, 1949.
7. The J. M. Ney Company: Ney Bridge and Inlay Book. Hartford, The company, 1958.

8. Phillips, R. W.: Studies on the density of castings as related to their position in the ring. J.A.D.A., *35*:329, Sept. 1947.
9. Coleman, R. L.: Physical Properties of Dental Materials. (National Bureau of Standards Research Paper No. 32.) Washington, U. S. Government Printing Office, 1928.
10. Hollenback, G. M., and Skinner, E. W.: Shrinkage during casting of gold and gold alloys. J.A.D.A., *33*:1391, Nov. 1946.
11. Hollenback, G. M.: Simple technic for accurate castings: new and original method of vacuum investing. J.A.D.A., *36*:391, April–May 1948.
12. Asgars, K., Mahler, D. B., and Peyton, F. A.: Hygroscopic technique for inlay casting using controlled water additions. J. Pros. Den., *5*:711, Sept. 1955.
13. Mumford, G., and Phillips, R. W.: Dimensional change in wax patterns during setting of gypsum investments. J. D. Res., *37*:351, April 1958.
14. Phillips, D. W.: A scientifically correct inlay technique. D. Digest, *39*:72, Feb. 1933. Controlled casting. J.A.D.A., *22*:439, March 1935. Present-day precision inlay investing and casting technic. J.A.D.A., *24*:1470, Sept. 1937.
15. Phillips, D. W.: Controlled casting. J.A.D.A., *22*:439, March 1935.
16. Phillips, R. W.: Relative merits of vacuum investing of small castings as compared to conventional methods. J. D. Res., *26*:343, Oct. 1947.
17. Lyon, H. W., Dickson, G., and Schoonover, I. C.: Effectiveness of vacuum investing in the elimination of surface defects in gold castings. J.A.D.A., *46*:197, Feb. 1953.
18. Phillips, R. W., ed.: Symposium on dental materials—their use and recent developments. D. Clin. North America, Nov. 1958.
19. Ryge, G., Kozak, S. F., and Fairhurst, C. W.: Porosities in dental gold castings. J.A.D.A., *54*:746, June 1957.
20. Ficaro, J. P., Lemire, P. A., and Kernodle, C. C.: Personal communications.

14

THE PONTIC

SELECTING SHADES FOR PORCELAIN FACINGS OR VENEERS

For an indirect method of bridge construction, the shades of the facings should be selected before the abutment teeth are prepared. Although approximating teeth are usually the most important, corresponding teeth in the approximating quadrant and occluding teeth must be considered also, even if this means a compromise, since a marked contrast with any one of these areas will be noticeable.

In the direct or semidirect techniques, shades should be chosen with the retainers on the teeth. The color of the intact labial or buccal surface of a prepared tooth will be relatively unchanged if cement powder, mixed with a combination of 50 per cent water and 50 per cent glycerin, is placed inside the casting to mask the metal. Repetition with different trial mixes will assist in finding a shade, or a combination of shades, in the cement that will restore the natural appearance of the abutment. A notation of the powder combination should be placed in the patient's record so that the same mixture may be used when the prosthesis is cemented permanently.

At least two shade guides should be used, in case the first choice of facing is not obtainable at the depot. This will necessitate fewer staining modifications.

The patient should face a north, natural light, if possible. Lipstick, amount and color of rouge, earrings, spectacle frames, and clothing, as well as the color of the office walls, can influence shade selection. If one particular shade of lipstick is habitually worn by the patient, it may remain; but if excessive make-up is used, generally it is advisable that it be removed and that the patient's clothing be covered with a neutral drape.

Incisors, cuspids, and bicuspids should be matched, first on the incisal or occlusal, then on the cervical. If, owing to a high lipline, all the facing will be exposed during speaking or smiling, the shade of the facing must coincide in its entire length with that of the approximating teeth. If the cervical will not be exposed, no more than the incisal or occlusal one-half or two-thirds need be of major concern. Customarily only the occlusal half of molar facings must blend with the approximating and occluding teeth.

Shade and Form

Facings that will harmonize with the approximating teeth without some reshaping and subsequent reglazing can seldom be procured. They cannot be manufactured to fit individual cases and must be thought of as "blanks" to be worked into form, position, and alignment by the operator. Many facings are more translucent or more shiny than the teeth they will approximate, but this lack of harmony is largely overcome by the metal backing and luting material. Even a facing of correct shade will look out of place if overglazed. Harmonious form in the facing will lessen, to a degree, the requirement for exact shade matching; however, the closer the shade match, the happier the patient.

TYPES OF FACINGS

The porcelain facings in common use are the pin, the flatback, the Trupontic,* the Sanitarypontic,* the porcelain biting-edge,* and the reverse-pin. Overjet and vertical overlap, length of the space inciso- or occluso-cervically, width of the space, and frequently translucence, shade, and shade distribution will have a bearing on the type of facing used in constructing the pontic (Fig. 202).

Pin Facings

Two types of pin facings are recommended: the Dentsply† and the Harmony.‡ The Dentsply, or long-pin, facing has a porcelain component similar in contour and bulk to the flatback, or Steele's,* facing. The pins are at right angles to the metal-contacting surface.

The Harmony facing has a built-on bulk of porcelain to be adapted to the ridge so that only porcelain will have a static relationship to the tissue.[1, 2] The pins protrude from the bulkiest portion of the facing in a

---

* The Columbus Dental Mfg. Company, Columbus, Ohio.
† The Dentists' Supply Company, York, Penna.
‡ Harmony Dental Products Corp., Pasadena, Calif.

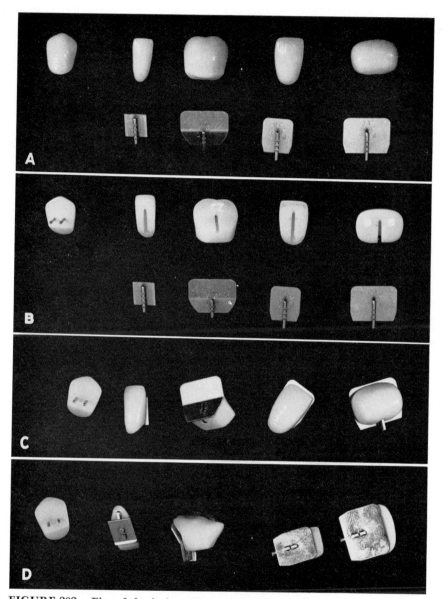

FIGURE 202.   Five of the facings discussed in this text.

A, Left to right: Long-pin facing (The Dentists' Supply Co.); porcelain biting-edge; Trupontic; Steele's flatback; and Sanitarypontic. (The last four are supplied by The Columbus Dental Manufacturing Co.) An appropriate backing is seen under each facing.

B, Same facings, same order, and their backings as viewed from the lingual and the occlusal.

C, Backings in position.

D, Backings partly removed.

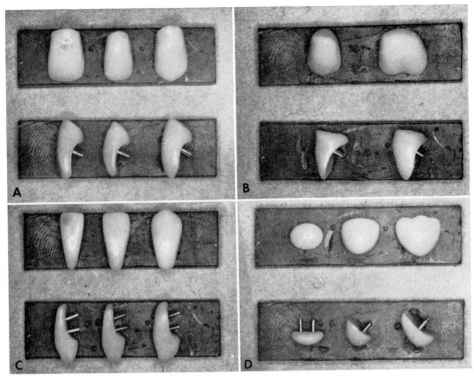

FIGURE 203. Harmony facings.
A, Maxillary anterior.
B, Maxillary posterior.
C, Mandibular anterior.
D, Mandibular posterior.

direction bisecting the angle formed by the two sections of the gold-contacting surface (Fig. 203).

The labial contour of the Harmony facing is not anatomic in an inciso-cervical direction. Two-thirds of the labial surface is natural; then the surface inclines somewhat toward the ridge. This is advantageous in a high percentage of cases. For irregular alignment with a high lipline, and when there has been more than average ridge resorption, the Harmony facing is superlative. It is adaptable in mandibular bridges when making bicuspid pontics with visible buccal surfaces and as a tip for contacting the ridge in molar areas.

Since the long-pin facing removes toward the labial or buccal, it can be adapted to almost all situations and types of occlusion. Excellent form can be produced. Contact porcelain, which already exists on the Harmony facing, can be added to the Dentsply. The pin facing may be hollow-ground and tipped incisally or occlusally, for protection, or to permit insertion in very short spaces, or when the vertical overlap is long without a corresponding overjet.

Flatback Facings

The flatback facing can be used advantageously when the space is average or longer inciso- or occluso-cervically, provided that the cusp or incisal edge contacts are normal or nearly so. In eccentric excursions there must be occlusal or incisal clearance to protect the porcelain. Usually esthetic contours can be fashioned.

The Trupontic facing is hygienic, but in many cases it presents exasperating difficulties in adaptation and shaping. The labial convexities and angles and directions of cusp arms cannot always be made correctly without displaying metal. The Trupontic facing, which also may be hollow-ground to shield the incisal or buccal margin, requires more length occlusally than the pin facing.[3]

Modifying a Pin Facing

A Dentsply pin facing can be altered so that when the pontic is built, the entire ridge-contacting surface will be porcelain. It must be ground to form and alignment, then shortened with a linguo-cervical bevel. A buccal plaster index is poured. The facing is grasped with a Graebner matrix* so that the pins are under the plate and the cervical half of the facing is exposed. Medium-fusing porcelain is built onto the lingual surface and over the cervical bevel of the facing with only minimal condensation (Fig. 204).

The facing is removed from the matrix and supported on a firing tray by a mound of silex. It is dried and fired to a low maturity. When placed on the working cast in the index, the contacting surface should have a plus contour. The facing is ground until contact with the ridge is continuous and the facing seats in the index. Embrasures must be formed and the cervical portion of the facing contoured to establish the correct contacting area. The facing is cleansed and fired to a suitable glaze (Fig. 205).

For this modified pin facing to be acceptable, the space for the pontic must have occluso-cervical height only slightly less than that for the Trupontic facing; if the span is long, there must be room for a greater bulk of metal in the beam.

Mandibular Sanitary Facings

Two lower posterior sanitary facings are in common use: the Steele's Sanitarypontic and the Harmony pin-tip. They are used on all lower posterior bridges unless occluso-ridge crest dimension is too short for both gold and porcelain or unless the space is so far to the anterior to necessitate complete buccal tooth form. When esthetic considerations are a factor with

---

* The Cleveland Dental Mfg. Co., Cleveland, Ohio.

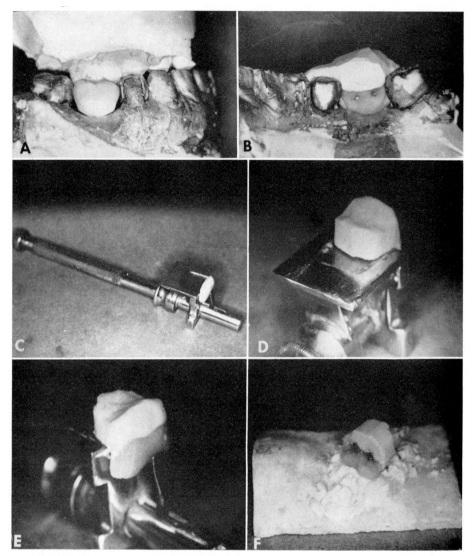

FIGURE 204.   *A,* Buccal view of pin facing ground to position on working cast.
B, Lingual view.
C, Facing held by Graebner matrix.
D, Porcelain powder built onto facing.
E, Showing porcelain powder carried onto buccal surface.
F, Facing on firing tray.
(Courtesy of Mr. Russell J. Jones, Cleveland, Ohio.)

the lower posterior pontic, either the regular Harmony facing (favored) or the Trupontic facing will be found superior.

Reverse-Pin Facing

The reverse-pin facing,[4] contrived from either a facing or a denture tooth, is very useful when pontics must be lapped or arranged irregularly, or when space width or occlusion is not appropriate for standard types. It does not have a universal application, but it gives beautiful results in many situations.

SELECTION OF FACING

A mold guide should be used if available. The kind and mold of facing may be selected using diagnostic casts. However, this is done more often

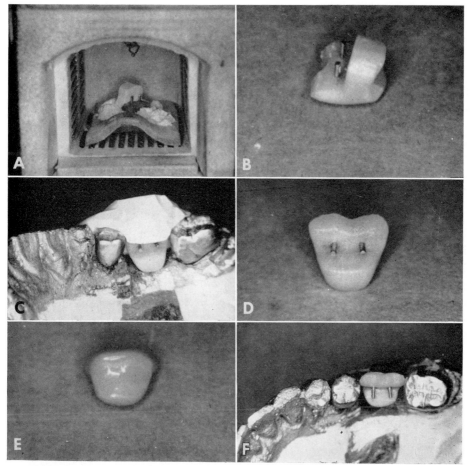

FIGURE 205. *A*, Facing in furnace.

B, Facing fired.

C, Facing contoured. Clearance between pins and added porcelain is sufficient to have bulk of metal in pontic for pinholes.

D, Facing glazed. Notice bevel along occlusal for protecting bulk of metal.

E, Highly glazed tissue-contacting surface.

F, Modified and glazed facing in position. (Courtesy of Mr. Russell J. Jones, Cleveland, Ohio.)

after the working cast has been articulated. If facings are selected and ground in on the diagnostic cast, they may be positioned in the space to determine the labial extensions of several types of retainer preparations.

Specific information concerning the facing should accompany the order. For example, it should read: "Steele's facing, upper right cuspid, mold 56G, New Hue shade 67." If the mold guide is not at hand, the order may read: "Steele's facing, upper right cuspid, 11.0 mm. long, 8.0 mm. wide at incisal, 6.0 mm. at cervical, New Hue shade 67." The facing chosen should be a little too wide and long so that there will be sufficient material for grinding to position and form.

GRINDING FACINGS TO PROPER POSITION AND FORM

Facings may be shaped and positioned on the working cast by (1) grinding to mesio-distal width; (2) adjusting to occluso-cervical or inciso-cervical length, which includes adapting the facing to the ridge; (3) forming the mesio-distal convexities and occluso-cervical contour; and (4) adjusting the long-axis inclination.

Width

The facing should be ground to the desired width with no attention being paid to mesio-distal contour (Fig. 206). The sides should be parallel inciso-cervically and labio-lingually, although, in some instances, not parallel with the long axis of the facing because of the effect that must be produced in the space. Only in an occasional case, to create an irregularity by overlapping an abutment or another facing, should a mesial or distal cut converge lingually. If there is more than one pontic and the space is not ideal, it must be decided in advance which pontic should have normal measurements and which should be constricted or made wider. Usually the one nearer the median line is given true dimensions (Fig. 207).

Length

With the articulator closed, the facings should be placed against the ridge with the incisal or occlusal edges as nearly in alignment as possible and with only the excess of porcelain needed for contouring extending beyond the occlusal plane. The length should be studied from the lingual to see how much of the retentive slot will be left if the facing is a flatback, how much of the cervical portion will remain if the facing is a Trupontic, or how close the retentive pins will be to the ridge if a long-pin facing is being used. Approximately half of the slot or half of the cervical porcelain

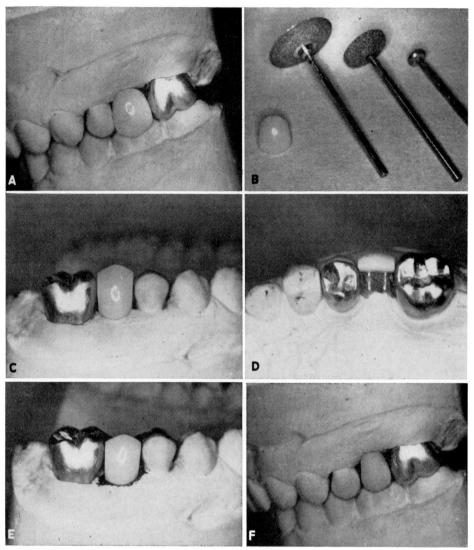

FIGURE 206. Progressive steps in shaping facings.

A, Facing selected is slightly wider and longer than the space.

B, Facing and stones to be used in shaping and positioning facing.

C, D, Cut to mesio-distal width, the facing is same width as distance between contact areas of retainers. Sides are parallel and do not cause facing to overlap abutments.

E, Facing shortened occluso-cervically. Ridge of working cast has been blackened with a pencil to aid in adapting facing.

F, Facing contoured and in alignment. Note embrasure form, convexities at cervical and occlusal, and grooves.

should remain. The retentive pins should be at a point at least one-third of the distance from the ridge to the occlusal or incisal, but preferably in the cingulum region in anteriors. There must be a clearance between the pins and the ridge of not less than 1.0 mm. If these conditions cannot be

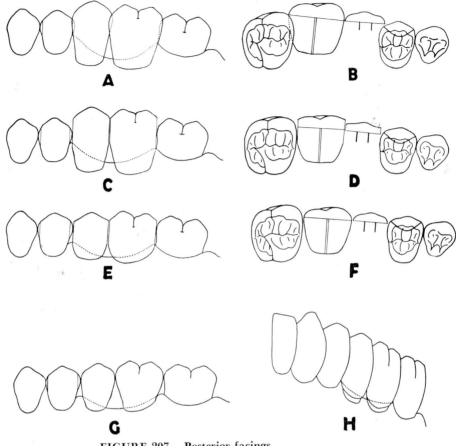

FIGURE 207. Posterior facings.
A, B, Facings chosen have excess width and length.
C, D, Cut to mesio-distal width.
E, Reduced in height.
F, G, Facings contoured.
H, Cementoenamel line and root form established.

met with the facings so positioned, they must be moved incisally or occlusally, and then be reduced in length on each end.

When adjusting the length inciso-cervically, the shade patterns of the approximating teeth will indicate whether to conserve the incisal or cervical of the facing. As a rule, the incisal or occlusal half will be ground less than the cervical.

The cervical is adapted to the ridge with the porcelain touching the ridge without interruption bucco- or labio-lingually. This fit may be realized by covering the ridge with black pencil markings, placing the facing in alignment against the ridge, and then grinding at the dark points of contact. This and the incisal reduction are continued simultaneously until adaptation, length, and alignment of the facing meet specifications. If the ridgelap of the facing is altered with care, allowing the lingual surface to angle in toward the ridge, it can be aligned so that very little of the labial porcelain must be lost. The facing may be supported by modeling clay or soft wax during the marking process.

Contour

Convexities mesio-distally must conform to the anatomy of the tooth being replaced and also must be in harmony with the abutment teeth. Inciso-cervically the buccal or labial contour of the facing should follow the outline of the abutments and should be compatible with the arch form. Similar labial or buccal markings and incisal or occlusal edge form should be incorporated.

On the ridgelap of a flatback or a porcelain biting-edge facing, the lingual two-thirds should be reduced further with a 30 degree bevel, to enable an apron of gold to cover the slot in the porcelain (Fig. 208).

The contour of the facing from the simulated cementoenamel junction to the ridge cannot continue the normal tooth root form. If this were done, the facing frequently would extend so far apically beyond the gingival lines of the abutment teeth that the effect would be unsightly and artificial. Beginning at the cervical line, the facing must be curved lingually until it meets the ridge at an obtuse angle. The V-shaped space created by the facing and the ridge must be greater than a 90 degree angle or it will form a food trap.

Grinding Harmony and Trupontic Facings to Form and Alignment

Harmony and Trupontic facings present problems in alignment dissimilar to those encountered with the flatback and long-pin facings. Adapting the porcelain-contacting area to the ridge so that the labial surface is

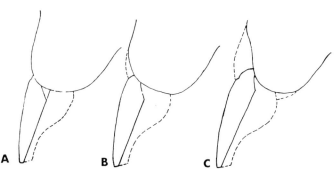

FIGURE 208. Ridge adaptation of anterior facings.

A, Ridge with minimal resorption. Cementoenamel junction ground into facing. Linguo-cervical beveled to make room for cast apron covering slot.

B, C, Progressive resorption. Facing is rounded into ridge. Incisal edge cannot be left exposed as shown here.

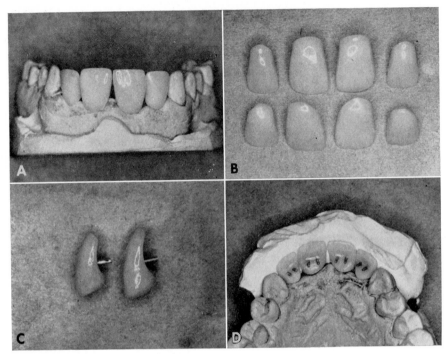

FIGURE 209.   Harmony facings.
A, Four Harmony incisors aligned on diagnostic cast.
B, Facings removed and in position under unground facings.
C, Proximal view of one aligned and one untouched facing. Note incisal bevel on left.
D, Facings aligned with labial index before being attached to resin base.

in alignment with approximating teeth, with minimal grinding on the labial surface, is more time-consuming than adaptation of the ridgelap of other facings. It must be done with more caution to avoid scarring the cast. The tissue-contacting area must be outlined by the lingual and prox-imal embrasures of the facing itself. Labial or buccal alignment must be established prior to inciso-cervical length, or a gap may occur at the linguo-gingival margin of the facing (Fig. 209). Irregular ridge form magnifies the difficulties of securing adaptation and contact without pressure. The recontoured surfaces must be reglazed (Fig. 210).

Grinding Reverse-Pin Facings to Form and Alignment

To construct a reverse-pin facing, either a porcelain denture tooth or a pin facing of appropriate shade and slightly oversize must first be selected. Denture teeth are popular for this purpose but it must be remembered that their shade distribution and translucence are less characteristic of human teeth than most bridge facings.

The tooth or facing is cut to width, length, and adaptation to the ridge, and is contoured following the designated sequence of operative procedures (see Fig. 211). The pins, if present, are cut flush with the facing

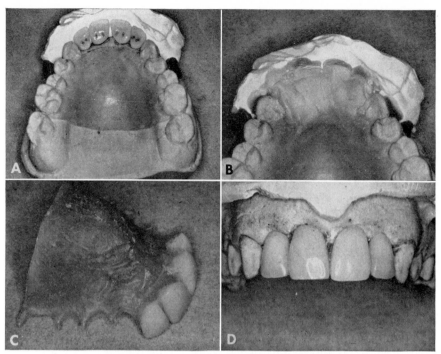

FIGURE 210. Harmony facings (continued).
A, B, C, Building and attaching base to facings.
D, Facings returned to cast.

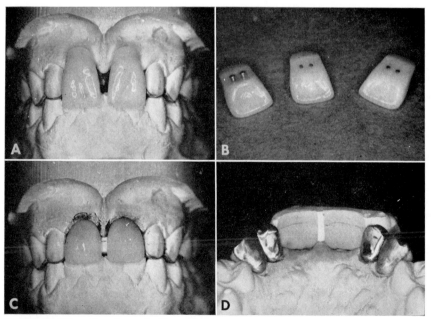

FIGURE 211. Showing grinding reverse-pin facings to form and alignment.
A, Denture teeth selected to be recontoured for facings.
B, With pins, and with pins cut off.
C, Ground to form and alignment.
D, Linguals showing adaptation to ridge and incisal areas which are hollow-ground for greater bulk of metal in casting.

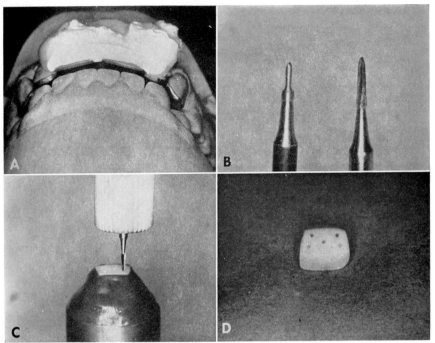

FIGURE 212. Showing grinding reverse-pin facings to form and alignment (continued).

A, Incisal clearance.

B, Drills made from carbide burs.

C, Facing mounted in compound. Holes are being drilled.

D, Facing prepared. Holes are widely distributed in bulky part of facing. Note concave incisal bevel.

and partially removed by grinding with a round bur. The facing is placed in aqua regia and the remaining metal is dissolved. The incisal third is beveled, or angled, and the edge is hollow-ground. The facing is set, labial surface down, onto modeling compound in a movable ring and taken to the drill press.

Drills, 0.025, 0.023, and 0.021 inch,* may be purchased, or they can be made from old carbide burs. The drill is lubricated with handpiece oil, and the holes, four or five in number and at least 1.2 plus mm. deep, are placed in the bulkiest part of the facing. They are distributed as widely as possible. For safety, the thickness of the porcelain should be measured before drilling, because a thickness of 1.0 mm. of porcelain should remain after the holes have been placed. If the facing is too thin, starting again with a new facing will save time (Fig. 212).

Protection

Facings must be protected on the incisal edge or bucco-occlusal margin.

---

* Williams Gold Refining Co., Inc., Buffalo, N. Y.

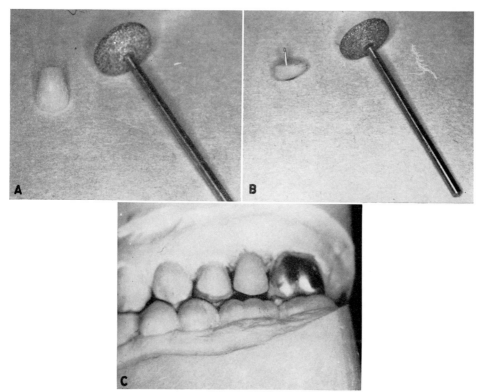

FIGURE 213.   Beveling pin facing for protection.
A, Facing and stone.
B, Beveled facing.
C, Facing in position, showing clearance.

Pin, reverse-pin, and Trupontics, when recontoured here, can be beveled or hollow-ground to be covered and reinforced by the casting. This need in no way affect the shape of the labial or buccal silhouette (Fig. 213).

However, when the flatback facing is reduced on the incisal edge or bucco-occlusal margin, the shelf of porcelain cannot be covered with metal and the facial surface must be recontoured to eliminate the table, one possible cause for future fracture of the facing. This must be done before the facing is conformed to the ridge. Recontouring the surface will force a new alignment and a new angle of approach to the ridge. If the ridge adaptation were done first, realignment would nullify facing contact and subsequent efforts might not correct the situation.

MANDIBULAR SANITARYPONTICS

The selection of a Sanitarypontic is not critical when constructing a lower posterior bridge. This facing comes in three shades: light, medium, and dark. Since it is used to further hygienic measures, rather than for esthetic reasons, the three shades are sufficient.

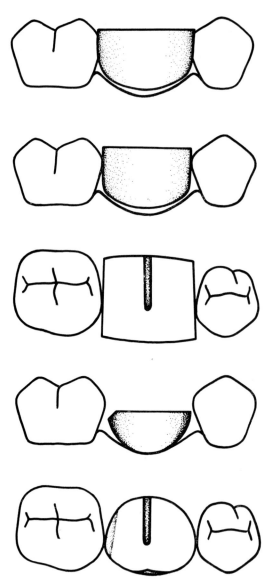

FIGURE 214. Steps in shaping a Sanitarypontic.

Top to bottom: Facing selected too wide and too high; facing reduced mesio-distally to permit placing between contact areas of retainers; facing contoured to give ample embrasure room and to approach ridge crest uniformly from all directions. Bevel will provide an adequate soldering surface; this may be done on each side. Buccal groove is indicated in porcelain.

If the facing is a little wider than the space, it can be reduced to size (Fig. 214). If it is slightly narrower than would be specific for the case at hand, the mesial and distal edges can be beveled and the occlusal casting contoured to accommodate to the space without resultant irregular form in the pontic.[5, 6, 7]

If the space is long occluso-cervically, the facing should equal that length minus the thickness of the gold occlusal. If it is extra long and narrow mesio-distally, it may be better hygienically if the facing does not contact the mucous membrane but stops about 3.0 or 4.0 mm. above the crest of the ridge. If the teeth and space are so short that the framework or facing, or both, would be weak, a facing may be contraindicated and a pontic fabricated of gold alone or one tipped with a Harmony pin-tip should be used (Fig. 215). When the space is near the median line and is long occluso-cervically, a Trupontic or a Harmony facing may have merit. (See Chapter 15, Pontic Form.)

Spaces of irregular ridge design compel irregular shapes in the underportion of the pontic (Fig. 216). There are no rules to set forth. Judgment must be used. However, if the space is malshaped because of tipped abutments, the apical section of the pontic should be no wider than the occlusal.

The height of the facing should allow for a minimal thickness of 1.0 mm. of gold in the thinnest sections of the occlusal casting, and it should touch the ridge with a rounded ridge-tip contact (Fig. 217*A*). The few exceptions almost always occur when replacing lower bicuspids. Sometimes here, because it is visible, the pontic must be contoured so that it will be aligned buccally with the incisal and middle thirds of the cuspid or first bicuspid.

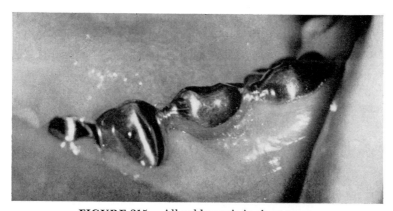

FIGURE 215. All-gold pontic in short space.

FIGURE 216. Pontics with irregular outlines to conform to configurations of ridges.

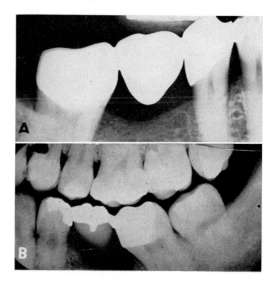

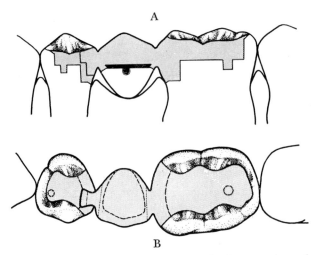

FIGURE 217. *A,* In the relationship between Sanitarypontic and ridge, contour should equalize mesial and distal embrasures; facing is beveled to increase soldering area on pontic casting and size of neck of occlusal rest shown here; backing is beveled toward facing to provide mechanical lock for wax and gold.

B, From occlusal, bucco-lingual width of the facing has been decreased with slight convergence toward mesial. Dotted line shows how backing is trimmed.

Except in the situation just noted, the convex underportion of the pontic should be centered over the ridge. The area in contact should never be more than one-third of the mesio-distal width of the space. The flat occlusal portion need not be parallel to the plane of occlusion. It can be tipped in any direction dictated by the positions of the opposing teeth. Viewed from the occlusal, the prepared facing should be widest mesiodistally in the areas that will be immediately below the connectors.

The mesial and distal surfaces of the facing should converge toward the lingual to form adequate embrasure areas (Fig. 217*B*). Its bucco-lingual width should be reduced from one-fifth to one-third, this reduction being greater in the mesial half of the facing. When a larger soldering area must be provided on the proximal surfaces of the occlusal casting, the mesial and distal margins of the facing should be beveled. These bevels should be angled toward the ridge at a little more than 90 degrees and should converge lingually.

For hygienic reasons, resin is contraindicated as a veneer for lower posterior pontics. The all-gold pontic must be perfectly cast and polished when used in this area.

MANDIBULAR PORCELAIN-INCISAL FACINGS

The esthetic appearance of a lower anterior bridge sometimes can be enhanced by the use of the porcelain biting-edge facing. It is adapted in the same way as other flatback facings, except that all reduction in length must be made at the cervical to conserve the bulk and strength of the porcelain at the incisal edge. The angle formed by the incisal porcelain and the flat lingual surface should be increased slightly so that the casting can give more support along the incisal. This facing is indicated in the construction of mandibular anterior bridges only and should not be used except when the relationship is such that minimal lingual forces will be directed against the pontic.

STABILIZING THE FACING

When the facing has been aligned and contoured, and is being held in position on the working cast with modeling clay or soft wax, it should be secured in this position by a small quantity of sticky wax applied to the exposed linguo-incisal edge and to the embrasures. The labial or buccal of the working cast should be coated with a separating medium or petrolatum, and a plaster index poured. This will be used to maintain the alignment of the facing during the waxing of the pontic. (See Fig. 218.)

The index is made of impression plaster or quick-setting stone, mixed to a medium thick consistency and applied to the buccal surface of the facing, the abutment teeth, and the ridge, working the plaster into the proximal embrasures without extending it over the incisal or occlusal margin of the facing. When the plaster or stone has set, it should be removed and trimmed to workable size, retaining enough length and height so that the index will seat accurately and easily on the working cast and hold the facing and subsequent individual casting securely in position.

THE BACKING

After the facing has been cleaned, if it is a flatback or a Trupontic, a

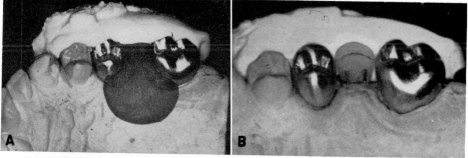

FIGURE 218. *A,* Facing stabilized with wax during making of buccal plaster index. *B,* Facing stabilized on working cast by plaster index. Index has been trimmed along occlusal to prevent interference with lateral excursions. Facing, pins, working cast, and index must be lubricated with Microfilm before wax is flowed into space.

backing must be adjusted. The backing, which supports the pin for the retention of the facing, should be trimmed short of the margin on the mesial, distal, and incisal or bucco-occlusal, and it should be beveled toward the facing. Thus the waxed pontic will hold the backing in position, and there will be a mechanical lock between the backing and the cast metal.

The backing should be removed and the lingual and cervical portions of the facing, the ridge, and the index lubricated so that molten wax will not adhere to these surfaces.

The backing is then replaced on the facing and the facing is returned to the working cast, to be aligned and supported by the plaster index.

If a broken-stress or nonrigid joint is to be used between the pontic and one abutment, it must be prepared at this time and be waxed with, or included in, the pattern for the pontic casting. Such connectors will be discussed at the end of this chapter.

WAXING AND CASTING

Against a Backing

Molten inlay wax should be flowed on the linguo-cervical of the facing, after which larger pieces may be softened, pressed to position, and attached. When the wax has been built to a sufficient height, the articulated casts should be closed and moved in eccentric excursions. The markings made in the wax will assist in carving the pontic to functional form (Fig. 219).

When more than one tooth is being replaced, pontics must be carved individually and to the exact dimensions required in the finished castings, with the wax surfaces free of flaws, and polished. Cast joints, to have resistance to deformation, sometimes must be so large[8] that embrasure form will be reduced and the underlying tissue overprotected. Acceptable size and form in the connector can be achieved more readily with solder or the subocclusal rest.

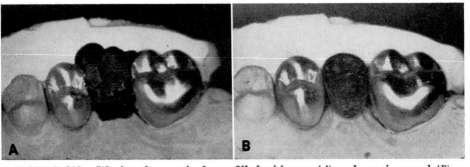

FIGURE 219. Waxing the pontic. Space filled with wax (*A*) and pontic carved (*B*).

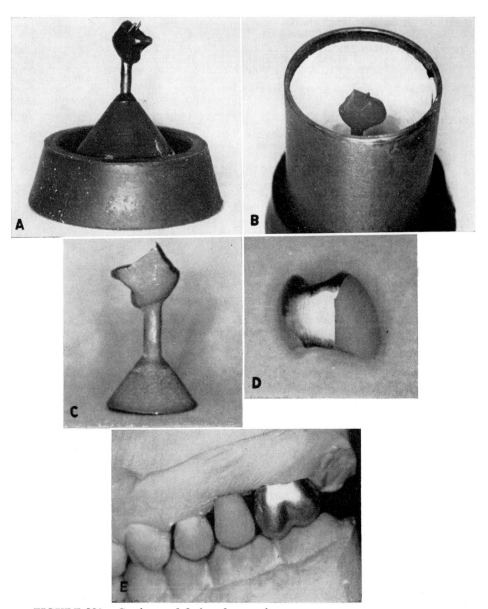

FIGURE 220. Casting and fitting the pontic.

A, Pontic pattern on sprue former. Sprue pin is attached to nonarticulating area at an angle that will cause the least turbulence in the molten gold. Carbon pins have been placed in pinholes. These will be drilled out after casting, and facing will seat.

B, Position of pattern in ring.

C, Pontic casting.

D, Pontic polished and facing seated. Margins should be polished and burnished around facing with a dull bur.

E, Pontic in position on working cast.

A large sprue pin is necessary to avoid porosity in pontic castings. It must be attached to the pontic at such a point and at such an angle that the attachment will not destroy occlusal carving, and so that the gold will flow along the surface of the backing instead of meeting it at right angles.

When Using Pin or Reverse-Pin Facings

When a pin facing is used, the pins must be checked to see that they are parallel and at right angles to the facing, and the lingual and cervical, as well as the pins, must be lubricated with one of several proprietary materials procurable.

The facing should be removed before the wax pattern is sprued and carbon rods must be placed in the holes left by the metal pins. After casting, the carbon can be removed with a bur and the facing will then seat on the casting (Fig. 220).

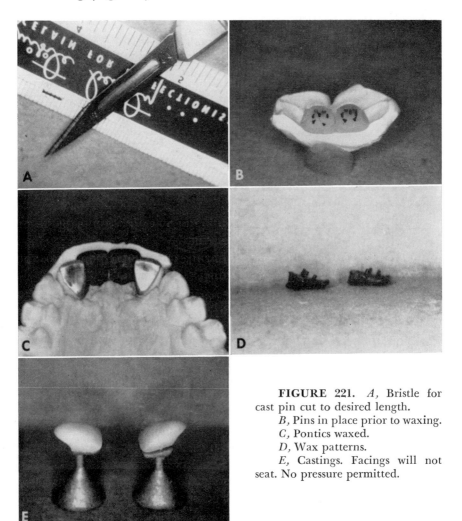

FIGURE 221. *A,* Bristle for cast pin cut to desired length.
B, Pins in place prior to waxing.
C, Pontics waxed.
D, Wax patterns.
E, Castings. Facings will not seat. No pressure permitted.

Special alloy pins that do not fuse to the pontic casting may be used in the pinholes made by Harmony facings. They can be removed with little difficulty.

The reverse-pin facing must be lubricated and nylon bristles or plastic pins (0.002 or 0.003 inch smaller than drilled holes) placed in the pinholes (Figs. 221 and 222).[3] The pontic is then built, contoured, sprued, and cast, as described earlier. The facing cannot be seated on the casting until the pins and contacting surface have been "stripped." This is done with a special deplating machine or by a reverse connection in an electro-plater. Usually less than 30 seconds at 1 ampere will effect the change in dimensions. The same result may be obtained by immersing the casting in aqua regia for tested periods of time. With either technique all margins, and surfaces not in contact with the facing, must be protected during the stripping process with a coating of lacquer.

It may be necessary also to countersink each hole slightly to allow complete seating of the facing on the casting.

If the space is short occluso-cervically and a facing cannot be ground

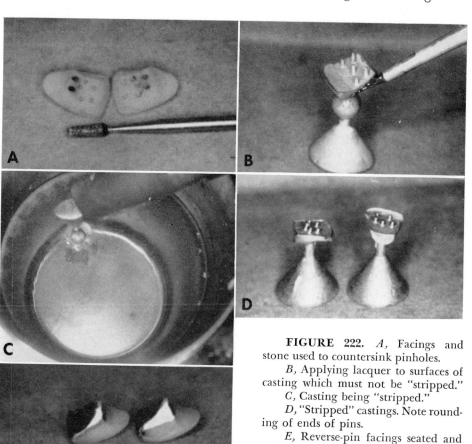

FIGURE 222. *A*, Facings and stone used to countersink pinholes.

B, Applying lacquer to surfaces of casting which must not be "stripped."

C, Casting being "stripped."

D, "Stripped" castings. Note rounding of ends of pins.

E, Reverse-pin facings seated and castings polished.

to position and form without spoiling its strength or shade, it may be helpful to cast a pontic and veneer it with resin. For biologic reasons, all of the pontic in contact with the ridge tissue should be metal. To secure uniform shading, this method of pontic construction is indicated many times when resin-veneered gold crowns are used as retainers.

The same alloy should be used in casting the pontic as was used in casting the retainers so that wear and contact shock during mastication will be equalized.

ASSEMBLY OF THE BRIDGE

After the casting has been cleaned and pickled, the sprue is cut off and that area polished to contour. The surface of the casting, against which the facing must fit, should be inspected closely for any bubbles or marginal burs that could interfere with seating the facing. These may be removed with a No. 700 bur. Any facing must be seated and removed from the casting without undue effort; otherwise there will be danger of cracking the porcelain.

When the facing has been seated, the pontic should be aligned on the working cast, using the plaster index. At this time the contacts, the adaptation to the ridge, the alignment, and the occlusion should be checked, and any needed corrections made (Fig. 223).

Although polishing may be postponed until after the bridge is assembled, better alignment and adaptation to the ridge will ensue if it is done before the bridge is rigidly assembled. The prevailing methods for polishing small gold castings can be employed if precautions are taken to prevent chipping the porcelain. Tripoli or rouge should not be used on the casting while the facing is in position, since these materials will stain the unglazed porcelain surface. Removal of the stain is practically impossible unless the facing is placed in an ultrasonic cleaner. After polishing the pontic, the proximal surfaces may be cleaned with a dull bur.

THE NONRIGID CONNECTOR

The nonrigid connector, or broken-stress joint, should be used in bridge construction only where the span is short and the supporting alveolus is not extensively reduced or actively receding. When trouble might be encountered in preparing the abutments for a mutual path of insertion, when inlays are indicated as the retainers, or when an inlay or crown has been made previously and is in good condition, one nonrigid connector may be suitable in building the bridge. For this joint to be successful and nondestructive, the replacement must have the same type of occlusion along its entire length; that is, either natural teeth or a tissue-supported prosthesis.

The need for a broken-stress joint is limited, and whenever possible it should be bypassed in favor of the solder or rigid connector.

Two forms will be discussed. The first and the best, because in action it must be considered as semirigid, has been called the "subocclusal rest." The second, indicated only when used in connection with an abutment already restored, is known as the "dovetail occlusal rest." Lingual rests, used to support cantilever anterior pontics, may be placed in this classification.

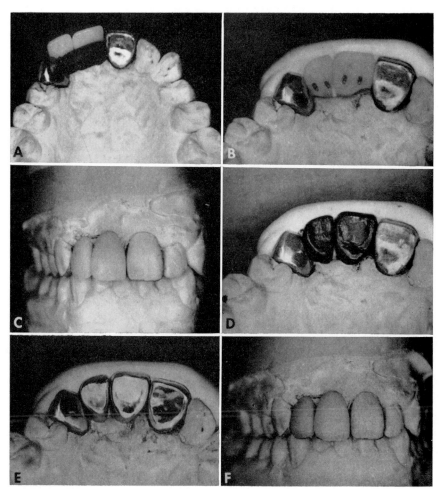

FIGURE 223. *A,* Facings selected.

B, C, Facings contoured and aligned.

D, Wax patterns for two anterior pontics. Note plaster index for keeping facings in alignment.

E, Pontics aligned on working cast with same labial plaster index.

F, Labial view of cast pontics.

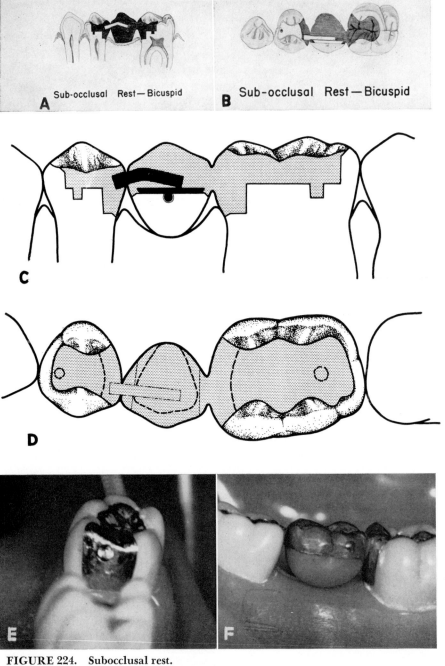

FIGURE 224.   Subocclusal rest.

A, B, Cross sections, maxillary bicuspid. Pin, 2.0 mm. long, angles from occlusal at 30 degrees and fits into hole drilled to give semisnug fit.

C, D, Cross sections, mandibular bicuspid. Pin need not come into contact with backing on facing but should be bent to clear occlusion.

E, Pinhole in mandibular molar is too high, since it includes beginning curve of marginal ridge.

F, Note desirable embrasure form at distal of pontic where subocclusal rest was used.

The Subocclusal Rest

The subocclusal rest is most often used when two inlays will act as retainers for the bridge. A solder joint will attach the pontic to the retainer in the stronger abutment (usually the posterior), and the subocclusal rest will be placed in the other inlay.

The subocclusal rest consists of a pin inserted into a prepared pinhole placed in the center of the contact area of the retainer. The pin should be 2.0 mm. long and may be made of 17-gauge high-fusing clasp wire. It must be square on the end, must closely fit the prepared hole, and should slant away from the occlusal at about 30 degrees (Fig. 224).

After the working casts have been articulated, or after the retainers have been cast in an indirect technique, the facing should be ground to position and form so that the center of the contact of the retainer on the weaker abutment will be on a level with the top of a Sanitarypontic, or behind a pin or flatback facing. The retainer is then removed from the cast, the pinhole is cut with a No. 35 inverted cone bur used as an end-cutting instrument, and the walls of the hole are smoothed with a No. 56 bur. Seventeen-gauge wire makes a serviceable pin, but 18- or 16-gauge may be substituted in smaller or larger surfaces. It should be bent cervically just outside the orifice of the pinhole, to parallel or touch the backing over the facing. The pontic is waxed around the wire and the gold is cast to it and the backing.

The subocclusal rest has several advantages over the dovetail occlusal rest. There can be no occlusal movement with it, and since it is placed in the center of the contact area, all embrasures are of normal size. It does not catch or retain food fibers, does not interfere in any way with the occlusion, and has maximal strength. There is one disadvantage: the retainers must be seated simultaneously and the preparations must approach parallelism.

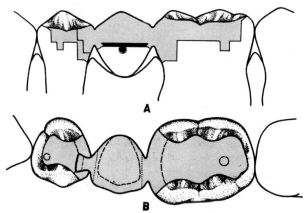

FIGURE 225. Dovetail occlusal rest, cross sections in bicuspid.

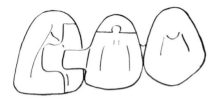

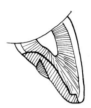

FIGURE 226. Lingual rest, maxillary central incisor.

The Dovetail Occlusal Rest

The dovetail occlusal rest is an extension of the pontic casting fitted into a dovetail-shaped rest seat prepared in the occlusal surface of the retainer (Fig. 225). The isthmus must be not less than 1.5 mm. wide and 2.0 mm. deep, and the rest at its extremity should measure 2.5 mm. at the widest point. A groove can be cut, 1.5 mm. wide, 1.0 mm. deep, and 2.5 mm. long, on the proximal surface of the retainer to receive a cast strut as a part of the rest. Theoretically, this will prevent occlusal movement of the pontic. This type of rest partially fills the embrasure areas, and all too often must be placed to the lingual of the normal contact point.

The Lingual Rest

The lingual rest on an incisor should be positioned far enough incisally to support the pontic under biting force and to free the embrasure by not forming a shelf under which food may lodge. The rest seat should be angular, deep enough for the rest to complement the lingual tooth form, and fashioned so that lingual movement of the pontic will be impossible. This seat should be placed in metal (Fig. 226). A proximo-lingual inlay will suffice for support and will not be visible from the labial surface. The indiscriminate use of lingual rests is not recommended.

REFERENCES

1. Smith, D. E.: Improved porcelain facing design for fixed prostheses. J. South. **California** D. A., *23:*34, April 1955.
2. Harmon, C. B.: Pontic design. J. Pros. Den., *8:*496, May 1958.
3. Johnston, J. F.: Pontic form and bridge design. Part I. Illinois D. J., *25:*272, May 1956.
4. Shooshan, E. D.: Reverse pin-porcelain pontic. J. Pros. Den., *9:*284, March–April 1959.
5. Adams, J. D.: Planning posterior bridges. J.A.D.A., *53:*647, Dec. 1956.

6. Boyd, H. R., Jr.: Pontics in fixed partial dentures. J. Pros. Den., *5*:55, Jan. 1955.
7. Klaffenbach, A. O.: Biomechanical restoration and maintenance of the permanent first molar space. J.A.D.A., *45*:633, Dec. 1952.
8. Dykema, R. W.: A study of the effects of certain variables on the comparative strengths of soldered and cast bridge joints. Master's thesis, Indiana Univ. School Den., June 1961.

Lucia, V. O.: Modern Gnathological Concepts. St. Louis, The C. V. Mosby Company, 1961.
Miller, C. J.: Inlays, Crowns and Bridges. Philadelphia, W. B. Saunders Company, 1962.
Moulton, G. H.: Esthetics in anterior fixed bridge prosthodontics. J.A.D.A., *52*:36, Jan. 1956.
Moulton, G. H.: Functional demands of a posterior crown or bridge. J.A.D.A., *66*: 534, April 1963.
Selberg, A.: An exposition of pontics and their construction for fixed bridges. Illinois D. J., *9*:440, Dec. 1940.
Tylman, S. D.: Relationship of the structural design of dental bridges to their supporting tissues. Internat. D. J., *13*:303, June 1963.
Tylman, S. D., and Tylman, S. G.: Theory and Practice of Crown and Bridge Prosthodontics. 4th ed. St. Louis, The C. V. Mosby Company, 1960.
Wilson, W. H., and Lang, R. L.: Practical Crown and Bridge Prosthodontics. New York, McGraw-Hill Book Company, Inc., 1962.

15

PONTIC FORM

The whole of fixed partial denture construction can be embraced by three fundamentals: namely, fit, form, and function. The one of predominant importance, which does most to improve the two others, is form. The resultants of these basic requirements are cleanliness, comfort, and concealment. These also are enhanced by form.

In the construction of a crown, a retainer, or a pontic, form need not necessarily mean a slavish reproduction in all dimensions of the tooth to be restored or replaced. It should imply that, in the topographic anatomy of the given restoration, the customary convexities, concavities, cusp forms, and groove outlines of the tooth have been included, and that these have been so placed, and so modified if necessary, that

(1) the contact areas will guard the interproximal gingival tissue, but at the same time permit the formation of embrasures that allow food to massage that tissue;

(2) the buccal and lingual gingival tissues can be stimulated as well as protected;

(3) the supporting alveolar process will not be subjected to disintegrating forces;

(4) the escape of food will be facilitated;

(5) masticating efficiency will be kept at a proper level; and

(6) oral hygiene can be sustained with minimal endeavor.[1]

All these requisites can be met without undue difficulty when restoring one tooth. With thought and some extra effort a retainer can be made that performs according to these specifications.

The pontic may present greater problems. In it, form must be combined with shade to assure esthetic appearance. Anatomic form must be reproduced to maintain function, but concomitantly modifications in form

278

may be necessary to reduce the forces and torque on the abutments, and to promote tissue health and hygiene. Such modifications must be controlled so that the pontic will not seem like a foreign body in contact with the tongue and other mobile tissue.

Form is observed, reproduced, and modified in two ways. The peripheral quadrilateral or pentagonal plane form of the pontic may duplicate the silhouette of the tooth being replaced, or it may be changed slightly to satisfy abnormalities in space width. The outline of the labial surface (Fig. 227), bounded by the incisal edge, the mesial and distal line angles, and the cementoenamel junction or the gingival line, is also a quadrilateral or a pentagon. It is smaller or narrower and inside the silhouette outline. The labial outline may copy the natural tooth or it may be altered in various subtle ways to suggest desired effects or harmonies with approximating and corresponding teeth. Plus or minus dimensions and long-axis

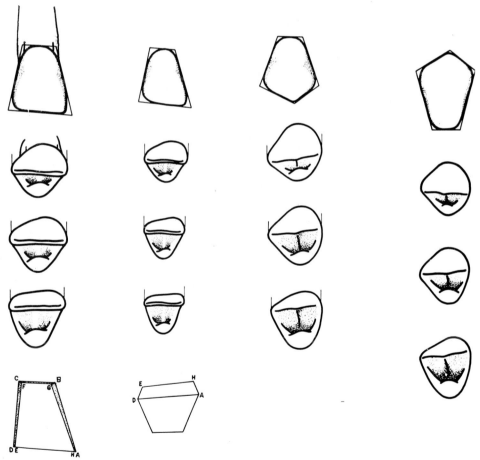

FIGURE 227. Geometric forms of silhouette (A-B-C-D) and labial surface outlines (E-F-G-H) of maxillary central and lateral incisors and maxillary and mandibular cuspids. Silhouettes of cuspids can be applied to bicuspids.

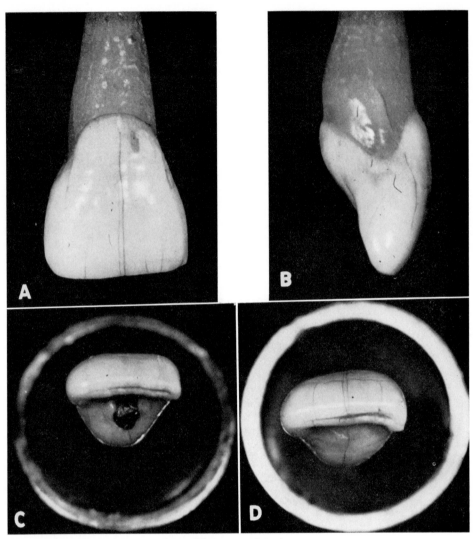

FIGURE 228. Contour of maxillary central incisors.

A, Labial.

B, Proximal.

C, *D*, Incisal.

A determined effort must be made to observe the convexities, concavities, and facets on associated teeth and to produce functional, harmonious form in crowns, pontics, and facings.

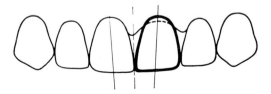

FIGURE 229. Form in the facing to harmonize long axes. The lines projected through the central incisors, which represent the visual long axes of the crowns, diverge cervically from the midline (broken line) to the same degree.

directions may be simulated by minor contour changes at incisal angles or along proximal surfaces.

The majority of modifications proposed in this chapter concern primarily alterations in the labial surface outline. Beginning at the median line and moving around the arch to the molars, form will be considered for the sake of esthetics.

THE MAXILLARY CENTRAL INCISOR

When replacing the upper central incisor, one must be influenced not only by the silhouette and labial surface outline, the labial mesio-distal convexities and concavities, and the inciso-cervical curve of the tooth being replaced, if pre-extraction diagnostic casts are available, but also by these same anatomic features on the approximating central (Fig. 228). The long axis of the clinical crown of the central present in the mouth must be projected too, as a guide in positioning and aligning the facing (Fig. 229). Form and angulation developed in the pontic should be the same as on the natural tooth.

Unless changes are demanded for esthetics, the contour of the mesial surface of the central incisor abutment tooth should be reproduced in the retainer casting or in the veneer crown. The same outline, although not necessarily the long axis or degree of rotation, must be transposed to the mesial of the pontic, studying the labial surface in sections before attempting to shape the facing for the expected effect. The facing *must* have sufficient bulk to make reshaping possible.

Incisal angles can be very expressive (Fig. 230). For instance, just a little too much rounding on the mesial can make an otherwise well-formed facing look out of place (Fig. 231). The illusion of decreased or increased width can be furthered to a degree by the form of the disto-incisal angle (Fig. 232) and the distal outline of the silhouette. When the space is wider, the incisal or occlusal edge should remain the same from the mesial angle to the beginning of the curve of the distal angle. The distal angle and the distal fourth of the facing will tend to have characteristics similar to the

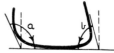

FIGURE 230. Areas of incisal angles which can add to or detract from esthetic appearance.

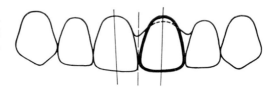

FIGURE 231. Excessive convexity at incisal angles changes the visual long axis of the pontic crown, destroying harmony.

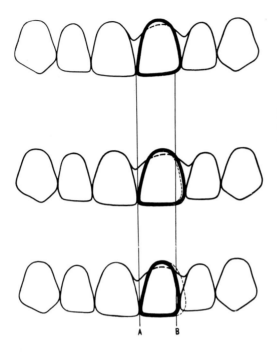

FIGURE 232. Treatment of silhouette in wide and narrow spaces when it is not feasible to alter abutment.

Lines A and B show the same mesio-distal length in the incisal edge of the replacement. Facings have been adapted to wider or narrower spaces by changing the convexity of the disto-incisal angle and the bulge of the distal contact area.

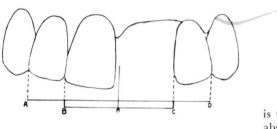

FIGURE 233. When single space is too wide, abutment and pontic can absorb equal amounts of excess.

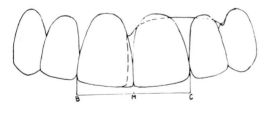

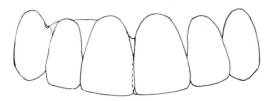

FIGURE 234. When single space is narrow, abutment and pontic may be reduced to absorb decrease.

distal of the abutment, but must be overcontoured to contact the approximating distal abutment or pontic. The major changes will be at the disto-incisal and disto-cervical, where the angles become arcs of larger circles.

When the space is narrow, the change in contour is on the distal also, where the curve of the angle will be more confined and the surface flatter but still suggesting the typal form of the natural tooth. (See Figs. 233, 234, and 235.)

The form in the same areas, and on the mesial too, affects the long-axis line. If the mesial and distal halves of a facing are the same, the long axis will be changed and the replacement will seem foreign to the environment (Fig. 236). However, if the mesio-cervical and disto-incisal segments of the facing have been given convex bevels, these will change the outline of the labial surface and increase the cervical divergence of the long axis (Fig. 237).

Other factors that help to fix the long-axis direction of the pontic facing are the angulation of the cervical half of the mesial surface outline, and the mesio-distal convexities of the mesio-cervical and the disto-incisal fourths of the labial surface.

Because of the usual resorption of the ridge tissue toward the lingual,

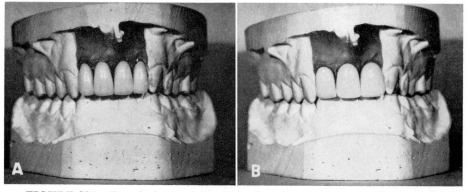

FIGURE 235. Four incisors missing. Four facings must be narrow individually (*A*); three facings may have too much width per unit (*B*). Usually wider facings will be more pleasing without its being obvious that (in number) one tooth has not been replaced.

FIGURE 236.

FIGURE 237.

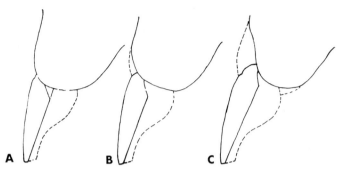

FIGURE 238. Ridge adaptation of anterior facings.

A, Ridge with minimal resorption. Cementoenamel junction ground into facing. Linguo-cervical beveled to make room for cast apron covering slot.

B, C, Progressive resorption. Facing is rounded into ridge. Incisal edge cannot be left exposed as shown here.

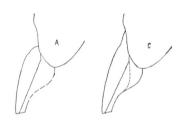

FIGURE 239. Cervical contour of labial surface. A—Correct. C—Incorrect.

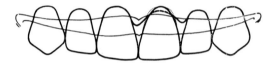

FIGURE 240.

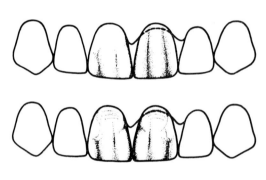

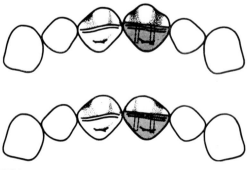

FIGURE 241. Labial ridge reduced.

284

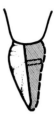

FIGURE 242.   Grooves placed in cervical third.

pontic facings many times will be longer than the abutment teeth. To achieve the maximum in appearance, the correct cervical outline should be ground into the facing, even if there is an extension of porcelain beyond this reproduction of the cementoenamel junction (Figs. 238 and 239). In a majority of cases, establishing the form will suffice, but occasionally the root of the facing must be stained yellow, brown, or pink, to accentuate the coronal portion of the pontic.

If the patient has a low lipline, exposing not more than the incisal one-half or two-thirds of the incisors, the interproximal embrasures can be widened discreetly in the gingival third (Fig. 240, heavy line) to allow easier access with the toothbrush and to permit a little more ridge coverage by the cingulum section of the pontic. If this is possible, the replacement will feel more natural to the tongue and perhaps will enable the patient to enunciate more clearly.

On many facings received from stock, the ridges running inciso-cervically the length of the labial surfaces must be removed. A facing with such ridges and grooves cannot be placed beside a tooth with a harmonious result (Fig. 241).

After the facing has been ground to position, form, and alignment, and the surface has been smoothed, markings must be made similar to those found on the labial of the corresponding tooth (Fig. 242). Such grooves, indentations, peculiarities in formation, abrasions, or eroded areas can be intensified or softened, as the case requires, by staining, and by glazing to produce a surface texture typical of the given mouth.

THE MAXILLARY LATERAL INCISOR

The replacement of the upper lateral incisor will present somewhat different problems. Usually this tooth has a very constricted neck. If this is accurately transferred to the facing, the interproximal embrasures may be so large that the effect will be bad. To prevent this, it often becomes necessary to alter the silhouette slightly by widening the neck of the lateral facing (Fig. 243). This can be done without encroaching on the form of the labial surface enough to destroy harmony of relationship and without copying the central in form and angulation.

Many upper lateral incisor facings placed in the mouth fail to meet

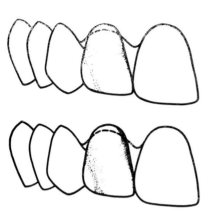

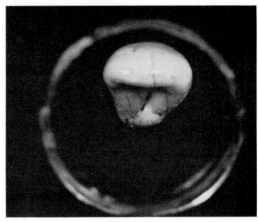

Fig. 243   Fig. 244

FIGURE 243. Neck widened, changing silhouette, but outline of labial surface remains constant.

FIGURE 244. Incisal view of maxillary lateral incisor showing the normal mesio-distal convexity of the labial surface. Lateral incisors vary in this convexity, but usually it is more pronounced than on centrals.

Fig. 245

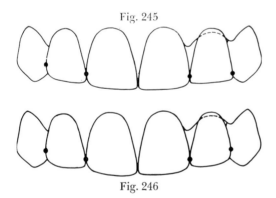

FIGURE 245. On left, contacts and form are normal; on right, facing is pyramidal and both contacts are close to incisal.

FIGURE 246. Contacts correctly positioned on each side.

Fig. 246

the requirements of form (Fig. 244) because (1) they are too flat mesio-distally; (2) they have almost square incisal angles, when the mesial angle should be less than 90 degrees and the disto-incisal angle 90 degrees plus; or (3) because straight mesial and distal outlines, with almost square incisal angles, are substituted for the ovoid type. This will bring the contact areas close to the incisal edge, whereas they should be well up toward the middle of the mesial and distal surfaces.

It is disconcerting, indeed, to see a lateral incisor replaced by a pontic that appears to be a pyramid, with contacts at the incisal angles (Fig. 245), when actually the typal form of the teeth in that arch calls for the mesio-incisal angle to be acute, with the contact at the angle, and the distal surface outline convex and contacting the cuspid much nearer the gingival line (Fig. 246).

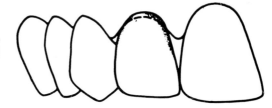

FIGURE 247. Mesio-cervical concavity suggested by subtle grinding and change in labial surface outline.

It can be difficult to increase the cervical width of an upper lateral incisor facing and also retain the semblance of the mesial concavity so often found on this tooth, but it can be done in the outline of the mesial edge of the middle third of the labial surface (Fig. 247). A "hint" is all that will be needed.

Increasing the cervical width of the lateral incisor may bring up still another problem when the typical mesio-distal convexity of that area must be formed for the sake of harmony. At times the mesial embrasure must be closed as desired, but the distal may be opened in accordance with the design of the tooth being replaced. This illusion of convexity must be created in the mesial half of the labial surface of the facing without distorting the long axis.

THE MAXILLARY CUSPID

Upper cuspid facings, as received from the manufacturer, will be more acceptable than the incisor facings. The incisal edge, commonly abraded on the natural tooth, must be copied and protected (Fig. 248). It should be remembered that the contact areas of many upper cuspids are much closer to the gingival line than those on the central incisors or the mesial surfaces of the lateral incisors. Often they must be moved cervically or incisally, or adjusted for the required long-axis angulation. If the mesial contact is shifted cervically, the distal contact will drop toward the incisal, the cusp will move mesially, and the crest of the cementoenamel junction will shift toward the distal. Many positions and forms can be suggested by the manipulation of these four points. (See Fig. 249.) This angulation of the crown in pontic construction can be regulated by the mesial embrasure and the mesio-labial convexities. (See Fig. 250.) The cuspid in the

FIGURE 248. Normal abrasion on cuspid. Facing is hollow-ground to make space for metal protection.

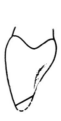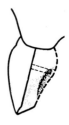

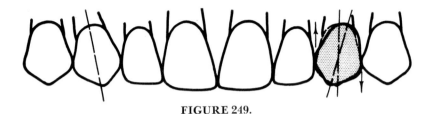

FIGURE 249.

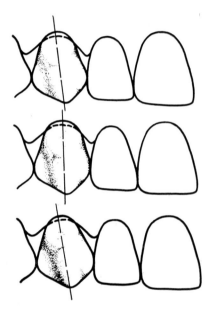

FIGURE 250.

approximating quadrant should be the guide, with minor attention being given to the adjacent lateral and bicuspid.

The height of contour of the cuspid is not in the center of the tooth mesio-distally, but is to the mesial of the midline of the labial surface (Fig. 251). Frequently there will be a definite concavity or groove to the distal of the height of contour, which curves distally to fade out on the distal surface short of the cervical line. This may be obliterated by wear, but if observation of remaining teeth or diagnostic casts shows it to exist, it should be incorporated in the pontic. While the mesial half of this pontic must retain the contour of the cuspid, the interproximal embrasure on the distal may be enlarged for purposes of hygiene.

FACTORS CONSIDERED IN MAXILLARY ANTERIOR PONTIC CONSTRUCTION

The contour of the lingual half of any upper anterior pontic will be governed not only by the length of span, quality and amount of the supporting structure, and inciso-ridge measurement, but also by one other factor, the height of the lipline. The higher the lipline, the less the cervical half of the interproximal embrasures may be opened. (See Fig. 252.) The use of less ridge coverage labio-lingually and wider lingual embrasures will

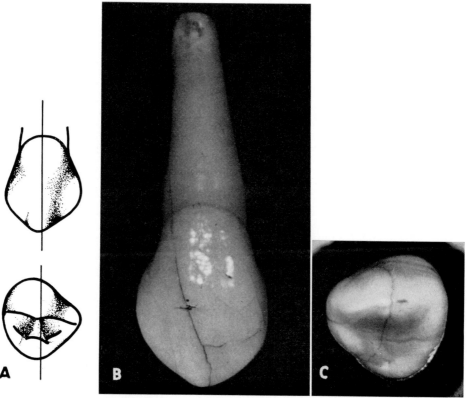

FIGURE 251.   *A*, Height of contour is in mesial half of maxillary cuspid. *B*, *C*, Labial and incisal views of maxillary cuspid.

FIGURE 252.   Dotted line shows how embrasures may be opened if lipline is low.

FIGURE 253.   Cross section showing reduced ridge coverage of central and lateral pontics.

Fig. 252

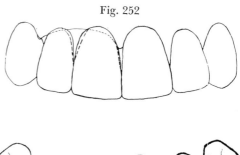

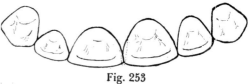

Fig. 253

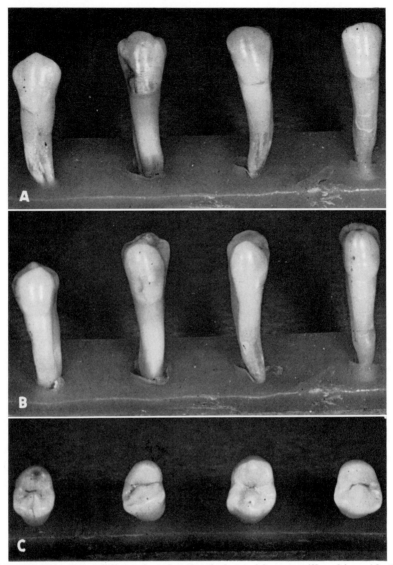

FIGURE 254. Buccal, lingual, and occlusal views of four maxillary bicuspids. Lingual cusps are off center, narrower, and more pointed. "Ears" and spillways must be reproduced in pontic construction.

give access for brushing, flow of mouth fluids, and stimulation of the ridge tissue.[2, 3] (See Fig. 253.)

The same type of construction is employed when the anterior pontic must be short inciso-cervically. The area of ridge covered is decreased at the expense of the normal cingulum contour. If the space is quite long from incisal edge to ridge crest, the ridgelap may become more ovoid if the lipline does not expose the contact. If that occurs, and all the incisors are missing, esthetic appearance might be improved with a removable bridge having a base to restore gingival contour.

MAXILLARY BICUSPIDS

When shaping an upper bicuspid pontic (Fig. 254), consideration must be given, first, to occluso-cervical contour; next, to the relationship of the bucco-occlusal margin with the opposing teeth. It will not be enough to position or grind the facing so that it clears the opposing teeth in lateral or protrusive movements. This must be done, but the position and form of the facing must continue the symmetry of the arch.

When using the flatback or long-pin, it is axiomatic that the middle third of an upper bicuspid facing must be recontoured occluso-cervically to remove excess convexity. However, with care in positioning the facing before adapting it to the ridge surface of the working cast, the amount of grinding on the buccal would be decreased, thus preserving the selected shade and reducing the amount of recontouring. (See Fig. 255A.)

The mesial of a bicuspid pontic should be a near-replica of the missing tooth, with some increase in the size of the interproximal embrasure through exaggerated contour in the cervical third. (See Fig. 255B.) On the distal margin, the contour may be changed to open the space and to reduce ridge coverage for better hygiene and tissue stimulation. Esthetic requirements in the upper bicuspid area rarely can be satisfied with a rounded pontic-tip, ridge-crest contact.

The mesial and distal developmental grooves on the buccal are two

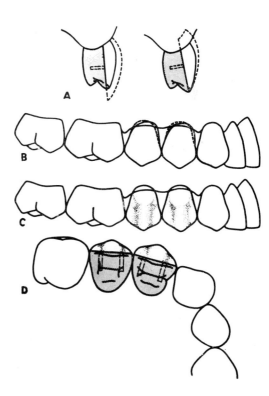

FIGURE 255.

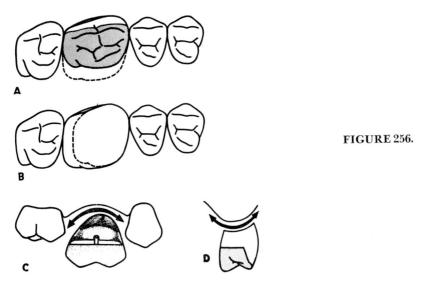

FIGURE 256.

landmarks frequently ignored when shaping upper bicuspid facings. Desig-nated by James Mark Prime[4] as the "ears" of the bicuspids, they are the boundary lines for small segments, buccal to and extending only a little way cervically beyond the contacts. The efficacy of such details must be stressed. (See Fig. 255C and D.)

MAXILLARY MOLARS

The upper molar pontic need not be so exact in its reproduction of form and harmony on the buccal surface as do those nearer the median line. With the exception of the occlusal, all embrasures can be enlarged (see Fig. 256A), even if the mesial outline must follow closely the pattern of the tooth being replaced. The surface next to the ridge can be reduced in all directions to make a narrower, almost rounded cone area. (See Fig. 256B, C, and D.)

The buccal cusp relationship with the opposing teeth should be in harmony with the teeth remaining in the quadrant, and the occlusal one-half or two-thirds of the facing should conform to the normal buccal sur-face contour. Facings that permit hollow-grinding of the lingual portion of the buccal cusps are preferable. (See Fig. 256D.) A flatback facing should never be used when it must be shortened unduly, or set out of alignment to accommodate either centric closure or lateral and protrusive excursions.

MANDIBULAR ANTERIORS

Lower central incisors can be made to look alike, but lower laterals must have a greater convexity in the mesial two-fifths. In many cases the

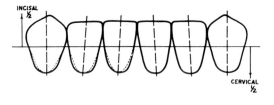

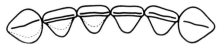

FIGURE 257. On left, dotted lines show outline of pontics with embrasures enlarged and ridge area reduced.

embrasures around lower anterior pontics can be opened below the incisal half with an ovoid tip at the ridge, without any ridgelap (Fig. 257).

When shaping lower incisor facings, it will be advantageous to observe and copy (1) the angles of the incisal edge from the lingual to the labial surface and from mesial to distal, (2) the flat or very slightly concave area in the middle half of the incisal third of the labial surface of the central, and (3) the long axis.

When a lower cuspid must be replaced, which fortunately is infrequently, it should duplicate its mate across the median line. Occlusion and space width sometimes will make an exact reproduction impossible, but similar characteristics, such as angles and directions of the cusp arms, the contour of the mesio-labial line angle, the long axis, and the mesio-distal and inciso-cervical convexities of the incisal third, can be "implied," whatever the situation. Success in this effort comes from experience. This statement applies equally to all replacements.

MANDIBULAR BICUSPIDS

With much of the occlusal half of the buccal surface occluding with the opposing teeth, it is difficult to make lower bicuspid pontics using facings adaptable to the previously discussed situations. Such a method of replacement is not often essential, but when a facing other than the Sanitarypontic is indicated, the buccal anatomy, complex in its arrangement, should be duplicated.

The facing selected, usually a long-pin or Trupontic, must be cut down from the occlusal toward the cervical so that metal may absorb and dissipate the forces of occlusion (Fig. 258A).

This protective metal should take the outline of an inlay that provides a full occlusal restoration. Depending on the degree to which the cervical area of the pontic will be visible, the adaptation of the facing to the ridge will conform to the pattern developed for upper bicuspids, including a wider interproximal embrasure on the distal. (See Fig. 258B.) When any display of metal is prohibited, the bridge must be fabricated using a por-

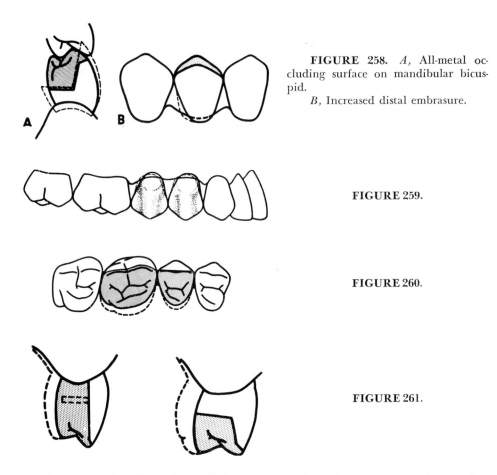

FIGURE 258. *A*, All-metal occluding surface on mandibular bicuspid.

B, Increased distal embrasure.

FIGURE 259.

FIGURE 260.

FIGURE 261.

celain veneer fused to the gold framework. A resin veneer would not be stable, and a base supporting tube teeth would not be tolerated by the tissue.

POSTERIOR PONTICS

When the form of a pontic has been modified (Figs. 259, 260, and 261) or exaggerated to promote self-cleansing, tissue stimulation and comfort, and to reduce torque, leverage, and pressure on the abutments, it should not be expected that, as an individual unit, it will function with the same masticating efficiency as the lost tooth. However, it will replace much that was missing, it will add to the total of the working surfaces, and the reconstruction of the abutments may improve their relationship with the opposing teeth.

Solder joints should be placed in the area of normal contact in the buccal or labial halves (see Figs. 262, 263, and 264), hence it follows that the buccal half of the posterior pontic should fill the space. When viewed from the occlusal or incisal, the buccal or labial half or two-fifths of any pontic should have normal form, with the remaining lingual part decreasing rather sharply in width as it approaches the lingual line angles. This will result in a much narrower and much more convex lingual surface.

The distance from the tips of the buccal cusps to the tips of the lingual cusps should be shortened from one-fifth to one-third, with the lingual cusps becoming more pointed and having smaller surfaces contacting opposing cusps (Fig. 265). This will lessen leverages and other forces on the abutment teeth, especially if the spillways are deepened and repositioned a little to the lingual. To eliminate the flat or concave areas that are found proximally on natural teeth and that would be food traps, the lingual

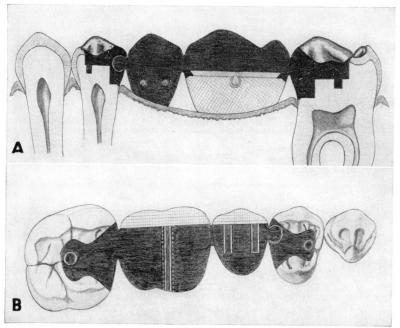

FIGURE 262. Buccal and occlusal cross sections of posterior pontics showing convex form, embrasures, and position of solder joints.

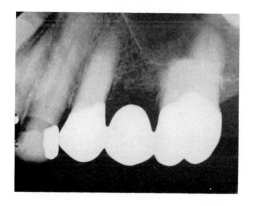

FIGURE 263. Cross sections of posterior solder joints. Placed at contact areas, they have a concave periphery.

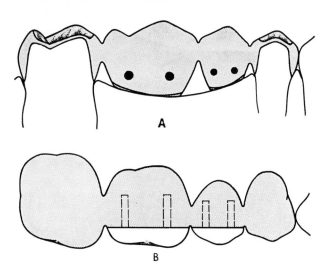

FIGURE 264. Cross section of solder joints.

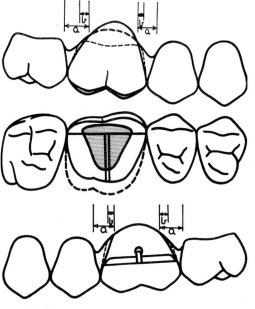

FIGURE 265. Reduced occlusal areas on the three pontics of a maxillary five-unit posterior bridge.

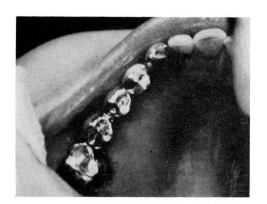

FIGURE 266. Reducing the area of contact between the pontic and ridge helps to establish convex surfaces on the proximals. Only the dark area in the center line will contact the ridge. This section becomes narrower as it approaches the lingual.

296

surface and those parts of the mesial and distal surfaces lingual to the contacts should be convex in form. (See Fig. 266.)

When the alveolar process is questionable or receded, but the fixed partial denture remains the restoration of choice, bucco-lingual width of the pontics may be diminished as much as one-third, the units as a whole being set slightly to the lingual in the final assembly of the bridge. The lateral cusp plane thrusts can be equalized in this way.

In any case in which the abutment teeth and the edentulous areas are short occluso-cervically, the amount of tissue covered by the pontic, and the resultant stagnation, will become a problem. Again at the expense of the lingual half, the occlusal surface of the pontic must be altered. Reduction of the bucco-lingual width, and much wider embrasures will partially rectify the situation, but its solution will depend largely on patient instruction and compliance with such instruction.

Governed Reduction

The amount of reduction of the lingual half of any posterior pontic will be governed by the length of the span, the quality and amount of the supporting structure, and the occluso-ridge measurement.

When the span is long, lingual modification of the individual posterior pontic will be mandatory to lessen the load carried by the abutment teeth during the closing of the jaws on a food bolus. This decrease in the length of the cusp plane will not bring about a lack of balance. Sufficient cusp plane surface will remain on the lingual portion of the pontic to continue the contact with the opposing teeth, because in lateral excursions cusp tips in such areas seldom, if ever, will move into contact with the cusp tips of the opposite jaw. Even then, balance would be continued by the occluding surfaces of the abutments.

RIDGE CONTACT

The contact of any pontic with the ridge tissue deserves special attention. If biologic acceptance and hygienic measures are to be possible, it must touch the ridge, but without pressure. In its over-all contour the pontic must conform to the shape of the ridge, yet it must never be concave in two directions (Fig. 267A and B). Bucco- or labio-lingual ridge form demands that the area approximating the ridge be concave, but mesio-distally it should be barely convex

There may be an occasional exception when the facing adapts to the tissue. The ridge contact should be in the form of an irregular "T" (see Fig. 267C), with the crossarm under the facing, or it may be only a narrow strip running at right angles to the crest of the ridge. The amount of con-

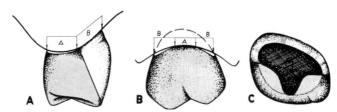

FIGURE 267. *A,* Shows slight space between pontic and ridge in area marked "A" but the facing is in contact.

B, Clearance is lateral to area "A."

C, Shows area covering ridge. Dark "T" will be in contact.

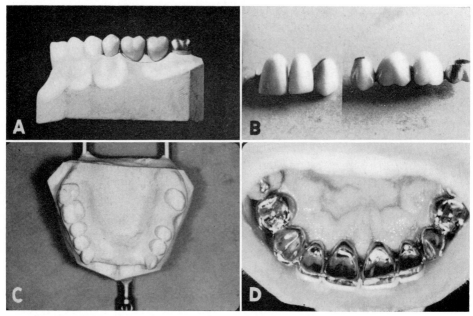

FIGURE 268. Ridge contact, area of coverage, and embrasure form of posterior and anterior pontics.

A, With less resorption, facings should lap ridge.

B, Embrasure form, anterior and posterior pontics.

C, Diagnostic cast for anterior bridge.

D, Anterior bridge, incisal view; excessive ridge coverage by central incisor pontics will make it more difficult to maintain hygiene and tissue tone.

vexity on either side of this contact area is minor (see Fig. 267*A* and *B*), but this will be enough to prevent a saucer-like food trap. Such form can be developed in far more than half of the pontics, making it easy to keep the tissue-contacting area clean by passing floss mesio-distally under the pontic. The area of contact of the pontic will be smaller than the ridge-lap, which in turn is much smaller in circumference than the outline of the pontic. Mesio- and disto-lingual segments of the ridgelap should be convex in form and peripherally should clear the tissue about 0.2 mm. for easier cleansing. If the pontic extends just over the crest of the ridge lingually (Fig. 267*A*), the tongue will be more comfortable.

There are no rules to govern grinding and positioning of facings that must be aligned irregularly. Trial, error, and imagination play major roles.

REFERENCES

1. Johnston, J. F.: Pontic form and bridge design. Part II. Illinois D. J., *25*:339, June 1956.
2. Klaffenbach, A. O.: Anterior fixed bridge prosthesis including acrylic resins. J.A.D.A., *34*:670, May 1947.
3. Moulton, G. H.: Esthetics in anterior fixed bridge prosthodontics. J.A.D.A., *52*:36, Jan. 1956.
4. Prime, J. M.: Lecture before Indianapolis Study Clubs, 1925.

Adams, J. D.: Planning posterior bridges. J.A.D.A., *53*:647, Dec. 1956.

Boyd, H. R., Jr.: Pontics in fixed partial dentures. J. Pros. Den., *5*:55, Jan. 1955.

Cunningham, D. M., and Dykema, R. W.: A case report (fixed bridge). Alum. Bul. Indiana Univ. School Den., Jan. 1956, p. 12.

Davis, M. C., and Klein, G.: Combination gold and acrylic restorations. J. Pros. Den., *4*:510, July 1954.

Gill, J. R.: Treatment planning for mouth rehabilitation. J. Pros. Den., *2*:230, March 1952.

Hagerman, D. A., and Arnim, S. S.: The relation of new knowledge of the gingiva to crown and bridge procedures. J. Pros. Den., *5*:538, July 1955.

Yock, D. H.: Indications for the use of plastic resins in crown and bridge prosthesis. J.A.D.A., *46*:505, May 1953.

16

SOLDERING

Solder is an alloy used to unite metal surfaces. Gold solder is similar in composition to a casting alloy, with the difference that tin is added to lower the melting range.[1] The requirements of a dental solder are numerous and rigid. It must flow readily at a temperature at least 100 to 150° F. below the fusing point of the parts to be joined, and must have strength to combat deformation or fracture. It should have a color and polished luster comparable to that of the cast metal, and should be as resistant to tarnish and corrosion as the cast alloys. These characteristics can be maintained by a knowledge of the fundamental factors that control the accuracy, properties, and clinical behavior of the solder joint.

The gold content of a solder is usually signified in reference to its fineness, i.e., 1000 fine is pure gold, and 700 fine is 700 parts gold and 300 parts other metals. Often, however, the manufacturer may designate solder in terms of carat, the carat referring to the carat of the gold to be soldered, rather than to the solder itself. For example, an 18K solder does not contain 18 parts in 24 of pure gold, but is to be used with an 18K gold alloy (Table 18).

The best, safest, and most sensible way to select a solder is from its melting range although traditionally the carat designations have been used. The upper limit of this range should be at least 100° F. below the lower limit of the melting range of the casting gold or plate on which the solder is to be used. Many people refuse to believe that occasionally 16K solder may require a higher temperature for fusing than 18K. Nevertheless this is true, because so much depends on the composition other than the gold content.

A soldering assembly is a mass of set soldering investment, trimmed and cleaned and holding the parts to be joined in the exact relationship that

300

Table 18. *Approximate Compositions of Dental Gold Solders*

	FOR 16K (.560 FINE)	FOR 18K (.650 FINE)	FOR 20K (.729 FINE)	FOR 22K (.809 FINE)
Gold	56.0	65.0	72.9	80.9
Silver	21.4	16.3	12.2	8.1
Copper	16.3	13.1	9.9	6.8
Zinc	4.8	3.9	3.0	2.1
Tin	1.5	1.7	2.0	2.1
Melting Range	1355– 1435° F.	1420– 1490° F.	1465– 1515° F.	1535– 1590° F.

should ensue following the operation. It should be poured to a minimal thickness of ½ inch, should extend not less than ⅛ inch beyond the terminal castings, and should be from ⅛ to ¼ inch wider than the widest casting contained in the assembly.

The requirements for successful and rapid soldering include stability and contact of the pieces to be joined, access, cleanliness, and controlled heating. Theoretically, there should be a clearance of 0.005 inch between the pieces to be soldered, which amounts to contact for all practical purposes. A good solder will flow into such minute openings by capillary action. The wider the space to be filled with solder, the weaker the joint, but even more important is the greater shrinkage during solidification of the metal, and the resultant distortion.

SOLDERING INVESTMENT

The composition of a soldering investment is similar to that of conventional casting investments, with quartz preferred to cristobalite as the refractory agent.[1] Quartz reduces the thermal expansion and thus the dimensional change during soldering. Just as the contraction of gold during casting must be compensated for, so the contraction of the solder must be balanced in part by the setting and thermal expansion of the investment. The compositions of soldering investments are adjusted accordingly.

ASSEMBLY OF THE BRIDGE

When the pontic has been polished, cleaned, and aligned, the plaster index should be luted to the working cast and the linguo-cervical of the pontic waxed to the ridge (Fig. 269). If all units of the bridge are posterior to the cuspid, the cervical half of the lingual of all units should be blocked out with modeling clay so that the occluso-lingual plaster index will not

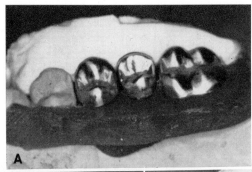

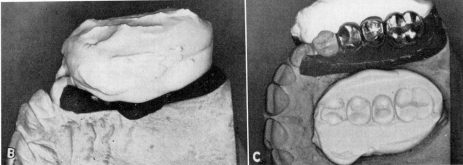

FIGURE 269.   *A,* Buccal index in position to stabilize pontic during making of occlusal index; modeling clay is used to outline area of occlusal index.

B, Occlusal index poured.

C, Index separated.

extend into undercuts. The individual parts of the bridge must be cleaned and assembled in the index and luted to position with the exact relationship that existed on the cast. The interproximal areas between all units must be filled with wax (Fig. 270). The exposed surfaces of the plaster of Paris should be painted with a separating medium, soaked in water to fill air pockets, and the soldering assembly should be poured, using an accepted soldering investment.

If the bridge is short, with no more than three joints to be soldered, this operation may be completed at one time (Figs. 271 and 272). If the bridge is longer, with more than three solder joints, one middle joint should be left unsoldered in the first assembly. Then the two parts of the bridge should be realigned, either in the mouth or on the working cast, another index made, and the soldering operation completed in the second assembly.

PREPARATION OF THE ASSEMBLY

Access for soldering may be secured by trimming the assembly to size, beveling the edges, and cutting spear-shaped grooves in the investment which lead to and expose the surfaces to be soldered (Fig. 274). These areas must be wide enough and deep enough for the flame to approach the surfaces from all directions. The wax, originally placed in the embrasures to help provide access and to prevent particles of soldering investment from falling between the surfaces during trimming, can be flushed away by a stream of boiling water. Any loose pieces of investment will be removed at the same time. Following the elimination of the wax and debris, and while the assembly is still hot, flux should be applied to the contact areas. The heat from the metal will melt the flux base and allow it to enter the embrasure. Minimal flux is required and excessive flux can be a nuisance. (See Fig. 275.)

FLUX AND ANTIFLUX

Flux, a borax-containing material, is a substance that maintains the cleanliness of the metals to be united and facilitates the flow and attachment of solder. It burns out during the soldering process, leaving negligible residue. Flux may be procured in either powder or paste form. The paste is easier to control. One of the best available is a paste manufactured

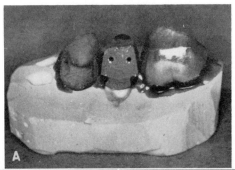

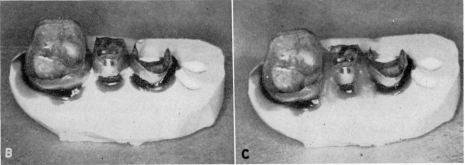

FIGURE 270. *A,* Bridge units assembled in occlusal index and secured with wax; index trimmed under pontic to enable poured investment to hold pontic securely.

B, Units luted on lingual.

C, Embrasures filled with wax to prevent soldering investment entering.

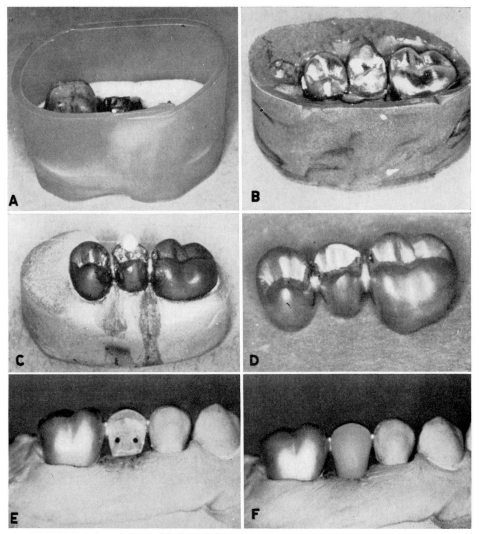

FIGURE 271. *A,* Assembly boxed for pouring.
B, Soldering assembly before trimming.
C, D, Soldered bridge; note size, form, and position of joints.
E, Bridge seated on working cast; metal contacts unscarred ridge.
F, Facing in position; it is barely narrower than space.

according to Dr. Cook's formula.* Any soldering flux with a petrolatum base should be stirred occasionally, especially if the jar is stored in a warm area, as heat will cause the suspended borax to settle and reduce the fluxing potential of the material at the top of the container.

An antiflux is any substance that precludes the attachment of solder. One of the best examples is gold rouge. It can be mixed with chloroform and painted on critical areas very near the joint and will hinder the union

---

* The S. S. White Dental Mfg. Co., Philadelphia, Penna.

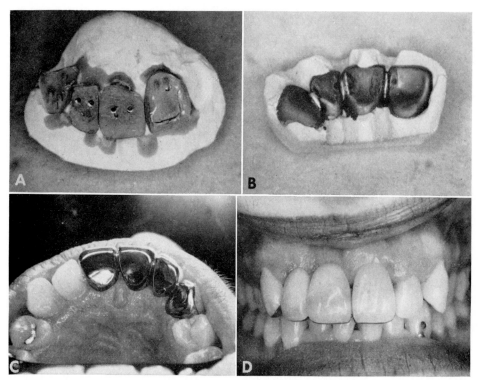

FIGURE 272.   *A,* Four units of an anterior bridge assembled for pouring soldering assembly. Joint areas are not yet waxed. Parts presumably are separated by correct distances. Spaces for retentive fingers of investment have been cut under incisal edges of pontics.

B, Soldered bridge. Joints are long and relatively thin. Observe investment holding incisals of pontics.

C, D, Lingual and labial views of cemented bridge. Joints do not encroach on embrasure form. Tissue is clear for massage by food. Solder is not visible from labial.

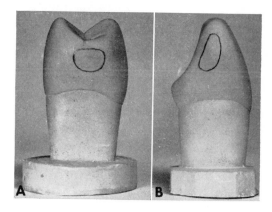

FIGURE 273.   *A, B,* Ideal location and contour of solder joints.

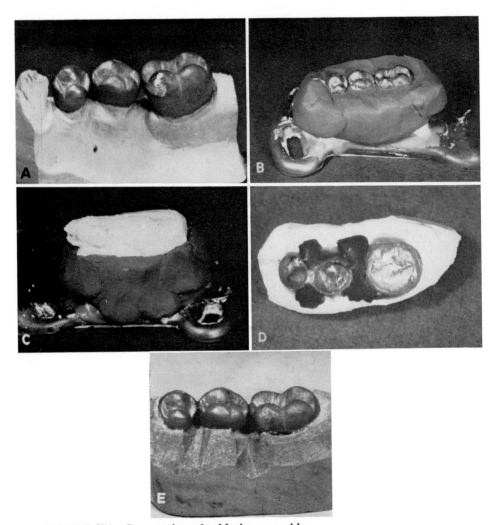

FIGURE 274. **Preparation of soldering assembly.**

A, Castings for splint on working cast.

B, All areas blocked out with modeling clay except those to be included in the plaster index.

C, Plaster index poured.

D, Castings assembled and secured to plaster. Areas to be soldered are protected from investment by wax.

E, Soldering assembly washed, trimmed, and fluxed. Since no facings are involved, surfaces to be soldered may be approached from either side. Joints can be smaller because no support will be required. Approximate contact, access, and cleanliness are demonstrated here. Correct application of heat completes the four requisites for soldering.

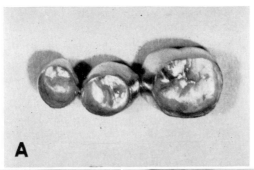

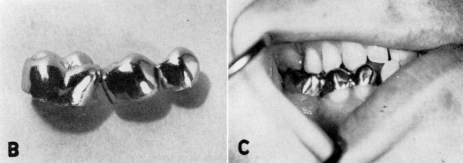

FIGURE 275. Soldering splint (continued).
A, B, Solder joints are about one-half the size required for a bridge; embrasures are not filled and hygiene should be easy.
C, Splint seated.

of solder with these parts. It must be kept away from the point at which the solder will be applied and from the crevice into which the solder must flow to create the joint. The need for it is limited.

HEATING THE ASSEMBLY

The soldering assembly should be heated to a temperature of 900 to 1000° F. in a furnace, or over a Bunsen burner flame, the block being supported by a wire screen. It should be placed to one side of the screen until it has dried, *not* directly over the flame. It is the belief of many operators that the assembly will be sufficiently hot when it has been dried, and that the torch is then needed only to heat the areas to be joined. However, experience proves that the assembly should be heated to a higher point, so that on application of the torch flame the castings held in the investment will become a dull red almost instantly.

WARNING: Overheating the investment may cause warpage and a breakdown of the ingredients, releasing elements such as sulfur and chlorine that can attack the metal. Chemical attack of the alloy will lead to brittleness and susceptibility to corrosion in the oral environment.

SOLDERING TECHNIQUE

Solder may be placed at the desired area in strips, but the size and form of the joint can be better controlled if the solder is cut into pieces and applied with tweezers.

Solder will accumulate at the hottest area of the metal. When a small pointed flame from the torch has brought the joint area to a dull red, a piece of solder should be placed in the embrasure and the flame should

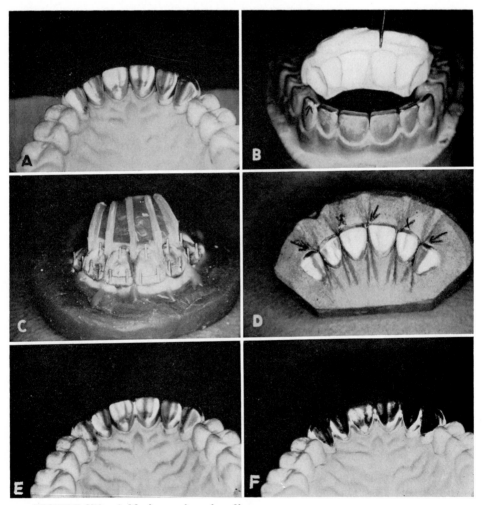

FIGURE 276.   Soldering a six-unit splint.

A, Six pinledges on cast.

B, Lingual plaster index.

C, Castings assembled in index; embrasures waxed.

D, Soldering assembly trimmed; arrows point to the three joints that will be soldered in first assembly.

E, Three double units returned to cast; a new index was made and a new assembly poured; two remaining joints were then soldered.

F, Six-unit splint with five solder joints.

be directed around the crevice into which the solder must flow. Only the reducing point of the flame should contact the metal. If the cardinal principles have been observed, the solder will flow at once into the contact area. Molten solder acts somewhat as a solvent for the surface of the casting and penetrates beyond the surface. However, contrary to popular opinion, a strong junction can be obtained without marked diffusion.

When lack of flux or contamination inhibits the flow of the solder, causing it to "ball" or "hang" on the surface of the metal, the torch flame should be removed and the unattached solder taken off, if possible. The castings are refluxed, a new piece of solder is applied, and the flame is again directed as described previously.

When the solder does not react quickly, it can become oxidized; the base metal constituents are then burned out and the melting range is raised. Much of the clinical success of a soldered bridge is dependent on maintaining the physical properties of the gold alloy in the abutment castings. These alloys are never inert. At elevated temperatures, induced by overheating in an attempt to cause solder to flow, the grain structure increases with an accompanying loss of ductility. The resultant brittleness can lead to fracture under masticating forces. Therefore care in soldering is important to assure maximal physical properties in the assembled bridge.

If the soldering assembly has been carefully heated and the torch flame correctly adjusted and applied, the time required for the soldering operation will be short. When molten metal solidifies, there is some shrinkage, which can be controlled well enough by having the units in contact, by properly heating the soldering assembly, and by producing no more than three joints in any assembly (Fig. 276).

When the soldering has been finished, the assembly should cool until the metal is black before being placed in water; the investment is then removed and the metal is cleaned. Rapid quenching from a high temperature will induce distortion.[2, 3, 4]

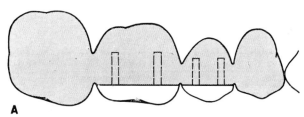

FIGURE 277. Cross sections of solder joints.

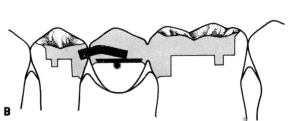

A good solder joint must have a complete and concave peripheral attachment, circular or elliptical in form (Fig. 277). No joint is acceptable if it has pits, irregularities, or open sections resulting from inadequate fluxing, debris, or insufficient heat. It should be centered at the contact areas of the castings, extending into the embrasures only far enough for strength. Solder must not extend to the margin of the retainer, because this can cause warping or rounding of the margin, and will interfere with finishing the cemented casting. There are no laws governing the size of solder joints other than those set up through the judgment of the operator. Ideally, the greatest measurement of the joint should never be at right angles to the line of force directed against the prosthesis. Since this rule must be violated many times in the construction of anterior bridges, joints in these areas must approach perfection.

PICKLING

The bridge should be placed in a porcelain pickling dish and a solution of 50 per cent hydrochloric acid* should be poured over it. The acid is heated until the surface of the gold is free of oxide; then the acid is poured off and the prosthesis is removed. Any greenish tint in the acid is evidence of copper or silver salts. If dirty acid is used for pickling, an electrolytic deposit of copper is quickly formed. This will lead to corrosion. Copper pans and iron tongs should not be used in connection with acid because they contaminate the gold alloy. The soldered bridge should never be pickled by holding it over a flame and then plunging it into acid, because of the possibility of a joint breaking during heating, or distortion occurring from the sudden change in temperature.[3] (See Fig. 278.)

If necessary, the solder joints may be contoured, using knife-edge stones

---

* Fifty per cent sulfuric acid may be used and it gives off less fumes. Hydrofluoric acid is excellent, but it is too dangerous for general use.

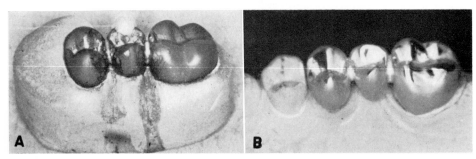

FIGURE 278.   Soldered bridge is black (A), but color and luster can be returned (B), by pickling and by using rubber wheels, pumice, tripoli, and No. 600 Carborundum powder.

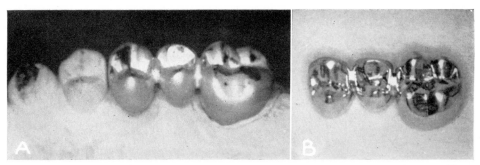

FIGURE 279. *A,* Equilibration of soldered, unpolished bridge on working cast. Note markings from articulating paper.

B, Bridge polished, washed, and ready for try-in.

or disks, and should be polished, using rubber wheels, pumice, tripoli, and No. 600 Carborundum powder (Fig. 279).

The prosthesis is now ready for trial in the mouth.

REFERENCES

1. Taylor, N. O., and Teamer, C. K.: Gold solders for dental use. J. D. Res., *28:*219, June 1949.
2. Steinman, R. R.: Warpage produced by soldering with dental solders and gold alloys. J. Pros. Den., *4:*384, May 1954.
3. Ryge, G.: Dental soldering procedures. D. Clin. North America, Nov. 1958, p. 747.
4. Perdigon, G. J., and Van Eepoel, E. F.: Minimizing solder joint warpage in fixed partial denture construction. J. Pros. Den., 7:244, March 1957.

Dykema, R. W.: A study of the effects of certain variables on the comparative strengths of soldered and cast bridge joints. Master's thesis, Indiana Univ. School Den., June 1961.

J. F. Jelenko & Co., Inc.: Crown and Bridge Construction. A Handbook of Dental Laboratory Procedures. The company, 1964.

Simpson, R. L.: Failures in crown and bridge prosthodontics. J.A.D.A., *47:*154, Aug. 1953.

Winslow, M. B.: Fixed splint and bridge assembly. J.A.D.A., *51:*47, July 1955.

17

GLAZING AND STAINING FACINGS

A ground, unglazed porcelain facing is rough, porous, and irritating, stains readily, and is an inviting area for plaque and bacterial growth. It should never be placed in contact with mucous membrane, either static or mobile. While some vacuum-fired facings can be given a semipolish after contouring, even these surfaces are not acceptable. "Any number of excuses may be made for using an unglazed surface, but the tissue will not accept any of them."[1]

Reglazing pontic facings can be done by rubbing dry porcelain powder into the pores and firing the facing to fuse the exposed ground surface, or by applying a coating of an overglaze and firing it at the temperature suggested by the manufacturer. The first method mentioned generally over-fuses the facing, thereby changing form and fit and reducing the physical properties.

Overglazes for restoring the surface texture and finish to ground porcelain facings have reacted favorably in accelerated solubility tests using synthetic saliva. When applied in a thin layer, never over 0.006 inch thick, they are transparent and do not alter the shade of the surface to which they are applied. Whether the overglaze is one that fuses at 1945° F.,* 1762° F.,* or 1600° F.,† if directions are scrupulously followed and if the glaze is adequately fired, it does not seem to dissolve, lose its luster, or change its surface texture in the oral environment. When the overglaze is fused at less than 1825° F., the holding period should be at least 1 minute.

---

* Steele's Super Glaze, The Columbus Dental Mfg. Company, Columbus, Ohio.
† The S. S. White Dental Mfg. Co., Philadelphia, Penna.

If the piece is overfired, the surface texture, although substantial, will be glassy and artificial-looking. Usually, however, this appearance can be improved satisfactorily by lightly rubbing the surface with a very fine sandpaper disk.[2]

APPLYING THE GLAZE

After the facing has been ground to form and alignment, it must be boiled in water to remove wax and grit, scrubbed with a detergent, washed, and dried with a clean towel (Fig. 280).

With the facing mounted on a facing holder, or prepared toothpick, and steadied with the finger, dry glazing powder, picked up on a clean napkin, should be rubbed into all ground surfaces that will not be in contact with metal later on (Fig. 281). If any powder is pushed inadvertently into the slot and lingual surface or gathers around the pins of a facing, it must be brushed off with a semistiff bristle brush.

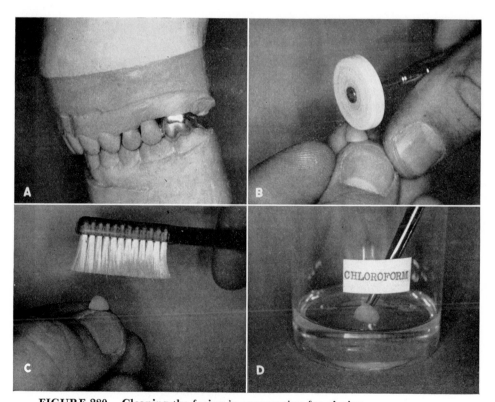

FIGURE 280. Cleaning the facing in preparation for glazing.
A, The recontoured facing on the soldered and equilibrated bridge.
B, Smoothing the facing with a rubber wheel.
C, Scrubbing facing with a detergent.
D, Dipping facing in chloroform to remove any remaining wax particles.

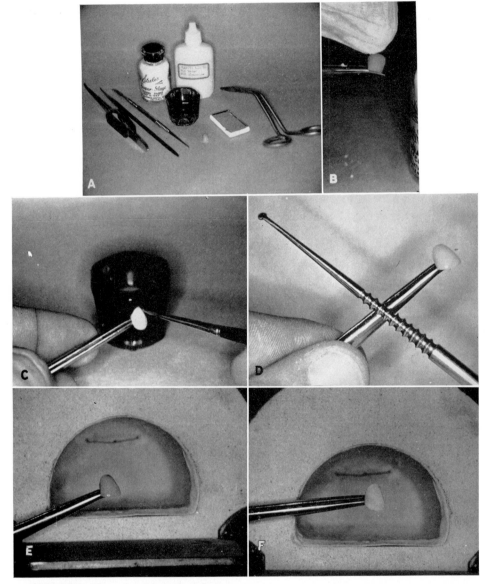

FIGURE 281.   Applying the glaze.

A, Armamentarium needed for glazing facings: tongs, brush, vibrator-spatula, glaze (one that fuses at 1945° F. or 1762° F.), Dappen dish, liquid, tray covered with platinum, furnace tongs.

B, Rubbing powder onto facing.

C, Applying glaze with brush.

D, Vibrating facing to spread glaze evenly.

E, F, Drying glaze before furnace door so that evenness of application, and quantity, may be verified.

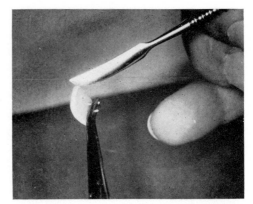

FIGURE 282. Removing misplaced glaze powder with instrument.

Glazing powder should be mixed to a creamy consistency, using the liquid medium found in the Glazing Kit.* A liquid made by placing equal quantities of glycerin and water in a bottle and heating the combination in a double boiler is suitable also. This mixture is complete in about 10 minutes.

The mixture of powder and liquid, mobile but not runny, is applied in a thin, even coat to all ground surfaces, again being careful to keep it away from, or to remove it from, the slot or any portion of the facing that will be in contact with the casting. The facing should be held before the furnace door to dry, or rotated above a clear-burning Bunsen burner flame, and should then be examined for evenness and thickness of the glaze. If any area has been missed or has a coating which is too thin, no attempt should be made to patch the spot. All glaze must be rubbed off and reapplied. To repeat: any powder on any surface that will come into contact with a casting surface must be removed with an instrument blade or fine brush (Fig. 282).

FIRING THE GLAZE

There are inexpensive furnaces having restricted upper-temperature ranges† (Fig. 283), which are suitable for glazing and for firing low-fusing porcelain. A burnout furnace should not be used, since the muffle will be contaminated by the gas from the wax.

The facing should be placed on a small firing tray, or sagger, which has been covered with a sheet of 0.001 platinum foil or which contains a mound of flint or fine silex powder. Platinum foil is preferable to ground silex because if the platinum touches the glaze, it can be peeled away,

---

* Steele's Super Glaze, The Columbus Dental Mfg. Company, Columbus, Ohio.

† K. H. Huppert Co., Chicago, Ill.; Barkmeyer, Redlands, Calif.

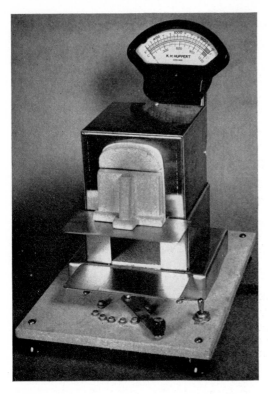

FIGURE 283. Glazing furnace (Huppert).

whereas silex must be broken off, sometimes spoiling the contour or glaze of the facing (Fig. 284).

After being preheated in front of the open muffle, the facing is placed in a furnace no hotter than 900° F., and the temperature is increased by 100° every minute. The current is turned off when the fusing point of the glaze has been reached. The furnace is allowed to drop in temperature to 900° F.; then the door is opened and the furnace is cooled to 500° F. The sagger is removed to the bench and covered with a glass beaker.

The first application of glazing material is expected to serve only as a filler for the pores of the porcelain; a second layer probably will be needed to provide a smooth, semiglossy surface. However, if characterization of the facing is required, the stains should be applied following the fusing of the initial coat. After the stains have been dried and examined, they should be fired at the designated fusing point, raising and lowering the temperature in the usual manner. Glaze is again applied, matured, and cooled, as previously described, although the fusing temperature must be lowered and the time increased in order to preserve the shade of the stains.

Facings should be resurfaced to have a luster harmonizing with approximating and corresponding teeth, except that the highest possible glaze should always be placed on Sanitarypontics and on porcelain surfaces to be clasped.

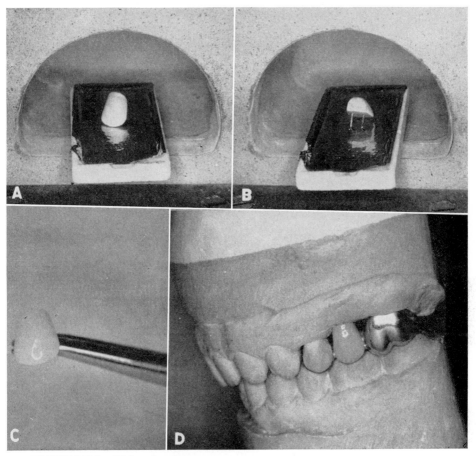

FIGURE 284. Firing the glaze.
A, B, Facing on firing tray in door of furnace.
C, Facing glazed.
D, Glazed facing returned to bridge.

STAINING

Two kits of stains are widely accepted. One fuses at 1762° F.,* the other at 1600° F.† The 1762° F. group must be used with the glaze that is fired at 1945° F. or 1762° F. The second type, which is fired at 1600° F., is coupled with the glaze that fuses at the same temperature; no holding time is used with this combination.[1]

Hairline Check

Stains must be applied to facings in a very subtle form, producing only

---

* Steele's, The Columbus Dental Mfg. Co., Columbus, Ohio.
† The S. S. White Dental Mfg. Co., Philadelphia, Penna.

a hint of the simulated object. A hairline check is made by using brown stain plus a very little black, with one part of the diluting agent added to four parts of stain. It should be neither thin nor ropy when mixed. It is applied with a very small brush in a rather wide strip; then, drawing the brush from cervical to incisal, alternately on each side of the stain, a narrow, hairlike, sometimes intermittent line is formed. It may be in the center of the tooth, and if so will follow the long axis; but if the check is nearer the margin, it probably will angle slightly toward the proximo-cervical.

Decalcified Areas

Decalcified spots are made from white stain with no diluting agent added. These are often in the cervical third and lateral to the center of the tooth, irregular in form, and frequently crescent-shaped, surrounding a pin point of caries which will show up as a brown dot. The white stain should be feathered around the edges.

Restorations

Silicate or resin fillings may be outlined with a fine brown line and shaded with white. Such a characterization is seldom desired by the patient, since it could denote a lack of pride in the upkeep or repair of the teeth.

Enamel Cracks

Cracks in enamel may be copied, and in an anterior bridge replacing one or two teeth are often of great help in establishing esthetic harmony. Gray stain is placed on the facing, with one edge a straight line and the remainder spread, thinned, and feathered toward the distal for a distance of 1.0 mm. plus at the incisal, narrowing as it reaches the end of the line,

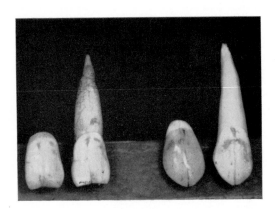

FIGURE 285. Stained facings.

which may be from 3.0 to 5.0 mm. long. To the mesial, the surface is shaded with white, not too heavily, thinning out quickly in about 0.6 mm.

After stains have been fused, they are covered with a layer of glaze, which is fired at the same temperature with a holding time of 1 minute (Fig. 285).

A reverse-pin facing and a pin facing in a light shade may be effectively stained along the incisal edge or proximal margins of the metal-contacting surface before the pontic is waxed. These stains do not require an overlay of glaze.

When staining bonded Ceramco porcelain veneers to simulate the appearance of separation between the individual units, a fine line of Steele's Superstain, made up of half brown stain and half diluent, will be painted at the junction of the units. A groove, made by a flexible diamond disk, should be provided. Since there appears to be some fluxing action at higher temperatures, inducing flow between the porcelain and the stain, this firing temperature should not exceed 1720° F.

SEATING THE FACING

When the facing has cooled and is tried on the pontic, the increased width produced by the overglaze may make it necessary to use a sandpaper disk on proximal edges to allow the facing to seat on the casting without interference.

Facings may check and have a tendency to be more friable if preliminary heating, or cooling, is not done with care.

REFERENCES

1. Pettrow, J. N.: Personal communication.
2. Kipp, R. P.: Personal communication.

18

CHECKING AND CEMENTING CROWNS AND BRIDGES

The occluding surfaces of the polished bridge should be dulled with a Burlew disk, after which the bridge must be washed before being placed in the mouth. Doubtless it will have been cleansed thoroughly beforehand, but repeating the process after the patient is in the chair will allay any suspicion of carelessness. In order that the patient may be more acutely aware of premature contacts, and more helpful in correcting them when the bridge is first placed in the mouth, it is an accepted practice not to anesthetize the abutment teeth at this time. Placing the metal in warm water before seating will tend to minimize discomfort.

SEATING AND CHECKING A FULL VENEER GOLD CROWN CASTING

The casting should be seated on the tooth with a mallet and orange-wood stick. If it does not seat, the inside must be scrutinized again for irregularities, which now will have a shiny, burnished appearance. If a plus-contact obstructs seating, it must be polished further, this process being repeated until the casting can be seated. When the contact is deficient, it must be rebuilt by adding solder.

With dental floss secured to the forefinger of each hand and with about a 2-inch length between the fingers, the floss is held taut and at a 30 degree angle to the occlusal plane. One finger, either inside or outside the arch, is kept stationary after the floss reaches the occluso-buccal embrasure, and the floss is forced through the contact area by downward pressure

320

from the other hand. Very often a bucco-lingual movement of the floss will hasten the entry into the cervical embrasure. A snapping-through should be avoided because of the probable injury of the gingival papilla.

Testing the Contact

The strength of the contact will be demonstrated by the resistance to the passage of the floss unless one (or both) of the approximating surfaces is rough or carious. If the interproximal soft tissue at the site chosen for testing is healthy, and if the alveolus is normal radiographically, the contact form and pressure may be considered correct for that mouth and the resistance to the floss can be accepted as a standard by which the contact strength of a restoration may be judged. An instrument has been built for making such a test,[1] but since it is not generally available, experience and judgment must suffice.

If the restoration seats, another check of the control or tested area should precede an appraisal of the newly established contact, adding or subtracting pressure until, after final shaping and polishing, the resistance to the floss is the same at the two contacts.

Checking for Overextension and Underextension

When the casting has been seated, an explorer point may be used for locating overextensions. After the occlusion has been registered with articulating paper, the casting is removed and occlusal and cervical alterations are made outside the mouth to escape overheating of the tooth and trauma to soft tissue. Marking, removal, and adjustment are continued until optimal occlusion has been reached, after which the contact areas and cervical margin must be re-evaluated for strength and position. If the casting is short and fails to cover the preparation, the crown must be remade since repair is impossible. The exposed tooth surface and its concomitant roughness will set up tissue irritation, which cannot be eliminated or controlled, and sensitivity and caries may develop.

Smith[2] writes:

"The fourth basic step in achieving a satisfactory crown is the fitting in the mouth. This amounts to a checking of the gingival fit and correction of the contact and occlusion. If the marginal fit is inaccurate, the crown should be discarded and the preparation re-evaluated, corrected if necessary, and a new impression made. Before the marginal fit can be checked, the crown must be completely seated. Excessive contour on the proximal contact areas will prevent the complete seating of the crown. This excess must be reduced, and normal contact must be developed. Final seating may be done by tapping the crown with a steel instrument and mallet. Positive seating may be sensed through the feel and ring of the instrument.

The margin of the crown may be examined then by using an explorer. An easily accessible point on the crown margin where the preparation margin is readily discernible by tactile examination is selected. With the point directed toward the gingival margin, the explorer is passed over the crown down onto the root surface. If the marginal fit is good, the passage of the point will be smooth. If the passage is interrupted by bumping over a prominence, it means that the preparation is not completely covered, and that the crown is not in place or that it is short. If the passage is interrupted by the point dropping off of the crown to the tooth, the crown is either too long or not in close apposition with the tooth. A further check of the marginal fit may be made by reversing direction of the point so that it is directed toward the occlusal surface, and is passed from the tooth surface below the crown margin up and over the casting. If the passage is smooth, the marginal fit is good. If the point catches under the margin of the casting, it is an indication that the margin is either too long, or is not in apposition with the tooth. If, in the passage, the point drops over an irregularity of the tooth, and then contacts the crown, it is an indication that the preparation is not completely covered.

"This procedure is repeated at a number of points around the gingival margin, and if any of the above irregularities are evidenced, correction is attempted. The seating of the crown is double checked, overextensions are reduced, and the margins are rechecked. The contour of the crown is checked, and the axial surfaces from the margin occlusally are shaped to be in harmony with the surrounding tissues. If the tactile examination is satisfactory, a bite-wing roentgenogram is taken as a check of the interproximal fit, and if this proves satisfactory, the marginal fit of the crown is accepted.

"*Summary.* The construction of cast crowns that possess accurate marginal fit requires: first, understanding; second, ability; and third, conscientious execution. . . . Crowns with accurate marginal fits should contribute to the preservation of teeth and the health of surrounding tissues."

INITIAL SEATING AND CHECKING FIT OF A BRIDGE

After the temporary coverings have been removed from the preparations and the abutments cleaned, the bridge should seat with little frictional resistance. If a long period of time has elapsed between taking the impression for the working cast and the completion of the bridge, a constant application of pressure to the seated bridge may be needed for several minutes so that the abutments will reposition themselves to conform to the path of insertion. There should be no permanent or marked change in the position of the abutment teeth or of the opposing teeth during this period of construction, although a slight temporary shift should have no adverse effect. A major discrepancy or extreme difficulty in seating will probably necessitate the breaking of one or more of the solder joints and reassembly and resoldering the segments.

After seating the bridge, the cervical adaptation of the retainers should be checked with explorers and bite-wing radiographs. Also, occlusion, strength of contact, alignment, pressure of the pontics against the ridge, and color matching must be examined.

Equilibration

Articulating paper or tape of one color will show the location and extent of any high spots in centric; another color should be used for eccentric movements. While it will color all surfaces that touch, the point of premature contact will be burnished and is the area to be altered. This routine must be continued until comfortable closure is possible in centric and in all excursions. If the working casts were accurately related on the articulator, and if carving and assembly were done with care, little adjustment should be necessary.

Considerable adjustment may be expected when a bridge has been constructed using casts related by a wax centric occlusion registration. Wax is notoriously inaccurate when the teeth are brought into contact and should not be used if the Kerr Bite Frame or some other equally satisfactory means of mounting is available.

A bridge constructed by the indirect technique should be returned to the working cast after soldering, and before polishing, for occlusal equilibration. If the opposing cast has been poured in stone, closure against the soldered bridge must be done with delicacy in order that the cast not be abraded. If the cast is worn or distorted, the bridge could be completed and polished with gross occlusal inaccuracies remaining.

After discrepancies in occlusion have been eliminated and the bridge has been polished, the facing may be glazed before the patient appears. This is psychologically advantageous; also, it is easier at this time to check the shade of the recontoured facing.

Contacts, Alignment, and Ridge Adaptation

The strength of contact must be checked with floss. If one of the retainers was inadvertently polished to a point where it no longer has the desired form or sufficient pressure against the approximating tooth, the bridge must be invested and the area recontoured by the addition of solder. A cemented bridge with a weak contact will be constantly annoying, owing to the packing of fibrous foods. As a consequence, not only is the

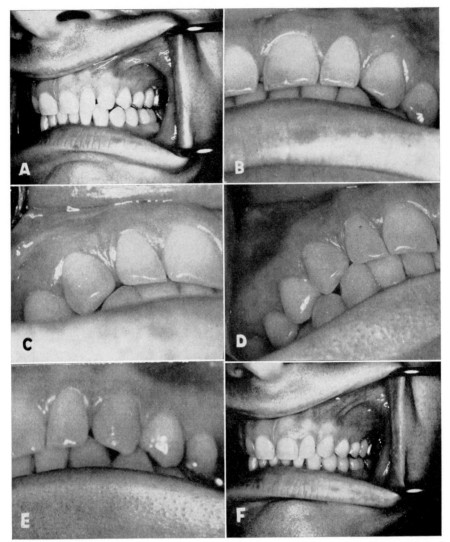

FIGURE 286.   Checking occlusion and alignment in the mouth before cementation.
A, B, C, Bridge in position; alignment correct but contact premature.
D, E, F, Occlusion corrected; teeth occluding.

patient unhappy, but, worse than that, a resorption of the supporting
structure around the abutment tooth may result. In order to maintain
alignment, the bridge must be reinvested.

In checking alignment, the relationship of the buccal cusps of the
prosthesis with the buccal cusps of the opposing teeth must be observed,
to ascertain whether the patient might bite the cheek or lip (Fig. 286).
This can happen in the posterior area wherever cusp tips or buccal margins approximate an end-to-end closure. The maxillary buccal cusps should
have an overjet, with the mandibular cusps curving slightly toward the
center of the opposing tooth. While errors in this relationship can be

corrected after the bridge has been cemented, to do so at this late stage may necessitate grinding a porcelain facing, which cannot be reglazed. Although the facing can be smoothed, the pores cannot be filled and the patient will be continually aware of a rough spot. Therefore this matter demands attention at the time the occlusion is being adjusted and before any cementation.

If the ridgelap of the metallic portion of the pontic contacts the tissue too forcibly, this must be recontoured and the ridge surface of the pontic repolished. Floss should be passed under the bridge, from front to back, to disclose the contact relationship with the tissue. A little clearance is acceptable, but contact without pressure is desirable.

When all changes have been made in occlusion, alignment, and contact, the metal parts that have been ground should be repolished. If stains are needed to add character or to enhance shading, or if adjustments in occlusion, ridge relationship, or alignment have included work on the facing, final glazing can be done while the patient is in the chair. Glazing is discussed in Chapter 17.

The facings should be fixed to the pontics, preferably with zinc phosphate cement; however, resin cement is an excellent material for luting porcelain to metal. The bridge is now ready for cementation.

CAVITY VARNISHES

Zinc phosphate cement, because of its satisfactory clinical behavior manifested throughout the years and its excellent handling characteristics, still remains the permanent luting agent usually recommended for the fixed gold alloy restoration.

There is, however, increasing evidence that the acidity of zinc phosphate cement may be somewhat greater, and that this type of cement may remain acidic longer, than previously believed. Every precaution should be taken to protect the underlying dentin and the pulp against the irritating effects of phosphoric acid; hence the possible role of the cavity varnish deserves careful consideration.

A number of commercial cavity varnishes are available and little difference generally exists in their composition. They are natural rosins or synthetic resins that have been dissolved in a solvent such as chloroform. The solvent rapidly evaporates to leave a thin, shellac-like film on the tooth surface. Other buffering salts, such as zinc oxide or calcium hydroxide, have been added in a few products, but these compositions have not proved to be superior to the usual inert rosin or resin-type varnish. Selection of a particular brand should be based on handling characteristics. The brand of varnish that will flow most evenly over the tooth surface and that is the most readily discernible is the preferred material.

A continuous, thin film of varnish, placed over the cut tooth surface, affords protection to the dentin and pulp in two ways. First, the varnish tends to minimize any seepage of deleterious fluids that may occur around the cemented restoration. Secondly, and more important, the varnish will minimize the penetration of any acid that may be present in the zinc phosphate cement. Thus the possibility of irritation to the pulp from leakage or acid is greatly diminished.[3]

From the foregoing discussion, it is obvious that the varnish is particularly indicated in a deep cavity preparation, where little dentin may remain to protect the tooth against thermal or mechanical shock or from irritants. In such a situation, the varnish may be helpful in maintaining both pulpal health and patient comfort. In a cavity preparation in which a minimum of at least 1.0 mm. of dentin remains, it acts as an insulator, and the use of varnish is of less consequence.

The varnish is painted onto the surface of the prepared cavity immediately before the restoration is to be seated. The tooth surface is dried and the varnish applied. Several methods of application are popular. The varnish may be painted on with a small camel's-hair brush, or a pledget of cotton may be employed to carry the varnish into the deeper areas of the cavity preparation. A small wire loop is supplied for application of one commercial product.

Regardless of the method favored, the varnish should be thin. Several thin layers are applied, and if the varnish becomes thick and viscous upon storage, it should be thinned by addition of some solvent such as chloroform or ether. A thick layer will *not* seal the margins. If, however, the film is thin and *continuous* over the entire cavity preparation, with no voids, maximal protection can be expected. The film thickness of the varnish is extremely low and retention of the restoration is not reduced.

CEMENTATION

Cementation will involve the following factors:
(1) a clean, dry crown or bridge;
(2) isolation of the area of operation;
(3) clean, dry tooth or abutment teeth;
(4) a saliva ejector in position;
(5) a cool, clean mixing slab and spatula;
(6) sufficient quantities of cement powder and cement liquid;
(7) an instrument for applying the cement to the inner surfaces of the castings and to the teeth;
(8) an orangewood stick and mallet;
(9) a cotton roll to cushion the biting pressure against the seated crown or bridge;

(10) cavity varnish; and

(11) brush or instrument for applying varnish.

Although discomfort from cementation is not prolonged,[4] many patients are grateful for anesthesia during this procedure, and some insist on it. The anesthetic has a tendency to decrease the flow of saliva, thus making it easier to keep the bridge and cement dry during the setting period.

After the abutment teeth have been isolated and dried, older operators may prefer to clean the prepared tooth surfaces with phenol, then to remove the phenol with a pellet of cotton soaked in alcohol and dry the abutments with warm air. The authors followed this technique with zinc phosphate cement for many years, and empirical observations indicated no ill effects. However, investigators now advocate that the teeth merely be scoured with pumice for the removal of any remaining fragments of temporary covering, washed, and dried with warm air.

Dental cements do not actually adhere in a chemical sense to the tooth surface or the metal. There is no attraction of unlike molecules. Therefore they must not be relied on to hold the casting in place. Such a concept can lead only to failure. The cement serves merely as a luting material to occupy the small space that exists between the restoration and the tooth. Even with a casting that visually fits perfectly, a minute crevice is present that must be occupied by the cement. It is true that close mechanical adaptation of the cement does exist between the irregularities of the cavity wall and the casting. In order to keep this intimate adaptation and avoid leakage, it is imperative that solubility be minimized and adequate strength maintained to prevent fracture of these small projections of the cement.

Zinc Phosphate Cement

There are many acceptable brands of cement, and selection should be based upon objective handling characteristics rather than inherent properties. Zinc phosphate cement, which is also used as a cement base, is made from a mixture of a powder and a liquid, the powder being essentially zinc oxide and magnesium oxide, while the liquid is phosphoric acid and water, with metallic salts used as buffers.[5] The water in the liquid is added in a definite concentration to control the setting time. This water balance is critical and every precaution should be taken to preserve it. Even minor deviations will markedly influence the setting time, and the consistency of the mix will vary accordingly. An increase in the water content accelerates the set, while a decrease retards it. If the liquid is exposed, it will either absorb or lose moisture from the air, depending on the humidity of the room. For this reason, the bottle should *always* be kept tightly stoppered and the liquid should *not* be placed on the slab until the operator is ready for mixing.

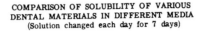

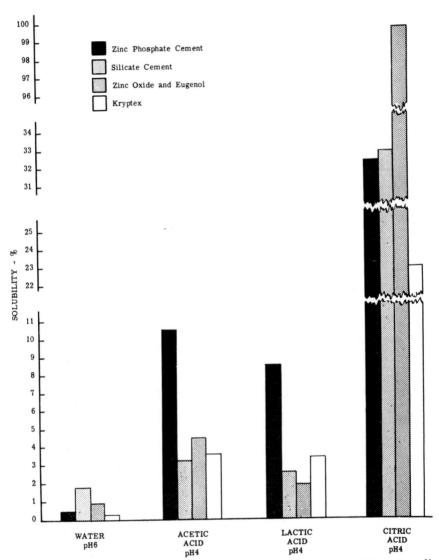

FIGURE 287. Solubility of various types of dental cement in different media. Although all show low solubility in distilled water, they are quite easily eroded in other acids that may be present in the oral cavity.

The neck of the bottle must be kept clean. Agitation of the liquid is not necessary and results only in a smeared cap. If a precipitate appears, the liquid should be thrown away. Precipitation or cloudiness in liquid may result from evaporation and from any crystallized liquid that is allowed to gather inside the cap or around the neck of the bottle. The last portion should be discarded also, because repeated opening of the bottle over a

long period of time alters the water content of the liquid through evaporation.

The importance, clinically, of careful manipulation cannot be over-
emphasized, since the present cements are the weakest link in the otherwise
strong chain of dental castings. At best they have a relatively low strength
and are somewhat soluble in mouth fluids, particularly the weak organic
acids commonly present in the oral environment (Fig. 287).[6] When handled
correctly, in conjunction with a well-fitting casting, they do their job;
however, improper manipulation of even the best commercial brands, of
which there are many, produces inferior chemical and physical properties
and invites subsequent failure.

Mixing Technique. The technique for mixing cement is easily
acquired, but it does demand attention to detail in the handling of the
materials. The main factor controlling the solubility, as well as the
strength, is the powder-liquid ratio. Solubility is directly related to the
amount of powder which can be incorporated into the liquid. The really
soluble portion of the cement is the crystalline matrix that forms around
the original particles of powder. With a greater amount of powder present
in the mix, less of this matrix will be formed and the cement will be

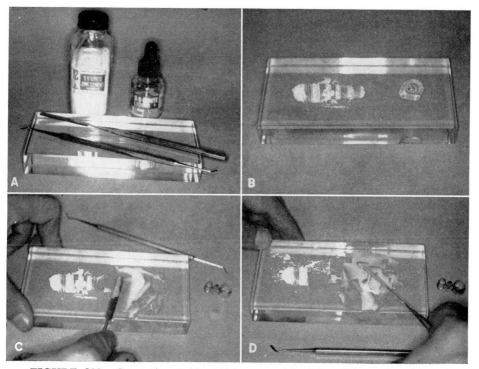

FIGURE 288. Cementing bridge with zinc phosphate cement.
A, Cement powder, liquid, slab, spatula, and instrument for applying cement.
B, Powder in separate piles, and liquid.
C, D, Mixing technique.

stronger and less soluble. Thus, for any consistency, as much powder as possible must be incorporated. Obviously, to seat a well-fitting casting, a thin mix and film of cement will be required; however, that consistency must contain a maximal amount of powder. The only way that this can be accomplished is by the use of a cool slab, approximately 60 to 75° F., although it must not be below the dew point. A warm slab will speed the chemical reaction and the cement will set before sufficient powder can be incorporated.

The mixing slab should be of heavy glass, clean, and free of scratches. When the powder is placed on the slab, it should be divided into five or six equal parts (Fig. 288). The liquid should then be measured and the first portion of powder thoroughly mixed into it. Before the second bit is added, the mass should be spatulated, using a rotary motion, until it is completely homogeneous. A good general rule is to mix each increment for approximately 20 seconds, with a total mixing time of 1½ to 2 minutes. The mix should be smooth and free of lumps or clots.

Cementing Procedure. A coating of cement is applied to the inner surfaces of the crown or retainers. After using maximal finger pressure, seating is completed using an orangewood stick or metal instrument and mallet (Fig. 289).

After the saliva ejector has been removed, a cotton roll should be folded and placed on the occlusal surface of the prosthesis and the patient should be asked to close in centric. This position is held without lateral or protrusive movement until the cement has set, which will be approximately 3 to 5 minutes. If the luting material is resin cement, any excess must be removed from the embrasures *before* setting takes place and *before* the patient is asked to close and apply pressure.

After the cement has set, the cotton rolls are removed and the patient

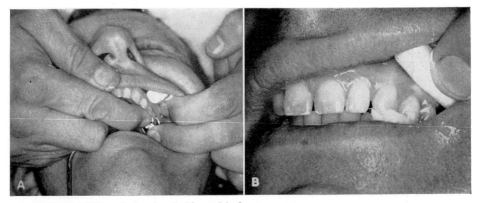

FIGURE 289. *A,* Seating bridge with finger pressure.
B, After bridge is tapped to place with a mallet and stick, patient is asked to close on cotton roll.

is permitted to rinse.* Excess cement around the margins of the retainers should now be removed, using scalers or chisels, and explorers. It must be stressed that no cement can be allowed to remain in the gingival crevices or the interproximal areas (Fig. 290). Occasionally the cement will be very hard to remove from the area just cervically to the contact. When this cannot be done with dental floss, vigorous lateral excursions by the patient will generally break the adhesion or locking of such cement fragments. After the oral cavity has been freed of debris, the occlusion should be rechecked and any corrected areas repolished.

If the abutment preparations are long and have parallel walls, it may be advantageous to drill a hole, with a No. ½ round bur, through the centers of the occlusal surfaces of the retainers to permit the cement to escape occlusally as well as cervically. After the cement has set and the bridge has been polished, a very small cavity can be prepared at the site of the occlusal perforation and the void can be filled with gold foil.

After cementation, any unfinished margins must be polished lightly

---

* Zinc phosphate cement may be considered as "set" when it is unyielding to an instrument, fractures under pressure, and has lost its surface luster.

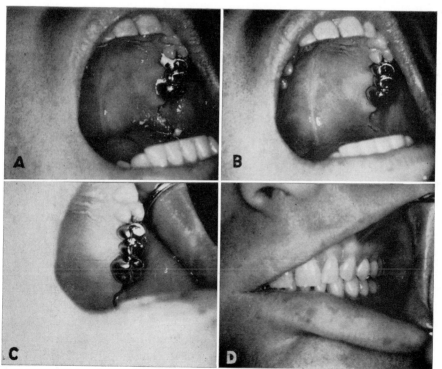

FIGURE 290. *A,* Cemented bridge before removing excess.
B, Cemented bridge—cement removed.
C, D, Two views of maxillary posterior bridge made six months after cementation. Occlusion and tissue tone are good.

with a finishing bur and flour of pumice and No. 600 Carborundum powder, applied with a revolving rubber cup.

Errors.   The most common causes of difficulty in use of zinc phosphate cement can be attributed to the use of liquid that has changed either through exposure to the atmosphere or by contamination or faulty mixing technique.

The probable causes of cement *setting too slowly* are (1) a mix that is too thin (that is, not enough powder has been incorporated); (2) a mix that has been spatulated too long (increased spatulation time increases setting time); or (3) a mix using liquid that has lost water because of improper care.

Mixing on a warm slab, insufficient spatulation time, or adding powder too rapidly will cause cement to *set too fast.*

If more powder than is needed for the mix was placed on the mixing slab, the surplus must never be returned to the bottle, as it may have come into contact with the liquid, and if so, it can influence the properties and behavior of subsequent mixes.

REMEMBER: Liquid is *never* added *to* a mix. Another mix must be made if the ratio of powder to liquid has resulted in a mix too thick for the intended use.

As previously discussed, it is recognized that zinc phosphate cement has inherent shortcomings of solubility and disintegration in oral fluids, and low strength. Furthermore, it is an acidic material that can engender pulp reaction unless adequate protection is provided for the underlying tooth structure.

Zinc Oxide-Eugenol Cement

Zinc oxide-eugenol cements are being advocated for use in the permanent cementation of fixed restorations. Certainly this type of cement has many attributes that would recommend it for such usage. It is kind to the cut dentin, adapts better to the walls of the prepared cavity than any other cement, and is less soluble in fluids present in the oral cavity. Unfortunately, it is not strong, having a compressive strength approximately one-fifth that of zinc phosphate cement. Likewise, it has poor resistance to abrasion and attrition. Contrary to popular opinion, the strength cannot be increased significantly by the addition of polystyrene. Only compounds such as ortho-ethoxy benzoic acid will markedly increase the strength, but solubility increases upon the addition of that chemical.

There is a great deal of interesting research in progress designed to develop a stronger zinc oxide-eugenol cement, but at the moment low strength still remains its recognized weakness. It is not possible to determine exactly what type of strength properties are essential in a cement that is to be used as a luting agent for the gold inlay or crown, nor is it possible to establish exactly what minimal numerical strength values are acceptable.

However, previous theories suggest that a certain minimal compressive strength is necessary in order to prevent fracture of the small cement projections which penetrate into irregularities in both the casting and tooth structure and thus tend to retain the casting. If this theory is accepted, then the use of the zinc oxide-eugenol cements that are currently available should be confined to restorations where undue stress will not be placed on the cement and where the margins would not be subject to an excessive amount of toothbrush abrasion or attrition.

There is some indication that the low strength, or some other property, does reduce the retentive powers of zinc oxide-eugenol cement. For example, approximately one-half the tensile force is required to remove inlays cemented with zinc oxide-eugenol cement as compared with those cemented with a conventional zinc phosphate cement. This would suggest that the case in which this material is to be used for permanent cementation must be carefully selected. Zinc oxide-eugenol cement may be a preferred material for cementation of the full cast crown, particularly on a tooth in which sensitivity might be a subsequent problem, since the margins in this restoration are well protected and adequate retention of the casting exists by virtue of the cavity design. On the other hand, universal use of this type of cement would be questioned in the cementation of three-quarter crown bridge retainers, because the margins in these restorations are exposed to possible abrasive action of food stuffs and tooth brushing, and the torque placed on the cement might in time lead to loss of retention.

Resin Cement

Resin cement has been introduced recently. Clinical experience to date has been mildly satisfactory, although evaluation over a still longer period of time is needed.[7]

The main advantage of this material lies in its somewhat lowered solubility.[6, 8] However, handling difficulties and lack of true adhesion to cavity walls have caused a pronounced waning in popularity.

POSTOPERATIVE TREATMENT

Whether the cemented unit be a crown or a bridge, an appointment should be scheduled within 24 to 72 hours, at which time occlusion, gingival crevices, tone of the gingival tissue, and mouth hygiene should be checked (Fig. 291). The occluding surfaces should be examined closely for premature contacts that may develop on marginal ridges, cusp planes,

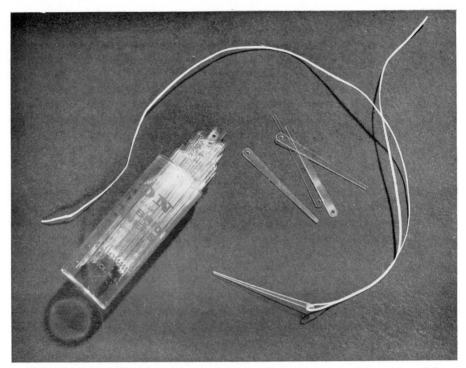

FIGURE 291. ZON Dental Bridge Cleaners. Very helpful for pulling dental floss or tape through embrasures of a bridge so floss may be moved from back to front, and also the reverse, between pontics and tissue. This is imperative in keeping surface clean and tissue healthy. (Johnson & Johnson, New Brunswick, N. J.)

or in sulci. After using articulating paper, only the shiny portion that does *not* retain a stain should be reduced with a round bur or stone. Then this reduction should be feathered into the surrounding surface. The occlusion must be checked again and the process repeated if indicated.

If, within a few days, there is complaint of soreness, sensitivity to cold or sweets, or slight sensitivity to heat, the occlusion should be checked again, because as a rule these symptoms indicate a premature contact or interference. It may be found that the occluding area must be constricted to reduce leverage, torque, or rotation, or that a cusp, marginal ridge, or sulcus must be reduced to prevent trauma in the direction of the long axis.

A few minutes should suffice to make any needed correction. However, the patient should be contacted within 48 hours to ascertain the effectiveness of the treatment. If the symptoms persist, the prosthesis and the abutment teeth should be re-examined.

At future visits crowns and bridges should be viewed critically at the cervical margins for caries, using sharp explorers or scalers. Radiographs may not disclose marginal lesions.

It appears that the profession now has three types of luting materials available, one of which, if used carefully, has established a record for adequate performance. With any one, emphasis is still on the maintenance of a dry field for seating, high standards of cavity preparation, and a meticulous fit of the casting.

REFERENCES

1. Lindquist, J. T.: A study of the intra-arch relationships in normal human dentures. Master's thesis, Indiana Univ. School Den., 1951.
2. Smith, G. P.: The marginal fit of the full cast shoulderless crown. J. Pros. Den., 7: 231, March 1957.
3. Phillips, R. W.: Cavity varnishes and bases. D. Clin. North America, March 1965, p. 159.
4. Lynn, L. M., and Ludwick, R. W., Jr.: Method to reduce pain during cementation of restorations. J.A.D.A., 53:563, Nov. 1956.
5. Skinner, E. W., and Phillips, R. W.: The Science of Dental Materials. 5th ed. Philadelphia, W. B. Saunders Company, 1960.
6. Norman, R. D., Swartz, M. L., and Phillips, R. W.: Studies on the solubility of certain dental materials. J. D. Res., 36:977, Dec. 1957.
7. Swartz, M. L., Phillips, R. W., Day, R., and Johnston, J. F.: A laboratory and clinical investigation of certain resin restorative and cementing materials. Part I. In vitro tests on adhesive characteristics. Part II. A twenty-eight month clinical evaluation of a resin cement. J. Pros. Den., 5:698, Sept. 1955.
8. Schouboe, P. J., Paffenbarger, G. C., and Sweeney, W. T.: Resin cements and posterior-type direct filling resins. J.A.D.A., 52:584, May 1956.

Baraban, D. J.: Cementation of fixed bridge prosthesis with zinc oxide-rosin-eugenol cements. J. Pros. Den., 8:988, Nov.–Dec. 1958.
Ewing, J. E.: Temporary cementation in fixed partial prosthesis. J. Pros. Den., 5:388, May 1955.
Gerson, I.: Cementation of fixed restorations. J. Pros. Den., 7:123, Jan. 1957.
Hedges, P. G.: Occlusion as it relates to fixed restorations. J. Pros. Den., 13:499, May 1963.
Schorr, L., and Clayman, L. H.: Cementing a large fixed bridge. J.A.D.A., 55:415, Sept. 1957.
Selberg, A.: A full cast crown technique. J. Pros. Den., 7:102, Jan. 1957.
Simpson, R. L.: Failures in crown and bridge prosthodontics. J.A.D.A., 47:154 Aug. 1953.
Sullivan, E. J.: Cementation and esthetic problems in crown and bridge procedures. J.A.D.A., 51:34, July 1955.

19

THE VENEERED GOLD CROWN

A veneered gold crown is a full cast crown having the labial or buccal surface and portions of the proximal surfaces faced with fused porcelain or resin. It may be used as a single-unit restoration or as a bridge retainer. In its capacity to harmonize with natural teeth, a veneered gold crown is inferior only to the jacket crown (Fig. 292).

To achieve this harmony and to maintain a healthy gingiva, it must be kept within the confines of the form, contour, and dimensions of the original tooth. There are exceptions when the malposition of a tooth, or the excessive width or narrowing of an edentulous space, cannot be improved by orthodontic intervention. However, the effect of altered contour on the health of the gingival tissues and the possibility of damage to the supporting structures by increased forces due to changes in occlusal form or by an increase mesially or distally in incisal width must be carefully appraised.[1]

The major items of concern associated with the construction of veneered crowns and bridges are

(1) tooth preparation;

(2) making castings which have fit, smoothness, minimal porosity, and resistance to deformation;

(3) building crowns to normal tooth form;

(4) matching human tooth shades;

(5) assembly of bridge units;

(6) durability; and

(7) maintenance or repair.

The extension of the veneer will be governed by

(1) the esthetic requirements of the individual case;

(2) whether porcelain or resin is to be used for the veneer;

(3) the relationship of the tooth to be restored with the adjacent teeth;

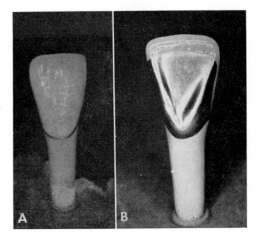

FIGURE 292. *A,* Labial view of porcelain veneered gold crown.
B, Lingual view.

(4) occlusion; and
(5) the amount that the tooth can be reduced.

INDICATIONS

The objective of any operative procedure on a tooth is, essentially, the conservation of tooth structure.[2] If this concept is accepted, the veneered gold crown cannot be considered a conservative restoration, since with it maximal tooth reduction and maximal contact with gingival tissue occur.[3, 4] Nevertheless, it is indicated on any tooth when a full crown is justified from a restorative or preventive standpoint, when it can be made to harmonize with its environment or its application will enhance esthetics, when maximal retention is needed and can be obtained, and when function will be assured.[5, 6]

The veneered gold crown may be used on any vital tooth if, after the cervical shoulder has been prepared, there is enough coronal dentin to resist fracture. It also can be used on a pulpless tooth[7] if a post can be placed in the root canal to support a cast core, or if the tooth can be rebuilt otherwise to prepared form. It may be substituted for either the porcelain or the resin jacket crown when the jacket might be broken or abraded in a short time owing to the occlusion, or when the length or shape of the tooth to be restored is such that only a well-fitting metal restoration will have prolonged retention.

CONTRAINDICATIONS

The veneered gold crown is contraindicated on a tooth with a pulp of a size that makes it impossible to prepare the tooth correctly, and on a tooth with a very short clinical crown, which will have insufficient retention and stability when it is reduced to allow space for metal and porcelain or resin.[8]

PREPARATION OF THE TOOTH

The problems of tooth preparation can be diminished in four ways:

(1) by close study of the radiographs and casts and an evaluation of possibilities;

(2) by recognition of the form and depth of the reduction needed in the prepared tooth crown to secure retention and permit reproduction of normal tooth contour and bulk of material for shading;

(3) by remembering that exposed labial and proximal contours may decrease very rapidly in diameter just inside the gingival crevice; and

(4) by realizing that insulted gingival and periodontal tissues do not always repair perfectly.

A certain bulk, at least as much as is needed for a porcelain or resin jacket crown, is necessary to produce the requisite color and translucence in a porcelain veneer or the desired shade in an acrylic or epoxy resin veneer. The preparation will be a combination of the jacket crown and the full veneer gold crown preparations if compatible form and color and a minimal display of gold are to ensue.[9, 10, 11]

To determine the receptivity of a given anterior tooth to a preparation for a veneered crown, the following factors must be assessed:

(1) length of clinical crown inciso-cervically;

(2) labio-lingual bulk in the incisal one-third;

(3) presence or lack of a well-defined cingulum;

(4) convexity of the labio-cervical enamel fold;

(5) width of the pulp horns in relation to mesio-distal width of the neck of the tooth;

(6) relation of the pulp to the incisal edge of the tooth;

(7) estimated relation of the pulp to the labial surface;

(8) position of contact areas (labially or lingually to normal position);

(9) depth of gingival crevice;

(10) incisal curves of gingival crevice on mesial and distal surfaces; and

(11) direction of dictated path of insertion.

Factors 1, 2, and 3 must be considered together if the tooth is to be used for a bridge abutment because of the necessity for a preparation which will resist torque and leverage. Inciso-cervically, the finished preparation should be more than half the length of the seated restoration and also should have metal encircling the cingulum without a shoulder encircling the tooth. On a short tooth or one that is thin in the incisal half, the stump generally will be incapable of resisting dislodging forces because of the incisal reduction needed for the framework and the porcelain incisal.

When there is no exposed convex cingulum, or when it is not expedient to expose it, a finishing line must be formed in the sulcus, and stability and retention obtained by two pinholes in the lingual (or cervical) third of the surface, parallel to the path of insertion and 1.5 mm. deep. If the stump is very short because of form or original measurement, these two pinholes, plus two others much closer to the incisal edge, will retain the casting following cementation. A No. 701 bur should be used for the holes whenever tooth and pulp size permit.

The mesio-distal measurement of the pulp horns may make the tooth impractical for a veneered crown preparation, especially if the neck is constricted. The tooth must be reduced enough for the crown to have shade and bulk without altering embrasure form, which may not be feasible if there has been no pulp recession. If such reduction is impossible, a veneered crown should not be used.

In order for an anterior veneered crown to be well constructed, there must be a clearance of 2.0 mm. along the incisal edge. This requirement eliminates some teeth which have pulp chambers irregular in contour and pulp horns extending quite far incisally.

The proximity of the pulp to the labial surface cannot be demonstrated radiographically but must be estimated. The probability that the pulp is too close to the labial surface for proper depth in the preparation of this area should be weighed, because labial exposures of the pulp are not uncommon. While endodontics is a valuable adjunct to restorative dentistry, every effort should be made to avoid it. The greatest possibilities for maximal service are still to be found with the use of vital teeth.

The more shallow the gingival crevice and the more convex incisally the proximal curves of the cervical line, the more difficult it is to prepare a tooth for a veneered crown with the expectation for satisfactory long range appearance. There is an alarming tendency, when using an ultraspeed handpiece, to make a flat labio-lingual seat on a veneer preparation at the immediate expense of proximal gingival and supporting tissue, and a heightened prospect of gingival tissue recession.

Protracted observation of cases in which preparations have been extended cervically to meet or go beyond the periodontal attachment has convinced the authors that this is bad practice, whether it be labially, lingually, or proximally. Regardless of the depth of the crevice or the area, 1.0 mm. under the gingival crest is far enough for any preparation, and 0.5 mm. will suffice for most. The extension of the preparation apically should not exceed one-half the depth of the crevice, especially if it is shallow.

Casts should be analyzed with a surveying instrument to determine a path of insertion most compatible to all abutments and to the criteria just set forth.

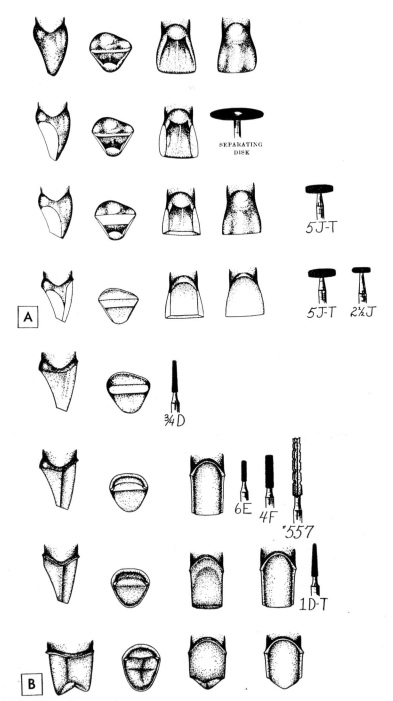

FIGURE 293.   Preparation.

A, Top to bottom: Uncut tooth; mesial and distal surfaces; incisal edge (this can pre-cede or follow reduction of labial and lingual surfaces); labial and lingual reduction.

B, Top to bottom: Corners rounded (if band impression will be used, band should be fitted at this point); shoulder prepared; all angles rounded and finishing line established. Preparation on a maxillary bicuspid.

Using Conventional Speeds

The steps in the preparation of either an anterior or posterior tooth are
(1) reduction of the mesial and distal surfaces,
(2) reduction of the buccal and lingual surfaces, and
(3) reduction of the incisal edge or occlusal surface (the order of 1 through 3 is not important);
(4) elimination of angles so that the cervical finishing line at this time has continuity and lies at or just under the gingiva;
(5) preparation of a cervical shoulder on the labial or buccal half; and
(6) modification of angles and smoothing irregularities. (See Figs. 293 and 294.)

Mesial and Distal Surfaces. The mesial and distal surfaces should be reduced with a disk, using the straight handpiece for better control. Started on or just inside the marginal ridges, these cuts must be carried cervically to the gingival line, or if the gingival line has receded, just beyond the cementoenamel junction, following the planes of the surfaces bucco-lingually. One proximal cut should be parallel to the path of insertion or converge only a few degrees toward the occlusal surface or incisal edge. The other must be compatible and should supply as much mechanical retention as is possible from the inclination of the tooth.

Buccal and Lingual Surfaces. The buccal and lingual surfaces are reduced in the same way as for a full veneer gold crown, except that the buccal must be cut deeper and be more convex in the occlusal half. Extension should be to the gingival line.

Incisal Edge or Occlusal Surface, and Axial Angles. A wheel stone is used for the reduction of the incisal edge, and wheel, inverted cone, and knife-edge stones and fissure burs for the occlusal surface. The preparation on the occlusal should duplicate roughly the contours of the original surface, except that the buccal cusp or the labio-incisal dimension should be shortened not less than 2.0 mm. The lingual cusp and marginal ridge areas should have clearance of at least 1.0 mm. in all excursions. The four walls are then connected at the axial angles to form a line at, and following the height of, the gingival crest, using sandpaper disks, a long taper diamond, or flat surface or concave diamonds. For a crown that is to be veneered with resin, incisal clearance need not be more than 1.2 mm.

At this point a copper band should be trimmed, marked for position, and laid aside if such an impression is to be taken.

The Shoulder. To make shading with normal contour possible, there must be a cervical shoulder (a chamfer is not sufficient) on the labial or buccal half or four-sevenths of the tooth. Terminations of the shoulder will be controlled by the width of the embrasure, the presence or absence of an interdental papilla, and the position of the tooth (i.e. labioversion, torsiversion, etc.). Almost always, however, to conceal the metal framework

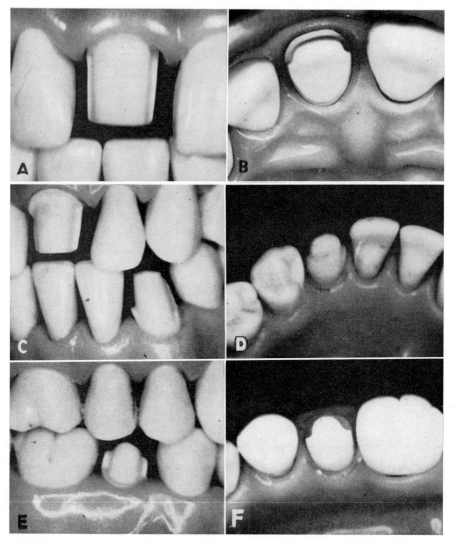

FIGURE 294.   Preparations suitable for cast gold crowns with bonded porcelain veneers.

A, Maxillary central incisor, labial view.

B, Maxillary central incisor, incisal view.

C, Maxillary central and mandibular cuspid; note extension of shoulders into inter-proximals on central and mesial of cuspid.

D, Mandibular cuspid, incisal view.

E, Mandibular bicuspid, buccal view.

F, Mandibular bicuspid, occlusal view.

effectively, this terminal point should be beneath or slightly lingual to the center of the contact area (Fig. 295).

The shoulder should be the same width as the diameter of a No. 557 bur, or approximately 0.7 mm., but if the tooth is large or if the pulp has receded, it can be as wide as 1.0 mm. This will entail further cutting in the cervical one-half or one-third, which may be done with a No. 557, 556, or end-cutting bur, or with a cylindrical or taper stone. Conversely, on small teeth or on those with constricted necks the shoulder may have to be less than 0.7 mm., which can create problems in shading the veneer. On each side it should end abruptly in a half-groove made parallel to the cervical half of the labial or buccal contour of the prepared tooth, even if it opens lingually to the incisal edge on an anterior tooth. It is important that the shoulder be just as wide at its proximal termination as it is on the labial surface so that the veneering material may have thickness for shade and contour in that area.

The shoulder and the remaining proximal and lingual margins should be extended uniformly at least 0.5 mm. under the gingiva. The chamfered cervical finishing line on the lingual should connect the mesial and distal of the shoulder, at the same time rounding the lingual angles. It should be made with a tapered, round-point stone.

On mandibular cuspids and first bicuspids, the mesial shoulder can be extended lingually onto the cingulum or lingual surface so that the metal frame will be hidden by the approximating tooth. The curvatures of the reduced labial or buccal surface should approximate the contour of the uncut surface until the preparation approaches the incisal or occlusal third, where it must curve more sharply toward the lingual surface. This must be rechecked after the shoulder is completed.

Using Accelerated Speeds

When using accelerated speeds, it is good judgment for the novice or the operator who makes veneered gold crown preparations infrequently

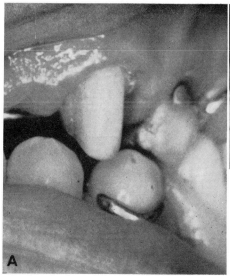

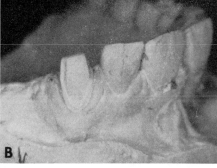

FIGURE 295. *A,* Maxillary cuspid prepared.

B, Cast of prepared maxillary cuspid. Shoulder on mesial extended lingually.

to reduce a contacting surface with a disk, since in this way there is less chance of scarring an approximating tooth. An opening made with a disk should be wide enough so that in cutting the tooth circumferentially with a No. 1D Densco diamond stone or a 700 R&R carbide it can pass freely through the opening. These are satisfactory rotating cutting instruments for use on all axial walls.

Anterior Teeth

Complete circumferential reduction of an anterior tooth may be completed using a No. 1D Densco diamond or 700 R&R carbide (or similar instruments of other companies), or the contact with an approximating tooth may be opened with a disk. If the diamond or the carbide is used, cutting may start on the labial surface as close as possible to an approximating tooth, and the reduction should be away from this tooth to the depth desired and should be extended across the tooth until the other contact area is approached.

The contact and proximal surface are cut with the stone, following a plane just inside the peripheral layer of enamel. Next the cervical area of the cingulum is reduced, and then the prepared surfaces are connected by cutting through the second contact area, again just inside the enamel surface. Fortunately, mesial and distal contours of anterior teeth are such that proximal surfaces may be reduced parallel to each other without extending the cuts cervically beyond the gingival line, and without forming shoulders on the mesial and distal surfaces.

The incisal edge is now shortened with a wheel stone to a clearance of 2.0 mm., making the cut surface at a right angle to the principal line of force directed against it. Many times this step is executed before circumferential cutting is begun. The incisal half of the remaining labial surface is checked to see that the contour has slightly more convexity than existed on the previously uncut surface. The remaining lingual is prepared with a round or round-edge wheel stone (123 SSW or 3½J Densco diamond) to have a minimal clearance in any position of not less than 0.6 mm.

The labial shoulder is cut with a cylindrical diamond, a carbide bur, or a conventional steel bur. On mandibular incisors, because of limited bulk, it may be impossible to cut the shoulder deeper than 0.4 or 0.5 mm., in which case the cutting instrument should be a No. 556 bur, or one of similar size.

Bicuspids and Molars

Reduction should start at the tip of the buccal or lingual cusp with a 1D diamond or a small torpedo-type stone, and at this point should be made approximately 1.0 mm. in depth, roughly following the contours of the buccal and lingual surfaces. Reduction should feather out at the gingival line on all surfaces and should stop at the gingival crest. The same stone or a larger cylindrical diamond or carbide bur can be used on the occlusal surface. The buccal shoulder may be made with a small cylindrical diamond, with a carbide bur, or a carbon steel bur. If the tooth is rotated, the shoulder should be cut farther lingually on the proximal surface which is exposed.

Connecting the proximal terminations of the shoulder around the lingual surface, the chamfered finishing line should be made with a round-point diamond or carbide bur. To facilitate impression-taking and pattern-investing, the sharp angles at the proximal margins of the grooves may be softened slightly.

Five programs of instrumentation for this preparation follow:

Table 19

INSTRUMENT	TO BE ACCOMPLISHED	R.P.M.
71L Premier "Ela" carbide	Peripheral reduction except lingual of anteriors. Occlusal or incisal reduction. Buccal or labial shoulder grossly outlined.	150,000
3½J Densco diamond	Lingual surface reduction of anteriors.	8,000 to 10,000
1D Densco diamond	Irregularities smoothed and angles rounded.	8,000 to 10,000
701 or 702 Premier "Ela" carbide	Shoulder positioned cervically and made square.	5,000

Table 20

INSTRUMENT	TO BE ACCOMPLISHED	R.P.M.
700 or 701 R&R carbide	Complete peripheral and incisal or occlusal reduction.	150,000
123 SSW diamond	Convex lingual surface reduction.	150,000
557 SSW steel bur	Shoulder extended into gingival crevice.	6,000
1D-T Densco diamond	Lingual chamfer extended into gingival crevice.	150,000
Sandpaper disks (any brand)	Irregularities smoothed and angles rounded.	6,000

Table 21

INSTRUMENT	TO BE ACCOMPLISHED	R.P.M.
1D or 2D Densco diamond	Peripheral reduction of posteriors. Labial, proximal, and incisal reduction of anteriors.	150,000 to 200,000
123 SSW diamond	Occlusal reduction of posteriors. Lingual reduction of anteriors.	150,000 to 200.000
701 SSW carbide	Buccal or labial shoulder.	150,000 to 200,000
1D-T Densco diamond (worn) or 44 SSW carborundum stone	Irregularities smoothed.	4,000

Table 22

INSTRUMENT	TO BE ACCOMPLISHED	R.P.M.
701 R&R carbide	Buccal, lingual, and occlusal reduction.	150.000 to 200,000
700 or 699 R&R carbide	Mesial and distal reduction.	150.000 to 200,000
1D-T or 1D-C Densco diamond	Location and contour of cervical margin.	150,000 to 200,000
170L SSW carbide	Finish labial or buccal surface and shoulder.	150,000 to 200,000

Table 23

INSTRUMENT	TO BE ACCOMPLISHED	R.P.M.
701 or 701-L Densco carbide	Occlusal or incisal reduction. Peripheral reduction of posteriors. Labial and proximal reduction of anteriors. Gross outline of shoulder.	150,000
1½J Densco diamond	Lingual reduction of anteriors.	150,000
¾D or 1D Densco diamond	Irregularities smoothed. Location and contour of cervical margin. Shoulder finished.	150,000
Sandpaper disks (any brand)	Preparation smoothed.	600

CONTROLLED DEPTH IN THE PREPARATION
OF A TOOTH FOR A VENEERED GOLD CROWN

Baker and Kondon[12] have devised a technique for pre-establishing and controlling the depth of cutting when preparing a tooth for a veneered or a coping crown. A Densco No. 330 carbide bur, which has a cutting head 1.5 mm. long, is used as a depth gauge for the initial steps (Fig. 296). Subsequent cutting may be done with the instrument of choice.

For a single tooth, the long axis is generally used to survey the buccal surface for the height of contour and the path of insertion of the crown. Before making multiple crown preparations for bridges or splinting, a common path of insertion must be selected for all the teeth and used for surveying the height of contour for each tooth that is to receive a veneered crown. At the height-of-contour survey line (not the gingival margin), the Densco 330 bur is used to make a cut mesio-distally like a Class V cavity, using the head of the bur as a guide for depth. The vertical portion of the "T" is made occlusally or incisally from this initial cut, maintaining an even depth in all areas of 1.5 mm. (Fig. 297).

The bur may then be used to cut across the cusps and into the occlusal grooves to ensure the same depth in the occlusal reduction.

The width of the finished shoulder at the gingival level is a result

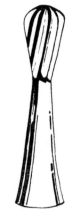

FIGURE 296.   No. 330 Densco carbide bur.

FIGURE 297.   Diagram of mesio-distal and "T" cuts. (Courtesy of Drs. R. E. Baker and P. N. Kondon, Tufts University School of Dental Medicine.)

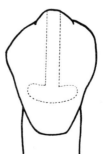
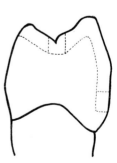

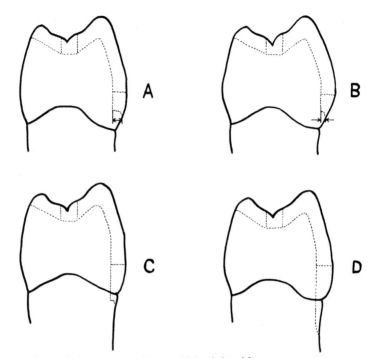

FIGURE 298. *A, B,* Contour affects width of shoulder.
C, D, Bulk of tooth affects length of preparation.
(Courtesy of Drs. R. E. Baker and P. N. Kondon, Tufts University School of Dental Medicine.)

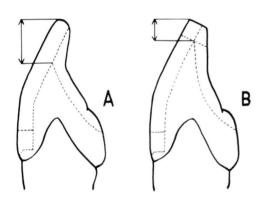

FIGURE 299.
(Courtesy of Drs. R. E. Baker and P. N. Kondon, Tufts University School of Dental Medicine.)

of the following factors and not necessarily the depth of the 1.5 mm. cut:

(1) the contour of the buccal surface of the tooth, curved or flat (Fig. 298*A* and *B*);

(2) the amount of gingival recession (Fig. 298*C* and *D*); and

(3) the path of insertion selected in multiple crown preparations for fixed prostheses.

Another favorable aspect of this technique is the amount of incisal

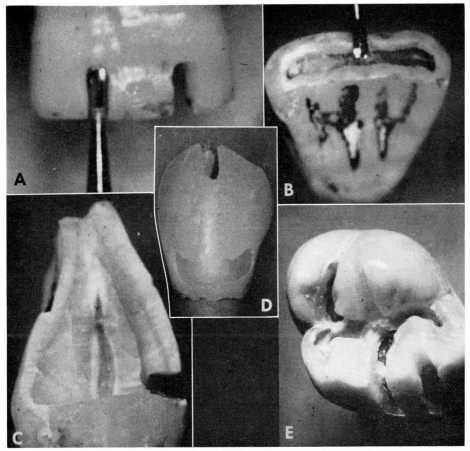

FIGURE 300. *A*, Cutting through incisal edge of maxillary central incisor with No. 330 Densco carbide bur.

B, Cutting into labial surface of central incisor.

C, Cut into labial height of contour showing its relationship to depth of enamel and to pulp chamber.

D, "T" cut on buccal and through buccal cusp of bicuspid.

E, Preliminary cuts on surfaces of molar. These guide further reduction of surfaces in preparation of tooth for veneered crown. All cuts are same depth as cutting portion of No. 330 bur. (Courtesy of Drs. R. E. Baker and P. N. Kondon, Tufts University School of Dental Medicine.)

reduction on anterior teeth and the manner in which it occurs. The minimal reduction is 1.5 mm.; the maximal reduction depends on the shape of the tooth. The labial portion is grooved to a depth of 1.5 mm. incisally from the height of contour. This is extended through the incisal edge. The lingual surface is reduced 1.0 mm. down to the cingulum, which is preserved for retention. As can be seen in Fig. 299*A* and *B*, a greater incisal reduction will occur on a long thin tooth than on a thick or worn tooth.

REFERENCES

1. Wheeler, R. C.: Complete crown form and the periodontium. J. Pros. Den., *11*:722, July–Aug. 1961.
2. Nuttall, E. B.: Personal communication.
3. Johnston, J. F., Mumford, G., and Dykema, R. W.: Porcelain veneers bonded to metal castings. Practical Dental Monographs. Chicago, Year Book Medical Publishers, Inc., March 1963.
4. Kahn, A. E.: Partial versus full coverage. J. Pros. Den., *10*:167, Jan.–Feb. 1960.
5. Wilson, W. H., and Lang, R. L.: Practical Crown and Bridge Prosthodontics. New York, McGraw-Hill Book Company, Inc., 1962.
6. Miller, C. J.: Inlays, Crowns and Bridges. Philadelphia, W. B. Saunders Company, 1962.
7. Abramson, I.: Role of endodontics in crown and bridge prosthesis. J. Maryland D. A., *1*:28, No. 1, 1958.
8. Hagerman, D. A., and Arnim, S. S.: Relation of new knowledge of the gingiva to crown and bridge procedures. J. Pros. Den., *5*:538, July 1955.
9. Dykema, R. W., Johnston, J. F., and Cunningham, D. M.: The veneered gold crown. D. Clin. North America, Nov. 1958, p. 653.
10. Brecker, S. C.: Crowns. Philadelphia, W. B. Saunders Company, 1961.
11. Pincus, C. L.: Esthetic variations in jacket crowns and bridge restorations involving periodontal and other deformities. Its application to oral rehabilitation. New York J. Den., *24*:132, March 1954 (Abstract).
12. Baker, R. E., and Kondon, P. N.: Personal communication.

Meadows, T. R.: Clinical comparison of cast gold crowns with acrylic and with fused porcelain veneer facings. J.A.D.A., *66*:772, June 1963.

20

PORCELAINS AND PORCELAIN FURNACES

For many years fused porcelain has been recognized as a restorative material that is compatible with oral soft tissues and that has superior esthetic qualities. Even though it is extremely friable and does not produce a mechanically sound restoration under an adverse occlusion, it has enjoyed continuing and growing popularity in the construction of jacket and veneered crowns and bridge pontics.

The Composition of Porcelain

Porcelain is formed by mixing and firing minerals, principally feldspar, kaolin, and quartz, plus fluxing substances and pigments.

Feldspar is a double silicate of aluminum and potassium, and at the normal firing temperatures for dental porcelains fuses and acts as a matrix, binding the small, irregularly shaped refractory crystals of kaolin and quartz together. It makes the porcelain vitreous and translucent when fired. Feldspar functions as a flux and surface glaze as well as a matrix.

Kaolin is a hydrated aluminum silicate resulting from the decomposition of feldspathic minerals. The name often is given to any porcelain clay that does not discolor when fired. The greater the quantity of kaolin, the more the opacity of the porcelain is increased.

Quartz imparts stiffness and hardness to the mass during and after firing. It acts as a refractory skeleton for the contracting kaolin and feldspar.

Fluxes are added to increase fluidity of the mixture and to absorb or remove certain objectionable impurities. Sodium and potassium carbonates, borax, glass, and occasionally lead oxide, are used. The fusing point of a porcelain may be varied by the quantity of flux incorporated.

The *pigments* used to color porcelain may be oxides of tin, nickel, cobalt, titanium, chromium, iron, or gold, or metallic gold and platinum. Fluorescence, as well as shade, may be a product of the pigmenting materials.

Porcelain Reactions to Firing

During the firing cycle in the construction of a crown all porcelains must go through several phases of physical changes. First is the biscuit stage, in which very little shrinkage has occurred; the mass is an opaque white with no color sheen, and it is easily contaminated by oil from the fingers or by other debris that may penetrate the excessively porous surface. Usually this stage is ignored in the laboratory. The porcelain is brought to a low maturity, erroneously referred to as a "high biscuit." Next is maturity, or vitrification, which may be divided into low, medium, and high phases. Third is a state of glaze. Fourth is coalescence, or the formation of an overglazed and rounded form.

Maturity will be recognized when true color and translucence can be seen, when shrinkage has occurred, and when there is a slight sheen on the surface of the porcelain. The degree of sheen and translucence will depend on the extent of maturity.

The state of glaze brings a light-reflecting luster to the surface. This stage may also be divided into low, medium, and high. Low is just over the border from maturity and might be esthetically desirable in some mouths. However, a low-glaze porcelain can be vulnerable to water sorption, which from a hygienic standpoint would be undesirable.[1] A medium glaze will be suitable in the majority of mouths. A high glaze is to be avoided, because it is very close to coalescence and results in an abnormal sheen, rounded corners, and loss of detail.

Porcelains may be divided into low- and high-fusing. Low-fusing porcelain is one that fuses under 1945° F., or the melting point of pure gold; high-fusing porcelain is one that fuses above 1945° F. The available commercial subdivisions are low (1600 to 2000° F.), medium (2000 to 2300° F.), and high (above 2300° F.) A high-fusing porcelain surpasses one in the low-fusing range in that the fusing temperature is not as critical, and staining, glazing, and repairing are easier, especially if done after the form, contact, and occlusion have been established. However, the many merits of some low-fusing porcelains should not be ignored.

Low-, medium-, and high-fusing dental porcelains are made for both air and vacuum firing. The most recent category includes those manufactured for the purpose of being bonded to metal structures. These also come in low and medium firing ranges and for both atmosphere and vacuum firing.

Air-Fired Porcelain

Air-fired porcelain has excellent physical properties, which are clinically comparable to those of vacuum-fired porcelain. Porcelain fired in atmosphere does have many air spaces between the particles to interfere with, or "scatter," light transmission.[2] Entrapped air or gas within a jacket or veneer creates or increases opacity.

Vacuum-Fired Porcelain

Vacuum-fired porcelain has some characteristics that differ from those of air-fired porcelain. It has certain claimed superiorities, some justified and some academic. There is a general increase in the strength of the porcelain, which probably is more significant in jacket crowns than bonded veneers.

The porcelain will have greater translucence. Almost without exception, vacuum-fired porcelains have an opaque shade to match each body shade, and this close match in color reduces variation in shade when the thickness of the veneer varies from area to area.[3]

When building a vacuum-fired jacket crown, it is necessary to cover the platinum matrix with an opaque. This is an integral part of the crown, and, as with the veneer, should duplicate or harmonize with the plotted shade pattern.

It is easier to obtain a smooth, nonpitted surface on the glazed porcelain. There will be more uniformity in color when several operators are using the same porcelain. Porcelain for vacuum firing can have a finer and graded particle size, thus increasing the wet strength of the material and making it less difficult to carve a built-up mass.

Shade is markedly affected by vacuum firing, and formulas must be worked out by each practitioner through experimentation. The lessened number of air spaces decreases the internal reflective surfaces. Thus, with opacity reduced and density increased, it becomes impossible to reproduce precisely the shades made with air firing.

The Furnace

The furnace has three important parts: the control system, the indicating system, and the heat chamber. The control system, or transformer, regulates the amount of electrical energy passing through the heating element, which in turn determines the amount of heat generated in the muffle. There can be fluctuations due to the amount of current usage on the lines. These are often seasonal, or they may vary depending on the time of day, which reduces the effectiveness and accuracy of automatic furnaces.

The pyrometer is a warning system in that it indicates the temperature within the muffle. It does *not* decide when the work is completed. The

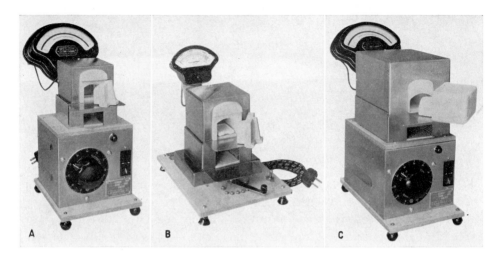

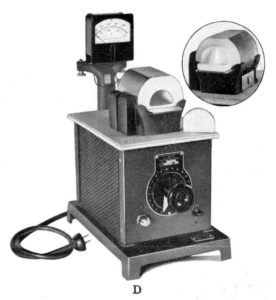

FIGURE 301. Furnaces.
A, B, C, Huppert.
D, S. S. White.

degree or extent of firing must be judged visually by reflected light, not by the temperature indicated by the pyrometer. Owing to its usual location close to or on top of the muffle, fluctuation in the temperature of the pyrometer itself leads to erratic readings. Pyrometers can be adjusted easily, and all should be checked routinely. If adjustment cannot be made to within 50 degrees of accuracy at 2300° F., then the instrument should be returned to the factory for examination.

In the muffle, heating is by convection and radiation. In vacuum firing, heating is predominately by radiation. Heating elements may be exposed or surrounded by refractory substances. Each furnace muffle develops its own spot or area of highest heat, and that spot can be at any place in the interior of the muffle. The major factors for premature burn-out of muffles are (1) too-rapid heating for the first 1000° F. (heating should be 50° F. per minute); (2) too-rapid or forced cooling of the muffle; or (3) firing over 2500° F. (just one such instance can reduce by one-half the potential life of the muffle). A new muffle, or one that has been repaired, should be degassed at 2450° F. from 2 to 4 minutes before the insertion of any porcelain ware.

Inside the muffle will be seen a protruding thermocouple, the end of which must be welded. A thermocouple is a combination of two dissimilar wires that generates a current as the welded end is heated. This current is then translated into temperature on the pyrometer. Various combinations of metals are used, depending on the temperature to which they are to be subjected. For high-fusing porcelain work, the wires are pure platinum and alloys of platinum; for low-temperature furnaces, the wires are base metal alloys. For the thermocouple to register the heat within the muffle accurately, it must be parallel to the roof. When checking temperature for accuracy, gold foil or a Tempil* pellet should be placed directly under the tip of the thermocouple. The pyrometer reading should always be correct for the highest temperature at which the furnace will be used.

Furnaces for vacuum firing are considerably more complex in design than those for air firing (Fig. 302). The furnaces available vary in the

* Tempil Corp., New York, N. Y.

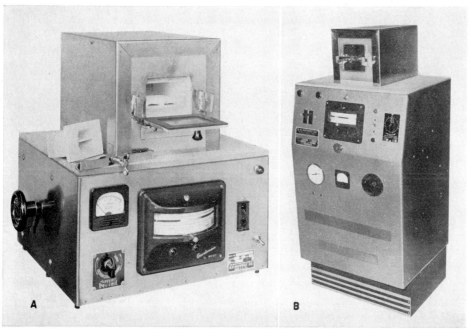

FIGURE 302. Vacuum furnaces (Huppert).

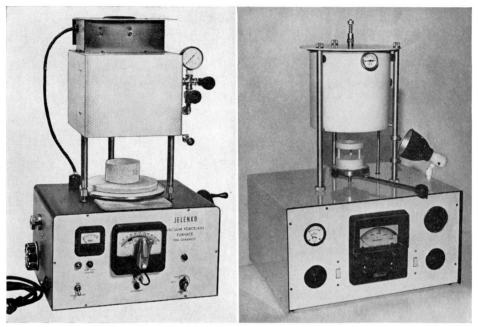

Fig. 303   Fig. 304

FIGURE 303.   Jelenko vacuum porcelain furnace.
FIGURE 304.   Dentsply Biomat porcelain furnace.

degree of automation and also in the orientation of the muffle. Furnaces that have vertical muffles, such as those manufactured by Jelenko* (Fig. 303) and Dentists' Supply Company† (Fig. 304), require lower firing temperatures than those with horizontal muffles, irrespective of whether they are being used for air or vacuum firing.

REFERENCES

1. Pettrow, J. N.: Practical factors in building and firing characteristics of dental porcelain. J. Pros. Den., *11*:334, March–April, 1961.
2. Vines, R. F., and Semmelman, J. O.: Densification of dental porcelain. J. D. Res., *36*:950, Dec. 1957.
3. Mumford, G.: Personal communication.

Hodson, J. T.: Preliminary study of dental porcelains. J. South. California D. A., *26*:334, Sept. 1958.
Hodson, J. T.: Some physical properties of three dental porcelains. J. Pros. Den., *9*:325, March–April, 1959.

* J. F. Jelenko & Co., Inc., New Rochelle, N. Y.
† The Dentists' Supply Company, York, Penna.

21

ESTHETIC CRITERIA IN A PORCELAIN RESTORATION

Three components of any porcelain restoration—form, surface characteristics, and color—are complementary to one another esthetically. Their importance to the success of a crown or veneer lies approximately in the order stated.[1]

Peripheral Form

A faithful duplication of the form of the patient's natural dentition generally leads to the most acceptable end result. While occasionally an increase or diminution in over-all size of the tooth is mandatory, the basic curves and angles present in the outline form should remain the same. The restoration should be viewed from one angle and the silhouette made to conform. The direction is then changed and the process repeated. This is done from the right side, front, left side, lingual, and incisal; if each stage is performed capably, the ultimate contour will be correct. It is almost impossible to arrive at this ideal form if the crown is shaped in a haphazard manner.

The working cast must record in detail the surfaces of the adjacent teeth, particularly in the embrasures, as little as possible of the cast representing the gingival tissue being removed. Areas that must receive concentrated consideration are the mesial and distal incisal angles, the concavities and convexities at the labial line angles in the gingival third of the crown, and the thickness of the incisal edge labio-lingually.

Causes and Effects of Gross Dimensions

Development of pleasing form in a veneered crown is absolutely dependent on sufficient reduction of tooth structure and the formation of a metal framework without excessive bulk in either the cervical collar or the incisal third. A great many veneered units have inordinate mesio-distal width in the cervical half because of shoulders that are too narrow, or that were not extended far enough into the proximal embrasures, or because a chamfer was substituted for the shoulder. The same situation may ensue, even though the tooth was correctly prepared, if the metal framework was made or left too thick in the labial half.

Crowns often have an exaggerated labial or buccal convexity inciso-cervically in the cervical half because of too little reduction of the tooth and too much metal. Incisal edges are frequently too thick labio-lingually, for the same reasons. Heavy incisal edges are especially obvious in mandibular incisors and from some angles in the uppers too, and they should be avoided for esthetic reasons even if function is not disturbed. All these abnormalities detract seriously from appearance.[2]

It may be out of the question to make a shoulder of desirable width on a small tooth. To compensate, the metal framework for a veneered crown can be made quite thin on the labial half, dispensing with the labial collar, the porcelain veneer to be built against the tooth itself in the manner of a porcelain jacket crown. This technique is also a good one to employ when the gingival crevice is shallow or when recession makes it impracticable to extend the preparation apically to meet the gingival tissue.

It should be remembered and emphasized that almost all teeth have flat or concave triangular areas at the cementoenamel junction on the proximal surfaces, with the apex of the triangle pointing toward and just under the contact. When a restoration is built that adds to the tooth contour in these proximal portions, the gingival tissue is displaced, probably both buccally and lingually, is abnormally stimulated during incising and mastication, and frequently reacts adversely.

The visual effect of overcontoured crowns is one of crowding, of a mass of material, and an accentuation of the darkness sometimes associated with embrasures. Overcontouring crowns on the labial surfaces in the cervical half or third makes the teeth appear too prominent, overprotects gingival tissue, and gives an appearance of grossness. This oddity in form does not change the contour of the lip while it is in repose but it creates a situation which is very noticeable when the patient is laughing or speaking.

Surface Characteristics

A tooth smoother than normal will give an impression of larger size, and the converse is also true. A glassy porcelain surface is always incompatible with enamel. Overprominent, exaggerated, and unnatural ridges and grooves on the labial surface of a veneered crown, doubtless associated with the forms of denture teeth and facings, add nothing to the beauty of a restoration and are seldom found on a human tooth.

Copying the heights of contour and existing irregularities on the surfaces of adjacent or corresponding teeth is recommended, although some latitude exists. Heights of contour are those areas from which a maximal amount of light is reflected. Vertical highlights suggest greater length, horizontal highlights an illusion of width. Changes in contour and the resulting highlights can be used to alter the apparent long-axis inclination of a tooth. For example, a vertical highlight running from near the mesio-incisal angle of an incisor toward the disto-gingival angle will suggest that the tooth has a mesial tilt.[3]

It is often obligatory to contour wax, resin, or the biscuited restoration in the patient's mouth, examining the moistened surface and comparing it with the adjacent teeth. This procedure is most significant when a single crown is to be placed among natural teeth. When a pair of central incisors or six anterior teeth in one arch are being restored, the dentist's knowledge of natural tooth morphology becomes of paramount importance.[4]

Color and Light

To make a veneer simulate the appearance characteristics, texture, and color of a tooth can be difficult, and matching natural teeth may be almost an impossibility. This stems from the fact that teeth are composed of a layer of enamel, usually translucent, which overlies a core of dentin, relatively opaque. A certain amount of light is reflected from the enamel surface, and the remainder either passes completely through, as in the area of the incisal edge of some teeth, or passes through to the dentinoenamel junction, where it is reflected back through the enamel. The light reflected from the outer tooth surface undergoes no change, but that passing into the tooth emerges having acquired the color attributes of the enamel and dentin.

Before these effects can be described and fully understood, the components of the visual sensation from a colored object must be explained. These are:

hue, that quality of sensation through which an observer is aware that one color is green and another red;

brightness, represented at its extremes by white and black, with gray as an intermediate, and indicative of the amount of light reflected from a matte-colored surface; and

saturation, that property which makes one sample of a pair of the same hue appear more intense or pure.

Since enamel is generally translucent, much of the light passes through it and is lost in the darkness of the oral cavity. Thus the incisal edges of many teeth lack brightness and will be gray in color. Toward the gingival one-third, the enamel becomes thinner and light is reflected from the basically yellow dentin core. Here the hue changes to yellow and becomes progressively more saturated. Directly at the gingival marginal area, some light is transmitted to the tooth through the red and translucent gingival tissues. This area then has a reddish hue superimposed on the yellow.

Psychological Primary Colors

The eye resolves all colors into a set of psychological primary colors: red, yellow, green, blue, black, and white. The basic color of the tooth being yellow, it can deviate only in one of three ways:

(a) in hue, by being a reddish yellow (orange) or a greenish yellow; (b) in brightness, either reflecting more or less light than a median gray; (c) in saturation, either by being a stronger or weaker yellow.

One other factor or effect is known as contrast enhancement. When a light and a dark color are juxtaposed (i.e., gingiva and tooth), each appears respectively lighter and darker than it would separately. When yellow and gray are approximated, the gray tends to take on the complementary hue to yellow (i.e., blue), so that in a strongly yellow tooth the incisal edge frequently appears blue gray. Red next to yellow often seems to make the red appear bluish red and the yellow a greenish yellow.

The fact that color has three basic attributes is of consequence in blending porcelain powders. For instance, if a yellow shade is correct in hue but is too saturated and needs dilution, then it must be diluted with a gray of similar brilliance rather than with a bright white modifying color.

Using a rating scale of 0 to 100 (0 being black and 100 white), the body colors of the New Hue shade guide vary in brightness from a maximum of 72 for shade 61 down to a minimum of 56.5 for a shade 87. The white modifier for Ceramco air-fired porcelain rates at 71 and would be suitable to modify the saturation of shade 61. However, for the other shades a mixture of the Ceramco white modifier with gray modifier, which has a brightness of 39, would be required.

If the nearest shade of porcelain powder to match a natural tooth is too orange (because it contains too much red), then the hue can be changed by the addition of a yellow-green porcelain of slightly greater brightness, since the green, in canceling out the effect of the red, forms a gray color. To change the saturation of a given specimen of porcelain, a modifier of the same hue and brightness but more intense or saturated in hue should be added.

These examples of the modification of hue, brightness, and saturation are indicative of the ways in which the color of a porcelain can be effected.

Additive and Subtractive Primary Colors

Two other sets of primary colors affect color matching. The first, or additive group, consists of red, green, and blue. If lights of these hues are mixed and the brightness and saturation are correct, a white light will be reproduced, the combinations of red and green giving yellow, and so on.

The second group, or subtractive primaries, are those which affect the admixture of pigments. In this case the pigment absorbs all the component colors in white light except one, which is reflected. These colors are yellow, magenta, and cyan (bluish green). When all these colors are mixed, all light is absorbed and black results.

As light falls on a natural tooth, yellow is transmitted to the middle third of the tooth from the gingival and gray is transmitted from the incisal. The two colors mix by the additive system and form the gradation found in this area. When this tooth is reproduced in porcelain by placing a tapered layer of gray over a yellow core of porcelain, the light reflected from the middle third area will be formed by the system of subtraction. As a rule, gray porcelain contains slight amounts of other colors, such as yellow or blue, and these will tend to give a color lacking clarity. The addition of red hues, such as are found in cervical blend stains, will counteract this.

Matching Natural Tooth Shades

Since the optical properties of dentin, enamel, and fused porcelain are dissimilar, it is in the main only by chance that an exact shade match is attained. The aim is to select and reproduce a shade that *blends* with the natural teeth.

Blending must be by eye and by instinct. No preblended shades match manufactured shade guides exactly, and it is difficult to match a natural tooth with the manufactured shade guides. The use of a denture tooth shade guide for veneered crowns predicates two errors in the color selection. It is recommended, therefore, that for veneered crowns a personal shade guide be made by using small castings of the metal and applying the appropriate porcelain to build a tooth-shaped unit (Fig. 305). For a jacket crown shade guide, tooth-shaped buttons of each powder and of some combinations should be fired.

The superior results attainable make this extra effort well worth while.

Adjuncts to Shade Selection

When the shade is to be selected, the patient should be seated with the head erect and at the operator's eye level. The operator should be able to stand between the patient and the light source, which preferably is

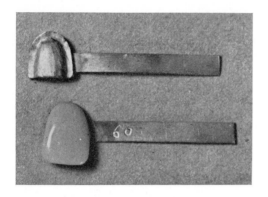

FIGURE 305. Suggested shade guide specimen for bonded porcelain veneer crowns.

a window with a northern exposure. A slightly overcast sky is best. A bright sky has light with a larger blue component, and early morning and late afternoon sunlight has a larger yellow component. The former would tend to enhance green color in the tooth, the latter yellow.

The room should have neutral gray walls or at least not be painted with brilliant colors.

Color Selection

The shade pattern for any crown should be worked out and recorded before the preparation is started. Tonal fatigue will start approximately 6 minutes after the operation begins on the tooth; after looking at an object closely for only a few minutes, it is no longer possible to differentiate color areas and variations accurately. Lipstick must be removed. When choosing the gingival color, the lips of the patient should be raised and the incisal covered. In selecting the incisal shade, the patient's lips should be in speaking position to give a more specific concept of the incisal shade and to eliminate any influence from the gingival third of the tooth. Then the selections must be verified with the entire tooth exposed.

The tooth and shade guide specimens must be positioned so that the minimum of light is reflected from the contours of the surfaces, and then observed quickly for match. If reflectance is a problem or if there are a number of different hues in the tooth, it is helpful to half-close the eyes and move away from the patient to gain an impression of the general qualities of the match.

Color Distribution Chart

Color selections and distribution should be charted after scrutinizing the tooth from frontal, profile, and standing positions, and with different sources or angles of light and environment. This will establish a reliable picture of the existing conditions.[5] To select the number from the series in a shade guide that is the closest match to the tooth will not give sufficient

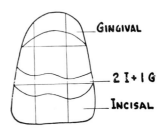

FIGURE 306. Color distribution chart.

information. It is essential that the distribution of the incisal and gingival shades and their overlapping combinations be designated on the color chart or prescription as they are seen on the tooth and the approximating and corresponding teeth.

The color distribution chart of the labial surface of the tooth, drawn to exact anatomic form, should be divided into thirds, inciso-cervically and mesio-distally (Fig. 306). This will assist in appraising and locating the irregular outline where the gingival color overlaps the mesial and distal surfaces and blends with the incisal shade, areas of incisal translucence, and also such characteristics as calcified areas, check lines, or stains. The chart should list or indicate everything seen on the tooth that must be included in the restoration to obtain an esthetic and harmonious result.

It is desirable to have duplicate shade guides, and if a laboratory is being employed to construct the jacket, to send with the order a copy of the color distribution chart and the specimens used in matching the tooth.[6, 7, 8]

Control of Shade

In the construction of a porcelain veneered crown, several factors combine to control the ultimate shade. The first is the color of the metal; the second, the opaque color; and the third, the color and translucence of the body and incisal porcelain.

If the tooth preparation and the metal frame have been correctly contoured, there will be enough room for an opaque layer that will obliterate the metal color. If space is at a premium, then some sacrifice in thickness of body porcelain and intensity of body color, rather than opaque, is necessary. Otherwise, in any combination the resulting crown would be gray in appearance.

To some extent the opaque color shows through the body color and influences the shade. When a crown is made with a variable thickness of body porcelain, the opaque shade must match the body shade exactly or there will be a variation in shade from area to area. The limited number of opaque colors in Ceramco air-fired porcelain causes some difficulties in this regard, and these colors frequently must be modified. It is somewhat easier to obtain consistent results with the vacuum-fired porcelains, which have a separate opaque shade matched to each body shade.

Of course, the fact that the opaque does affect the color of the veneer can be used to advantage when grayness of the incisal (or apparent translucence) must be increased or when yellowness in the cervical one-third must be enhanced. Modifiers can be added to the opaque to achieve these effects.

Staining

Where single crowns or a number of anterior crowns on one side of the arch are being made, staining may be mandatory to attain a degree of blending with the natural teeth. With a knowledge of available modifiers and stains, an accurate prescription for the color can be made and recorded on a diagram of the tooth. The authors often have found it necessary, especially in veneer construction, to modify body and incisal porcelain colors and to resort to surface staining in order to realize the maximal esthetic result.

Steele's stains, when fused to Ceramco porcelain, have a low-fusing temperature of approximately 1720 to 1740° F.

REFERENCES

1. Johnston, J. F., Mumford, G., and Dykema, R. W.: Porcelain veneers bonded to metal castings. Practical Dental Monographs. Chicago, Year Book Medical Publishers, Inc., March 1963.
2. Johnston, J. F.: Porcelain veneers bonded to precious metal castings. J. Canad. D. A., 26:657, 1960.
3. Mumford, G.: Recent studies in porcelain and porcelain jacket crown construction. Paper read before the Partial Prosthodontics Section, American Dental Association meeting, Philadelphia, Oct. 1961.
4. Shelby, D. S.: Practical considerations and design of porcelain fused to metal. J. Pros. Den., 12:542, May–June, 1962.
5. Theofilis, B. G.: The porcelain jacket crown. Senior thesis, Indiana Univ. School Den., June 1955.
6. Jones, R. J.: Personal communication.
7. Dunton, H.: Personal communication.
8. Moskey, M. S.: Personal communication.

Clark, E. B.: The color problem in dentistry. D. Digest, 37:499, 571, 646, 732, 815, 1931.
Committee on Colorimetry, Optical Society of America: The Science of Color. New York, Thomas Y. Crowell Company, 1953.
House, M. M., and Loop, J. L.: Form and Color Harmony in the Dental Art. Copyright 1939 by M. M. House.

22

THE CONSTRUCTION OF BONDED
PORCELAIN VENEER CROWNS

As early as 1887 dental restorations utilizing bonded porcelain veneers were constructed by Dr. Charles Land after his observation that the platinum matrix has an affinity for porcelain. For a number of years following 1907, frameworks for crowns and bridges were made of an iridioplatinum alloy over which a high-fusing porcelain was fired.[1] Later came swaged, brazed, and cast platinum cores and ferrules.

The resulting veneered restorations and prostheses were failures because of lack of fit, brittleness of castings, and poor bonding of the porcelain.[2] Platinum lacked the requisite physical and working properties for good dental restorations and it was frangible and easily contaminated when alloyed with iridium, rhodium, and palladium.[3, 4] Adding to these difficulties were casting investments that could neither compensate for the increased metal shrinkage nor withstand the high burnout temperatures necessary to assure complete castings.

Since 1950 investigation and clinical testing of restorations veneered with porcelain have been intensified and expanded by manufacturers, teaching institutions,[5] and independent practitioners. Wain, Coleman, Klaus, Taylor, Shell, Vining, and many others from the research laboratories of several manufacturers of dental alloys and porcelains have contributed notably to the progress made thus far in porcelain veneered restorations. Mumford, Brecker, Lyon, Vu thi Thin, Hobo, Teteruck, Jones, Kramer, Moskey, and Dunton are among those who have assisted in the evaluation of the materials used and in the stabilization and rationalization of methods of application.

With the techniques developed, building and bonding or fracture of the porcelain veneer should not be listed as problems. It may be said that bonded porcelain veneer crowns are now acceptable in most respects to a great number of people, are only partially successful in quite a number of cases, and are frustrating to the inept and less persevering segments of dentistry and the technicians' craft.

The techniques described in detail in this chapter are designed for use with Ceramco porcelain and Ceramco No. 1 Improved alloy. Supplementary information will be given about other porcelains and alloys.

Ceramco porcelain,[a]* manufactured for both air and vacuum firing, is specifically designed for use with Ceramco No. 1 Improved alloy.[b] However, in practice, it has been found that Harmony P. G.[c] and P16[d] gold alloys, and Ceramaloy,[e] a cobalt-chromium alloy, have a satisfactory balance† with this porcelain.

Other combinations of porcelain and alloy are obtainable in both high-fusing and low-fusing ranges and for either air or vacuum firing. Among these are Thermalite porcelain[f] and P16 alloy. This porcelain is available in three types: 1950° F. vacuum-fired, 1650° F. air-fired, and 1650° F. vacuum-fired. Microbond porcelain,[g] high fusing and for vacuum firing, is used with Microbond, an alloy of palladium, silver, and ruthenium.[6]

WORKING DIES AND CASTS

Polysulfide rubber impressions are excellent for making dies and working casts.[7, 8] (See Chapter 10.) Gingival displacement can be achieved efficiently with Westwood alum yarn and Hemodent. Only one full mouth impression need be made. The areas of the prepared teeth are poured with Vel-Mix[9] or a similar improved stone; the set stone is removed after 1 hour and a complete arch working cast is poured into the same impression. The first cast is sectioned to make the dies; the intact working cast is used to contour and align an individual crown or to assemble a splint or fixed partial denture (Fig. 307).

The opposing casts must be related with care and mounted on an adjustable articulator. When the dentist is demanding of himself in this

---

* The materials mentioned in the text that follows, indicated by superior letters, can be obtained from the following manufacturers:

   [a] Ceramco, Inc., Woodside, N. Y.

   [b] J. F. Jelenko & Co., Inc., New Rochelle, N. Y., and Julius Aderer, Inc., Long Island City, N. Y.

   [c] Williams Gold Refining Co., Inc., Buffalo, N. Y.

   [d] The J. M. Ney Company, Hartford, Conn.

   [e] The Niranium Corp., Long Island, N. Y.

   [f] Distributed by The J. M. Ney Company, Hartford, Conn.

   [g] Austenal Company, Division of Howe Sound Co., Chicago, Ill.

   † Veneering porcelain and alloy are said to be in balance when the contraction of the two materials has been synchronized so that the alloy, after the veneer has been fired, contracts just enough more to place the porcelain under compression. This reduces checking and increases strength.

matter, he will have suitable "tools" and can fashion crowns or bridges requiring minimal corrections.

CASTINGS

The next step in bonded porcelain veneer crown construction is producing the casting. A cast restoration, to be worthy of cementation, must fit, must have surface smoothness and density, and must be capable of resisting deformation either through bulk or inherent physical properties.

"Fit" in a casting may be defined differently by different people. To the authors, it means a snug adaptation of the metal to the entire cut surfaces of the tooth, covering all the prepared tooth surfaces after polishing but with no extension of the casting beyond the margins of the preparation, and correct contour and adequate bulk in the cervical fifth. To others, it may mean close adaptation of the casting to the tooth structure only in the cervical fourth or fifth, with the remaining area etched to provide more freedom for seating and flow of cement. However, a cast framework for a bonded porcelain veneer crown cannot have the same degree of frictional retention as a well-fitting partial veneer crown. It must seat without undue pressure. When the pattern is lined with soft wax, removal and seating will abrade the inner surface and help establish the desired type of fit.

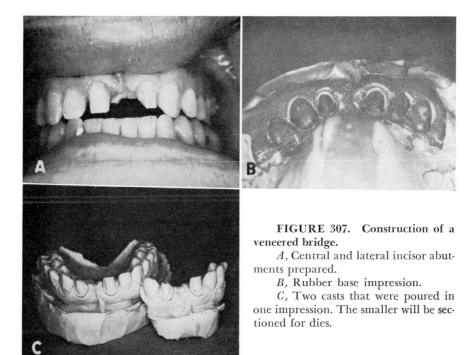

FIGURE 307. Construction of a veneered bridge.

A, Central and lateral incisor abutments prepared.

B, Rubber base impression.

C, Two casts that were poured in one impression. The smaller will be sectioned for dies.

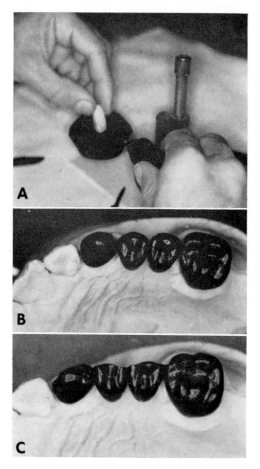

FIGURE 308. *A,* Dipping lubricated die into molten sprue wax to give inner surface of pattern a smooth, unblemished surface.

B, Wax patterns for a crown and two pontics carved to full contour. Each of these three units will be veneered with bonded porcelain.

C, Wax patterns cut back to best form for veneering.

Forming the Wax Pattern

A casting that fits must duplicate the form and dimensions of a wax pattern which also fits. The metal frame must support the porcelain bonded to it, and, since any flexure of the metal will cause checking or outright fracture of the veneer, it is essential that the wax pattern have no internal creases. If this is attained, it matters little how the pattern is formed. The authors use stone dies, lubricated and dipped in a dish of molten Kerr's blue sprue wax, which gives a smooth, well-adapted inner surface to the pattern. Also, because of the softness of this inner layer, the investment can more effectively expand the pattern during setting. The contour is built up with a wax which meets the specifications for indirect inlay waxes.

The wax pattern for a casting to be veneered should be carved to full form first, then the area to which the veneer will be bonded is cut back to the form most desirable for veneering (Fig. 308). This cutback should be at least 1.0 mm. deep toward the center of the tooth at every point on the labial or buccal surface, but as the incisal edge is approached, the depth must be increased for a minimal clearance of 1.5 mm. between the wax pattern and the opposing teeth. Clearance over the buccal cusp and occlusal surfaces of any posterior unit should be approximately 1.5 mm. On a maxillary bicuspid or molar crown, the surface to be veneered preferably will terminate halfway down the lingual slope of the buccal cusp or cusps.[10]

There should be no sharp or right angles within the area to be veneered; however, there should be an invisible right angle where the surface of the veneer meets the flat face of the casting. The bucco-cervical collar in the wax pattern should be left approximately twice as thick as it will be after the casting is prepared for veneering. When the pattern is finished, all surfaces that will be exposed should be as smooth as possible.

A porcelain veneered gold crown is built with the incisal edge "unprotected" by overlying metal. This is an esthetic virtue and a mechanical necessity. The only incisal edge fractures seen by the authors have occurred when an attempt was made to protect the incisal edge with a lingual metal veneer, indispensable for the Hollenback and Hagen crowns.

Although the incisal edge should be reproduced in porcelain, it is advisable that the areas on the lingual surface, making contacts in centric occlusion and the beginnings of the eccentric movements, should be metal. This permits subsequently some occlusal adjustment without leaving a rough, unglazed porcelain surface. For the same reason, the occlusal surfaces of posterior crowns or pontics are left unveneered unless the absolute in esthetic results is requested by the patient. (For selecting shade and shade pattern, see Chapter 14, The Pontic.)

Spruing

To make castings without voids, the patterns must be sprued in an unorthodox manner. When investing a posterior pattern, a 10-gauge or 12-gauge (never less than 14-gauge) sprue is attached to the tip of a cusp, perpendicular to the plane of the occlusal surface. An 18-gauge vent is extended from a point diagonally across the occlusal surface to the face of the crucible former, about 2.0 mm. from the casting ring (Fig. 309). The gold will enter the mold and circulate in a manner that ordinarily might cause turbulence. However, the air will be forced ahead of the gold and out into the vent, assuring a complete casting.

If there is a thin area in the pattern, possibly on the labial or buccal surface, another 18-gauge vent is run from there to the crucible former, also very close to the casting ring.

Investing

Three satisfactory investment materials[11] are available: Ceramigold*

---

* Whip-Mix Corporation, Louisville, Ky.

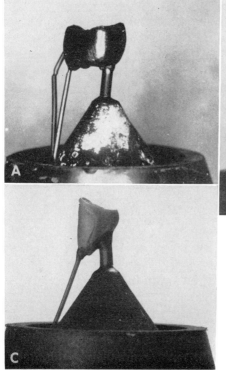

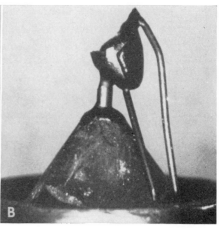

FIGURE 309. Three wax patterns sprued for casting Ceramco No. 1 Improved alloy.

Ceramvest,* and HFG.† Clinically, HFG investment seems to give routinely the best results for full coverage restorations. With it a water-powder ratio of 10 ml.:50 gm. is used. While this proportion tends to yield a casting that is slightly looser than the ideal demanded in full and partial veneer gold crowns, this looseness is necessary to avoid any deformation of the underlying casting when placing a veneered restoration on the tooth. Expansion control with HFG investment is effected by changes in the water:powder ratio. For example, when splinted units are used on abutments and when partial veneer crown retainers are used in conjunction with porcelain veneer crowns, the ratio of water to investment powder is increased to 11 ml.:50 gm. for the partial veneer crown. The resulting casting will have frictional retention.

A vacuum investing technique is used, and, because HFG seems to have a higher surface tension than regular gypsum investments and traps bubbles against the wax surface much more readily, the pattern should be painted with a surface tension-reducing agent.‡

Mixing Technique. The water is placed in the mixing bowl, the powder is added, and the mix is stirred by hand until the powder is wetted.

---

* Kerr Mfg. Company, Detroit, Mich.
† The Ransom & Randolph Co., Toledo, Ohio.
‡ Kerr's Vacu-Film or Jelenko wax pattern cleaner.

The mix will be quite stiff, but because water forms during the chemical reaction which occurs, it will become thinner as the mechanical spatulation is continued.

The investment is mechanically spatulated from 10 to 20 seconds and then vibrated around the pattern for at least 30 seconds. The investment is allowed to bench-set for not less than 1 hour. The ring is then placed in a cold furnace and over a period of 1 hour is heated to 1300° F. It is heat soaked at this temperature for an additional 30 minutes, when it is ready for casting.

Casting

A special Wesgo* high-heat crucible is used in a centrifugal casting machine which is wound to give a slightly higher casting pressure than is normal. A gas-oxygen torch† is employed for melting the alloy. The crucible is preheated, but neither flux nor an asbestos liner is used in it. The metal in the crucible is heated in that part of the flame just beyond the end of the light blue zones.

As the alloy melts, a scum appears to form on its surface. With continued heating this scum disappears, the button becomes shiny, and the metal is in condition for casting. After the casting ring has bench-cooled until the button becomes dark, it is quenched in water and the investment removed. These investments are difficult to break off, but by grooving the sides of the investment block, it can be split, facilitating exposure of the casting. The casting is soaked in hydrofluoric acid to hasten elimination of the investment from the inner surface.

Finishing

Prior to fusing the porcelain, those surfaces of the casting which are not to receive porcelain are finished with stones and rubber wheels. Then the occlusion should be rechecked and corrected on the articulated working casts, and also in the mouth, if possible. This is important because only minimal alterations should be made in the contour of the frame after the veneer has been glazed. After adding and glazing the porcelain veneer, final polishing of the metal is accomplished with tripoli, or Shure Shine,‡ followed by Amalgloss,§ No. 600 Carborundum powder mixed with water, or Buehler's AB Alpha polishing Alumina, No. 2,|| mixed with a few drops of a liquid detergent.[8]

---

* Western Gold and Platinum Co., Belmont, Calif.
† Linde Oxweld torch #W17 with a 125 M4 multiflame tip, Linde Co., Div. of Union Carbide Corp., Speedway, Ind.
‡ Aurora Dental Specialties Co., Hillside, Ill.
§ The L. D. Caulk Company, Milford, Del.
|| Buehler, Ltd., Evanston, Ill.

Ceramco alloy, as well as all other alloys used to support bonded porcelain veneers, can be finished to an exceptionally high luster, and all resist tarnish in the oral environment as well as standard crown and bridge alloys. Each will remain clean if the patient maintains a satisfactory level of oral hygiene.

PREPARING THE FRAME FOR VENEERING

After all exposed surfaces of the casting have been smoothed with rubber abrasive wheels, the area to be veneered with porcelain is roughened with a coarse wheel stone. Then the casting must be pickled in hydrofluoric acid for 8 hours. This time can be reduced to 30 minutes if the acid container is placed in an ultrasonic cleaner. The casting is washed and heated in the furnace for 15 minutes at a temperature about 25 degrees above that at which the porcelain will be fused. This will remove any gas contamination resulting from the casting process and will obviate one possible cause of porosity in the porcelain veneer. If a metal conditioner* is to be applied, the temperature would be 1950° F.; if the opaque is to be fused directly on the casting, it would be 1825° F.

The metal conditioner is mixed to a thin, creamy consistency with a special nondrying liquid and a minimal thickness is painted on the surface of the casting. It is dried before the open muffle and placed in the furnace at 1200° F.; by raising the temperature 100 degrees per minute, it is heated to 1925° F., or until a sheen appears on the surface. The casting is removed from the furnace immediately and placed under a cover until cool (Figs. 310 and 311).

Britecote† and Culvergard,‡ which give a bright gold color to the surface, are fired at 1945° F. They are similar except that Britecote gives a more lumpy surface.[12] Britecote can be "set" on the casting with a torch.

The Opaque

The opaque is mixed with water to a consistency of thick cream and applied to the surface of the casting. By alternately vibrating and drying the surface, a layer 0.35 mm. to 0.4 mm. thick is built up. The surface is brushed smooth, the opaque is dried, and the casting is placed in the furnace at 1200° F. The temperature is increased 100 degrees per minute until 1800° F. is reached. This same firing schedule is used for all subsequent bakes. The casting is withdrawn from the furnace immediately on reaching 1800° F. and placed under a cover to cool. The opaque

---

* Ceramcote, Ceramco, Inc., Woodside, N. Y.
† Ceramco, Inc., Woodside, N. Y.
‡ The Wilkinson Company, Santa Monica, Calif.

material will have shrunk during the firing so that it is now 0.3 mm., or slightly less, in thickness (see Fig. 311*D*).

The Body Porcelain

The crown is now ready for the application of the veneering porcelains. The body porcelain is mixed to a consistency of very thick cream and applied to the casting with a spatula. By alternate vibrating and blotting, the crown is built to a slight overcontour in all dimensions to compensate for the anticipated shrinkage. Sufficient excess must be added near the

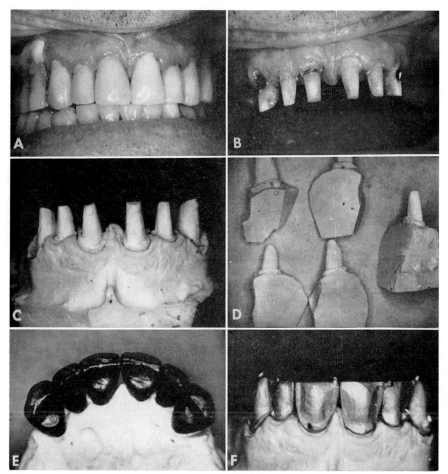

FIGURE 310. *A,* Six maxillary anterior teeth with abraded resin veneered gold crowns.

B, Crowns removed, showing excessively prepared teeth. No further cutting was done.

C, D, Stone cast and sections for dies.

E, Wax patterns on working cast. Cast and dies were poured in the same polysulfide rubber impression.

F, Castings seated on working cast. Heavy sprue pins were attached to lingual surfaces; vents to other surfaces. Labio-cervical collar is heavy.

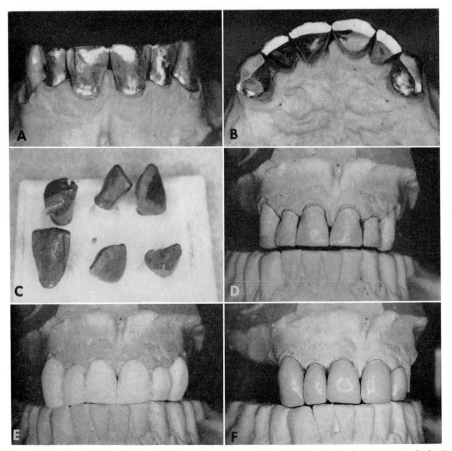

FIGURE 311. *A,* Castings contoured for veneering. Incisal angles are rounded. Cervical collar is thinned. Surfaces to be veneered have been stoned.

B, Incisal view of castings. Labial margins round; lingual margin precise.

C, Castings degassed and metal conditioner (Ceramcote) fired.

D, Opaque fired.

E, Body porcelain applied ready for first firing.

F, First application of body porcelain fired.

margins to prevent the porcelain from pulling away from the metal. The incisal and labial surfaces of the crown are trimmed with a sharp blade to create space for the incisal or the enamel-colored porcelain. The amount removed will depend on the shade distribution of the natural tooth to be matched. Margins must be feathered to avoid a distinct line of demarcation between the two porcelains (Fig. 312).

The Incisal Porcelain

The incisal porcelain, because of its coarser particle size, is mixed to a thin consistency and flowed onto the surface with a brush. It is built up in layers to correct contour and the surface is smoothed with a large soft brush. The crown is dried in front of the open muffle. After the firing cycle has been repeated, the surface of the porcelain should have a semi-glazed appearance. If more porcelain must be added in spots to complement form, the glaze should be removed from the surface of the crown before this is done (Fig. 313).

Again it is dried and fired as before. Final alterations in contour and topographic anatomy are made at this stage, using small, mounted carborundum stones. The surface is smoothed with white abrasive disks or a Dedeco* white rubber porcelain polishing wheel; otherwise, it will be necessary to subject the porcelain to the glazing temperature for such a length of time that contours and anatomic detail will be obscured or rounded.

---

* Dental Development Mfg. Corp., Brooklyn, N. Y.

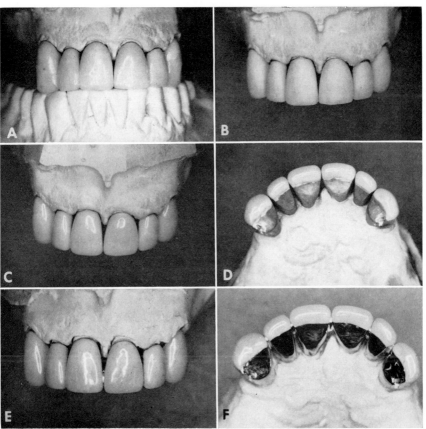

FIGURE 312.   *A,* After second firing. Body and incisal porcelain were added. Contour incorrect.

    B, Contoured for third firing.

    C, After third firing, labial view.

    D, Incisal view.

    E, Six-unit splint soldered.

    F, Lingual view after being polished.

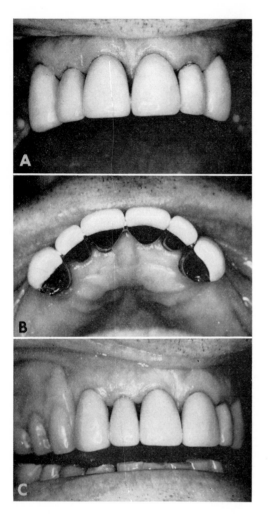

FIGURE 313. *A, B,* Six-crown splint cemented.

C, Supporting a Class I precision attachment partial denture.

Glazing

Before the crown is glazed, all debris must be removed from its surface. This may be effected by (1) placing it in an ultrasonic cleaner* (Figs. 314 and 315), (2) boiling it in chloroform, or (3) brushing it under running water. It is dried and preheated in front of the furnace for 2 to 3 minutes, then placed in the furnace at 1200° F. and carried to 1800° F., raising the temperature 100 degrees per minute. The degree of glaze desired will not be the same for all patients, and there will be dissimilar effects if the glazing temperature is varied between 1780° F. and 1810° F. The higher the temperature, the more glossy the surface becomes. When the application of surface stains will assist in blending and harmonizing the color or shade pattern with the adjacent teeth, it is done at this stage, using normal staining procedures. (See Chapter 17, Glazing and Staining Facings.)

* Williams Gold Refining Co., Inc., Buffalo, N. Y.; L&R Mfg. Co., Kearny, N. J.

Fig. 314

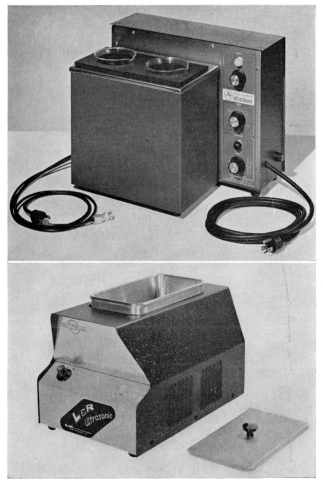

Fig. 315

FIGURE 314.   Williams Ultracleaner.
FIGURE 315.   L&R Ultrasonic Cleaner.

After the porcelain has been fused, the casting is pickled in 50 per cent hydro*chloric* acid (not hydro*fluoric*). Any small pieces of porcelain adhering to the exposed metal surface are removed with stones, and the scratched surface is finished with a fine rubber wheel, followed by tripoli applied with a brush until the surface is completely free of any blemishes.

CROWN WITH PORCELAIN SHOULDER

When the crown is to be made without a labio-cervical collar of gold, a somewhat different technique is employed for the wax pattern. A

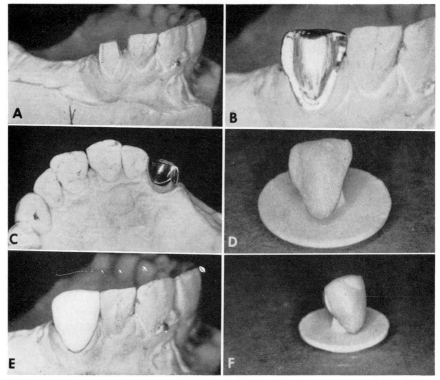

FIGURE 316. *A*, Working cast.
B, Cast framework ready for veneering.
C, Casting, lingual view. Sherer rest seat. Cingulum contoured for cast retentive arm of clasp.
D, Opaque fired.
E, Body and incisal built.
F, First firing; shrinkage along margins.

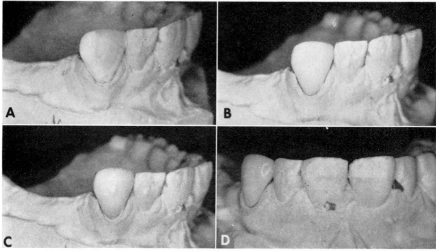

FIGURE 317. *A*, Porcelain added to plus contour before second firing.
B, Veneer contoured after second firing.
C, D, Veneer glazed.

piece of 0.001 platinum foil is burnished to overlap the shoulder cervically and incisally about 2.5 mm. Adaptation to the shoulder should be close. The pattern is waxed and carved to form but is not extended labially over the platinum foil (Fig. 318). Spruing is the same as described before except that, to ensure casting over the platinum foil, an auxiliary sprue, or vent, must be attached very close to the cervical of the labial wax wall. The casting is cleaned, polished, and conditioned for veneering.

The opaque is applied to the surface of the casting, but not to the foil collar, and fired. The veneering porcelains are built up to oversize form and then a V-shaped ditch is cut at the cervical, exposing the platinum. After firing, the crown is contoured, porcelain being added to complete its form. The ditch is overfilled and the crown is fired for the second time. If more porcelain is needed, it is added and the crown is again contoured and glazed. Before cementing, the platinum is peeled off the porcelain (Fig. 319).

This method of construction is indicated when recession has gone beyond the cementoenamel junction, when recession is anticipated, or

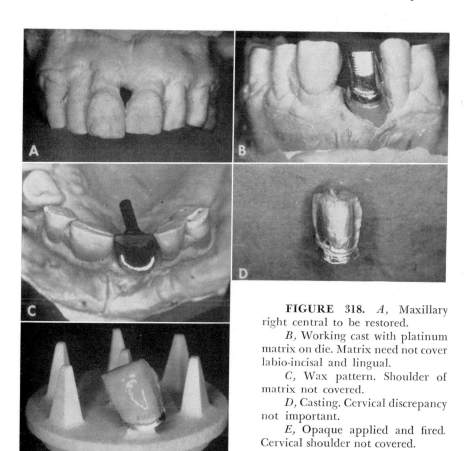

FIGURE 318. *A,* Maxillary right central to be restored.

B, Working cast with platinum matrix on die. Matrix need not cover labio-incisal and lingual.

C, Wax pattern. Shoulder of matrix not covered.

D, Casting. Cervical discrepancy not important.

E, Opaque applied and fired. Cervical shoulder not covered.

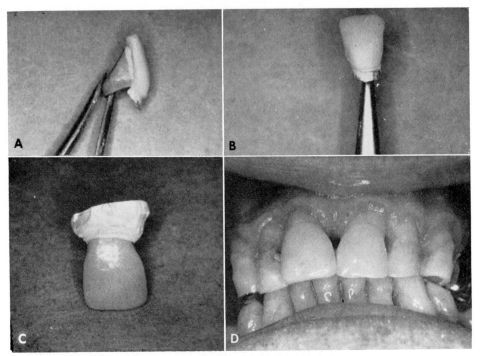

FIGURE 319. *A, B,* Cervical ditch and marginal shrinkage.
C, Crown supported by ceramic investment for glaze firing.
D, Porcelain veneered crown without labio-cervical collar of gold on maxillary right central incisor. Crown fits against prepared tooth as a jacket crown.

In any situation when esthetic considerations are paramount. Strength and retention are not sacrificed in the single-unit restoration. However, if the crown were a retainer for a bridge, subject to leverage or torque, the frame might not withstand deformation and the veneer could be checked.

This technique demands more care in handling during construction, especially if the crown is used as a retainer. It is an excellent restoration esthetically and possibly is less irritating to the gingiva. Certainly, if recession did occur, it would be longer before dissatisfaction with appearance would require the tooth to be reprepared and another crown constructed.[13]

VACUUM-FIRED VENEERS

Regardless of the combination of materials used, certain factors remain constant for all vacuum-fired porcelains fused to metal. The metal should be degassed in the vacuum. Each addition of porcelain opaque, body or incisal, should be vacuum fired *except* the glaze firing, which is *always* done in air. Vacuum firing increases considerably the intensity of the color and the translucence of the porcelain; therefore a shade guide of vacuum-fired porcelain is mandatory. Porcelain powders designed for air firing cannot be used for vacuum firing unless they are modified by the addition of opacifiers and pigments.

The degree of vacuum used and the time of application vary from porcelain to porcelain. Water will boil at room temperature under reduced pressure, and so will some of the veneering porcelains near their fusion temperature. Because this would increase the porosity of the porcelain rather than decrease it, the last part of each firing of these porcelains must be completed in air.

When building a Ceramco porcelain veneered crown, the casting is degassed in a vacuum of 27 to 28 inches of mercury, and this pressure is constant for all firings. If Ceramcote is applied, it is dried and fired in a vacuum to 1825° F., the vacuum is released, and the firing is continued in air up to 1925° F. The opaque is fired to 1750° F. in a vacuum, the vacuum is released, and the firing is continued to 1825 to 1850° F. There is a slight variation in the firing temperatures of the different colored opaques. They should be fired until a sheen appears on the surface.

The body and incisal porcelains are fired to a temperature of 1700° F. under vacuum, which is then released and the firing continued to 1800° F.

Glazing must be carried out at normal atmospheric pressure.

VENEERS WITH INTRACORONAL ATTACHMENTS

A porcelain veneer can be built around the female section of a precision attachment that has been positioned and soldered to the casting. A little distortion will occur, but this can be dissipated with a sizing tool (Figs. 320 and 321).

Formerly a solder was supplied that flowed more freely, was more the color of gold, and had a lower fusing point than standard Ceramco solder, and it was preferred when precision attachments were to be soldered in the units, because it would run into the joint area more readily. The incidence of ruined crowns was high, and its manufacture has been discontinued, since

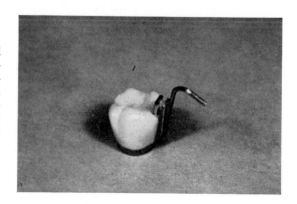

FIGURE 320. Molar gold crown with complete porcelain veneer built around precision attachment. In the construction of a small percentage of clinical cases, a discernible warping of this attachment was noted. Adjustment was done quickly.

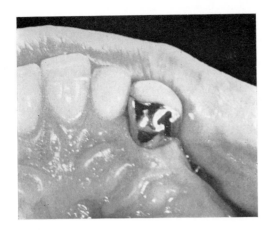

FIGURE 321.   Cuspid crown with veneer and precision attachment.

the metal structure could not be heated above 1800° F. during the firing of porcelains. This is regrettable; it was very useful.

VENEERS UNDER CLASPS

When a porcelain veneer crown is being built to support a clasp, the designed rest seats or ledges and any lingual retentive undercuts and proximal guiding planes are surveyed and carved into the wax pattern for the frame. Heights of contour and retentive undercuts are surveyed and ground into the porcelain just prior to glazing. When a crown is to be clasped, the glaze should be higher than is needed on many other restorations because the smoother surface has less abrasive action on the inner surface of a clasp. With a lesser glaze, occasionally a wrought wire retentive arm will leave a faint gray metallic mark on the crown surface. The porcelain veneer crown is quite helpful in the preparation of mouths for clasp-retained partial dentures (Fig. 322).

CEMENTATION

The dentist may use the cementing technique of his choice, but it should be noted that temporary measures should be employed for only short periods of time. When an abutment tooth must be slightly repositioned because of movement from its original alignment, a petroleum jelly and cement powder luting material may be used, but for just a few hours. Removing a cemented prosthesis or having it loose on a tooth may result in an internal pressure that will check the veneer. The authors strongly recommend immediate permanent cementation. Teeth are seldom sensitive if they have been prepared with care and covered so that they were not subjected to premature contacts, lateral movement, or torque. A cavity

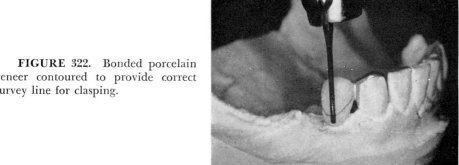

FIGURE 322. Bonded porcelain veneer contoured to provide correct survey line for clasping.

varnish, such as Copalite, should be used since it has no adverse effect on cementation and does afford some protection to the pulp against the acid in the cement mix.

REFERENCES

1. Brecker, S. C.: Porcelain fused to gold. J. California D. A. and Nevada D. Soc., *36*:425, Dec. 1960.
2. Perlman, T. H.: The use of platinum and porcelain in dental restorations. D. J. Australia, *26*:118, June 1954.
3. Perlman, T. H.: Further observations on cast platinum and baked porcelain restorations. D. Digest, *56*:298, 1950.
4. Brecker, S. C.: Porcelain baked to gold—a new medium in prosthodontics. J. Pros. Den., *6*:801, Nov. 1956.
5. Johnston, J. F., Dykema, R. W., and Cunningham, D. M.: The use and construction of gold crowns with fused porcelain veneers—a progress report. J. Pros. Den., *6*:811, Nov. 1956.
6. Vining, R., Austenal Company: Personal communication.
7. Phillips, R. W., and Schnell, R. J.: The use of rubber impression materials. Practical Dental Monographs. Chicago, Year Book Medical Publishers, Inc., May 1962.
8. Johnston, J. F., Dykema, R. W., Mumford, G., and Phillips, R. W.: Construction and assembly of porcelain veneer gold crowns and pontics. J. Pros. Den., *12*:1125, Nov.–Dec. 1962.
9. Dykema, R. W., Johnston, J. F., and Cunningham, D. M.: The veneered gold crown. D. Clin. North America, Nov. 1958, p. 653.
10. Johnston, J. F., Mumford, G., and Dykema, R. W.: Porcelain veneers bonded to metal castings. Practical Dental Monographs. Chicago, Year Book Medical Publishers, Inc., March 1963.
11. Schnell, R. J., Mumford, G., and Phillips, R. W.: An evaluation of phosphate bonded investments used with a high fusing gold alloy. J. Pros. Den., *13*:324, 1963.
12. Mumford, G.: Personal communication.
13. Jones, R. J.: Personal communication.

Hagen, W. H. B.: Combination gold and porcelain crown. J. Pros. Den., *10*:325, March–April 1960.
Lund, M. R., and Bonlie, D. R.: Baked porcelain restorations without the use of the platinum matrix. J. D. Res., *40*:94, 1962 (Abstract).

Lyon, D. M., Cowger, G. T., Woycheshin, F. F., and Miller, C. B.: Porcelain fused to gold—evaluation and esthetics. J. Pros. Den., *10:*319, March–April 1960.

Morrison, K. N., and Warnick, M. E.: Investment compounded specifically for ceramic procedures. J. D. Res., *38:*762, July–Aug. 1959 (Abstract).

Morse, F. F. E.: Porcelain fused to metal. Comparisons of the air-fired and vacuum-fired porcelain jacket crowns and porcelain fused to precious metal. Dental Practitioner and Dental Record, *13:*99, Nov. 1962.

Mumford, G.: The porcelain fused to metal restoration. D. Clin. North America, March 1965, p. 241.

Mylin, W. K.: Present status of porcelain fused to metal restorations. J. Kentucky D. A., *14:*152, July 1962.

Pruden, K. C.: Abutments and attachments in fixed partial dentures. J. Pros. Den., *7:*502, July 1957.

Pruden, W. H., II: Porcelain veneer crown. J. Pros. Den., *10:*955, Sept.–Oct. 1960.

Shell, J. S., and Nielsen, J. P.: Study of the bond between gold alloys and porcelain. J. D. Res., *41:*1424, Nov.–Dec. 1962.

Thin, Vu thi: A study of the Brinell hardness of metals used in conjunction with the porcelain fused to metal technic. Master's thesis, Indiana Univ. School Den., June 1962.

Warnick, M. E., and Morrison, K. N.: Porcelain-faced crown technique. D. Digest, *68:*60, Feb. 1962.

Wheeler, R. C.: The implications of full coverage restorative procedures. J. Pros. Den., *5:*848, Nov.–Dec. 1955.

23

THE CONSTRUCTION OF BRIDGES
WITH BONDED PORCELAIN VENEERS

Bridges with bonded porcelain veneers may be fabricated either before or after the veneers are fired. If this is done *prior* to the application of porcelain, the solder must have a melting point high enough (in fact, very close to that of the casting alloy) so that the bridge will not warp or come apart during the firing of the veneer.

If bridges are soldered *after* veneering, air-fired veneers seem to tolerate the operation with no ill effects. With vacuum-fired Ceramco units, a great number of fine bubbles may appear on the surface, and while their tops can be removed by polishing with a rubber wheel, the natural glazed surface of the porcelain is thus destroyed and pits remain which may collect debris.

When veneered units are to be assembled (either for bridge construction or splinting), the proximal surfaces which will be soldered must be contoured to provide enough area for the joint, larger for bridges, smaller for splinting. The longer the span, the larger the joints must be. Also, joints formed with the special solders must be larger if the frame for a bridge is assembled before veneering, as clinical experience and critical observation show such joints to be less perfectly formed and therefore more liable to break.

PONTIC DESIGN

Pontics may be designed to have an alloy, porcelain, or both, in contact with the ridge tissue. The authors prefer a pontic frame similar to that used

385

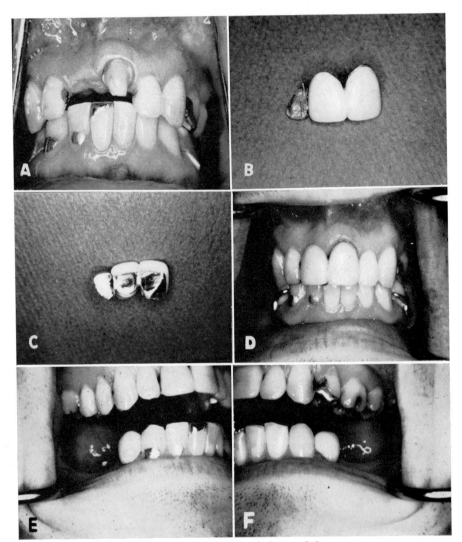

FIGURE 323. Bridge and crowns with bonded porcelain veneers.

A, Maxillary central incisor missing. Central incisor abutment prepared for veneered gold crown; lateral incisor prepared for pinledge.

B, Fused porcelain veneers on central incisor retainer and central pontic.

C, Lingual showing unsupported incisal edges of porcelain.

D, Bridge cemented. Gingival tissue covered cervical gold collar in eight days. Clasped mandibular bicuspids are restored with gold crowns with fused porcelain veneers.

E, F, Crowns with clasps removed.

with a long-pin facing, where the greater part of the ridge-contacting surface will be highly polished and correctly contoured metal, with a labio- or bucco-cervical rim of porcelain. An all-porcelain ridgelap entails a more complicated technique.

The incisal edge of an anterior pontic should be reproduced in porcelain, but the lingual section, which will occlude in centric and in the begin-

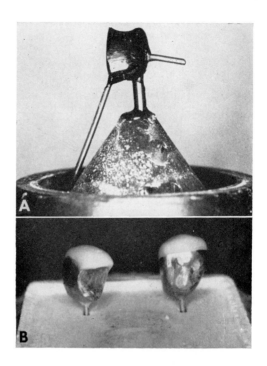

FIGURE 324. *A,* Pontic pattern sprued. Handle extends from lingual surface.

B, Handle supports pontic in firing tray.

nings of eccentric movements, should be metal in order to make future equilibration easier and repolishing possible. The occlusal surface of a posterior pontic usually is not veneered except on a portion of the lingual inclines of the buccal cusps. The outline and area of the veneer on any pontic should simulate that of a veneer crown without a labial collar of metal on the tooth being replaced. In thickness, the pontic veneer should approximate that of the veneers on adjacent retainers so that the shades will match or blend (Fig. 323).

Before investing the pattern for a pontic, a section of 18-gauge wax rod, 2.5 or 3.0 mm. long, is extended to form a handle, at right angles from near the center of the lingual surface but at a point that will not interfere with occlusion (Fig. 324). Pontics, before assembly, are hard to control, and this handle will expedite not only the application and firing of the porcelain but also the assembly of the fixed partial denture for soldering.

FABRICATION OF BRIDGE PRIOR TO BAKING VENEERS

Soldering Assembly

The castings are finished with stones and burs and polished with a rubber wheel. The units to be soldered are assembled on the working **cast** and an occlusal or linguo-incisal plaster index is formed. The units are

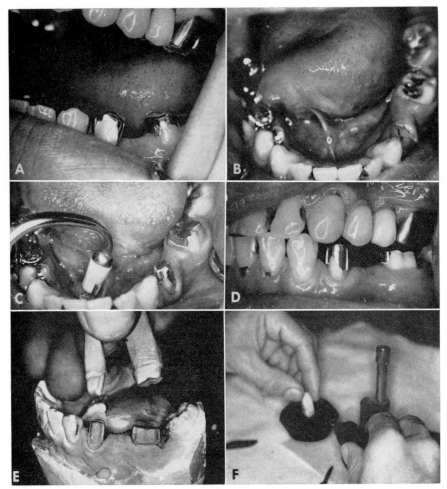

FIGURE 325. *A,* Mandibular posterior space.
B, Restorations removed from abutments.
C, D, Abutments rebuilt to prepared form with castings.
E, Working cast and dies. One rubber base impression.
F, Dipping lubricated die prior to waxing pattern for retainer.

seated in the index, and to facilitate its easy removal after the soldering assembly has hardened, any plaster past the heights of contour should be cut away because difficulty in removal may fracture the soldering investment. The units are luted to the plaster and the embrasures are filled with wax (Figs. 325 and 326).

Whip-Mix* high-heat soldering investment, which will stand the shock of rapid heating without cracking, is mixed to a stiff putty and vibrated into the retainers and around the projections on the lingual surfaces of the pontics until a base of investment ¼ inch thick is formed. After setting for at least 30 minutes, the assembly is boiled in carbon tetrachloride or chloro-

* Whip-Mix Corporation, Louisville, Ky.

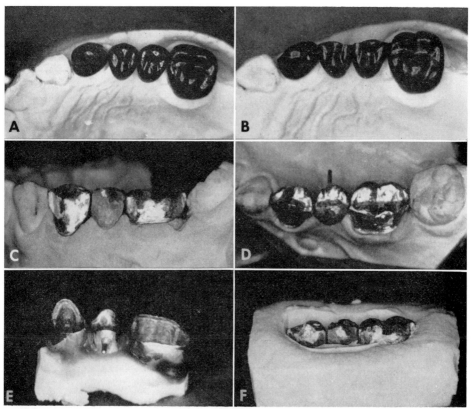

FIGURE 326. *A, B,* Wax patterns for opposing bridge. First waxed to full contour, then cut back to form for veneering.

C, Cast retainers and pontic for mandibular bridge.

D, Occlusal view of castings showing handle on pontic. This will secure it in soldering assembly.

E, Ready to pour soldering assembly. Contacts and embrasures protected by wax.

F, Soldering assembly.

form to melt and dissolve the wax. The index is removed and the investment block is trimmed. (Hot water may be used to remove the index, but cautiously, inasmuch as water will further soften an already weak investment.)

Soldering

There is no need to enlarge the embrasure areas of the soldering block, as the intense, small flame of the soldering torch (Torit #77 with an A tip)* will heat the area readily (Fig. 327).

A small amount of Ceramco flux is mixed with water to a paste and the joint areas are fluxed. The assembly is placed in a cold furnace, rapidly heated to 1300° F., and removed. A gas-oxygen torch is adjusted so that the

---

* Torit Mfg. Co., St. Paul, Minn.

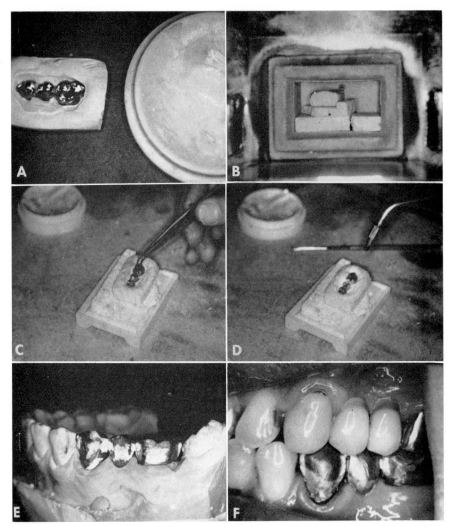

FIGURE 327.   *A,* Soldering assembly fluxed.
B, Drying.
C, Placing small pieces of solder.
D, Soldering.
E, Soldered and prepared frame on working cast. Cervical collar has been reduced and surfaces stoned.
F, Occlusion adjusted in mouth.

flame measures about 3 inches, with a blue inner cone 3/8 inch long. The castings are heated to a bright red and pieces of Ceramco No. 1 solder are applied. The solder is heated until it slumps into place, at which stage the castings will have taken on a glossy appearance. A greater quantity of solder seemingly is needed to form a joint of specific size than is required to form a joint of similar size with a standard gold solder.

The assembly is bench-cooled before being placed in water to aid in the removal of the investment. It is pickled in 50 per cent hydrochloric acid to remove the flux. The cast handles are cut off and the castings are repolished to the rubber wheel stage. The veneering areas are ground with a coarse stone. The frame is equilibrated on the working cast, but it may be tried in the mouth also, to determine fit and to check the occlusion further. Prior to the application of the veneering porcelain, the bridge is placed in hydrofluoric acid and then degassed.

Veneering

Basically, assembled units are veneered in the same way as a single unit, except that the pontics must be built to fit the ridge. Following the opaque bake, a piece of cigarette paper is cut to fit over the ridge area, moistened, and adapted to the cast. The framework is then placed on

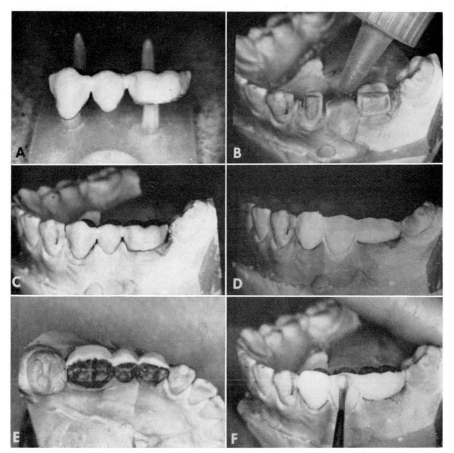

FIGURE 328. *A,* Prepared and degassed assembled frame with opaque applied and fired.

B, Cigarette paper adapted to ridge of working cast.

C, Frame seated over paper separating medium.

D, Body porcelain applied.

E, Occlusal view. Body porcelain tapered toward occlusal to make space for incisal porcelain.

F, Adding incisal porcelain.

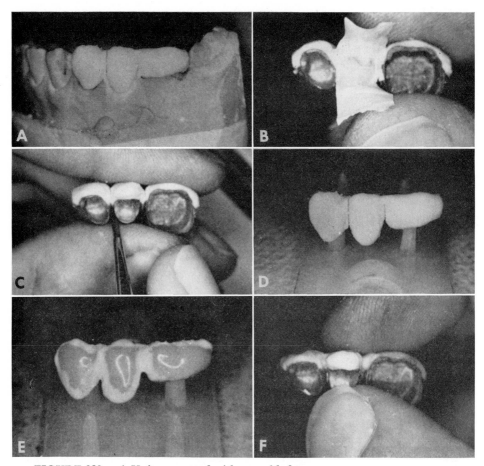

FIGURE 329. *A,* Units separated with razor blade.

B, Cigarette paper attaches to pontic and must be removed.

C, Cleaning embrasures and casting surfaces not to be veneered.

D, Bridge on firing tray. Being divided, porcelain will shrink toward three centers.

E, On firing tray for second baking. Porcelain added to lines of separation, to contacting surface of pontic, and to other areas lacking contour.

F, Excess porcelain on pontic.

the working cast over the cigarette paper, which will act as a separating medium between the stone and the porcelain to be built to contour against the cast (Fig. 328).

The veneers are built to full contour with body porcelain, with some excess to compensate for shrinkage. The area for the incisal (or occlusal) color is cut away and the incisal porcelain is applied. After being carved to form, the unit veneers are separated by a razor blade. The cut must be made in the embrasure down to the already bonded opaque layer to allow shrinkage of the porcelain toward several centers. Thus warpage of the framework can be avoided (Fig. 329).

The bridge is removed, and the cigarette paper, which usually remains attached to the porcelain, is peeled away. Porcelain that has flowed into the proximal embrasures is removed with carvers and a moist brush. The

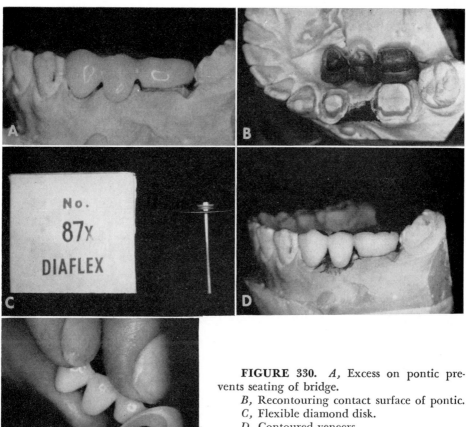

FIGURE 330. *A,* Excess on pontic prevents seating of bridge.
B, Recontouring contact surface of pontic.
C, Flexible diamond disk.
D, Contoured veneers.
E, Smoothing veneers before glazing.

bridge is placed on a firing tray with the supports fitting up inside the abutment castings. A wide selection of trays should be at hand from which to choose one with suitable spacing between the points. At times muffle repair clay must be used, or a heavy piece of nichrome wire must be bent to form a custom-made support.

After firing, shrinkage will be found where the razor blade was used for separation and at the gingival area. Another layer of porcelain must be added to the lines of separation and the cervical must be overcontoured enough for a small surplus of porcelain to remain after the second firing.

The ridge area of the working cast is blackened with a lead pencil so that, with the graphite acting as a marking agent, the bridge can be ground to fit the ridge intimately. The general contours of the buccal or labial surfaces are produced, using a Busch Silent stone.* The interproximal surfaces and the contact areas are shaped with a Horico No. 87X diamond

* Pfingst and Company, Inc., New York, N. Y.

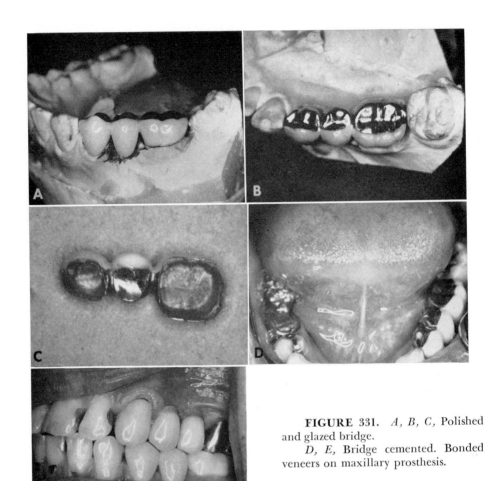

FIGURE 331.   *A, B, C,* Polished and glazed bridge.
   D, E, Bridge cemented. Bonded veneers on maxillary prosthesis.

disk.* This disk, being flexible and very thin, makes it possible to satisfactorily form fine grooves between the units, which may be stained to heighten the effect of separation. (See Chapter 17.) After contouring and smoothing, the porcelain is glazed and the finished bridge is polished, as described previously (Figs. 330 and 331).

FABRICATION OF BRIDGE AFTER BAKING VENEERS

Soldering Veneered Units

Veneered units can be assembled and soldered without damage to the porcelain or to its surface texture, provided that neither the soldering investment nor the flux contacts the veneer (Fig. 332). The fixed partial

---

* Pfingst and Company, Inc., New York, N.Y.

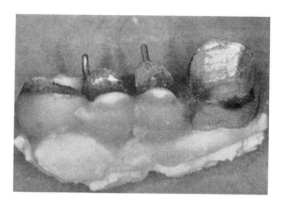

FIGURE 332. Glazed veneers covered with wax to protect surface from soldering investment.

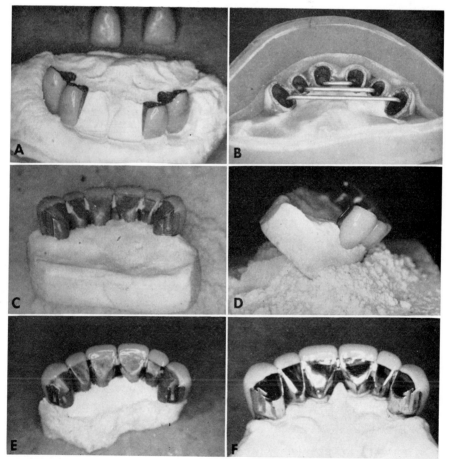

FIGURE 333. *A*, Units of a splint being assembled in plaster index.

B, U-shaped stainless steel supporting rods in place, ready for pouring soldering assembly.

C, Units fluxed.

D, On firing tray to be placed in furnace for heating.

E, *F*, Six units soldered and polished.

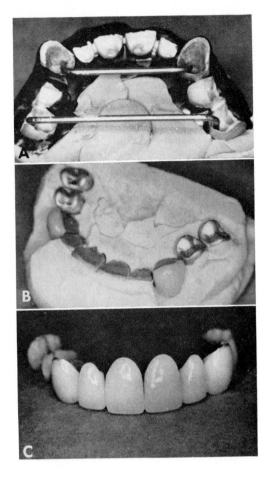

FIGURE 334. *A*, Ten-unit bridge. Cuspid retainers are veneered crowns with porcelain bonded prior to assembly of prosthesis. All other units cast from standard crown and bridge alloys. Solder joints to be made from standard gold solder.

B, Soldering assembly trimmed so that no investment will touch porcelain veneers. Bicuspid units and incisor pontics soldered before this assembly. Four joints to be soldered.

C, Assembled bridge.

denture units or those to be splinted are assembled in a plaster of Paris index and baseplate wax is flowed over the porcelain surfaces to prevent contact with investment. The soldering assembly is poured with Whip-Mix high-heat soldering investment, which must set for a minimum of ½ hour. This high-heat investment has little strength; therefore it must be reinforced to prevent fracture of the assembly, particularly when long spans are to be soldered. U-shaped stainless steel wire rods, with the tips placed inside the crowns, and extending from one side of the assembly to the other, are used for reinforcements.

The soldering assembly is placed in warm water and the index is removed. Any investment covering the wax on the porcelain surfaces is very carefully cut away and any minute particles of wax must be removed by boiling the assembly in chloroform. To avoid any overflow onto the porcelain when the assembly is heated, only minimal amounts of Ceramco flux are used. The fluxed soldering assembly should be dried in front of the open furnace muffle for 20 minutes or more, after which, during a 10-minute interval, it is slowly introduced into the furnace (Fig. 333).

A .560 fine (or 14 carat) solder, which will fuse at about 1435° F., is the most practical for this operation. Regular crown and bridge solders are preferred to the higher-fusing solders used to unite the parts prior to the application of porcelain veneers, because they fuse at lower temperatures, will fuse much more rapidly, will flow more readily, and according to clinical observation the joints are superior, especially as to form and the absence of blemishes. By comparison, the solders designed solely for use with the veneering alloys are sluggish and have a very high fusing range. Many of these joints have discernible defects.

When a .560 fine solder is to be used, the furnace should be heated, and when a temperature of approximately 1550° F. is reached, the assembly is removed and the solder is applied to the joint areas in small pieces and in such quantity as judgment dictates. It is replaced in the furnace until the solder flows and the parts are well joined. The bridge or splint is allowed to cool under a cover to room temperature before being placed in water to free it from the investment.

It is then pickled in 50 per cent hydrochloric acid to remove the flux and is polished, using the polishing Alumina (mixed with a detergent liquid), Amalgloss, or No. 600 Carborundum powder. Each will give a very high gloss to the surface of the metal.

See Chapter 17 for a discussion of cervical and incisal staining.

REFERENCES

Johnston, J. F., Dykema, R. W., Mumford, G., and Phillips, R. W.: Construction and assembly of porcelain veneer gold crowns and pontics. J. Pros. Den., *12*:1125, Nov.– Dec. 1962.

Johnston, J. F., Mumford, G., and Dykema, R. W.: Porcelain veneers bonded to metal castings. Practical Dental Monographs. Chicago, Year Book Medical Publishers, Inc., March 1963.

24

THE PORCELAIN JACKET CROWN

A single-unit restoration held in high esteem today by the profession and the discriminating public is the jacket crown.[1] The word *jacket,* although not highly technical, has been used by the profession at large to denote a porcelain or resin restoration that covers the clinical crown and terminates at or under the gingiva. It can preserve the vitality and health of the individual tooth and associated structures and maintain or satisfactorily re-establish esthetic appearance. It is used on fractured, carious, discolored, malaligned, or abraded teeth, and when constructed over a balanced preparation, it has a long life (Fig. 335).

The jacket crown is contraindicated on very short teeth, which would have minimal retention when prepared, or on maxillary anteriors when

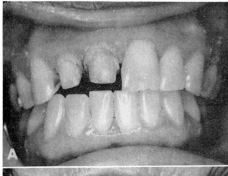
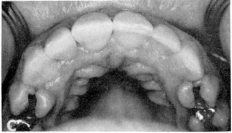
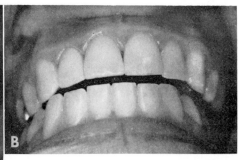

FIGURE 335. *A,* Maxillary central and lateral incisors partly prepared for jacket crowns. Because of fractured incisal edges, teeth had been restored with resin crowns when patient was an adolescent. Following normal gingival recession, margins were exposed.

B, C, Teeth rebuilt with porcelain jacket crowns. Teeth were reprepared; shoulders were placed in gingival crevice.

the opposing teeth occlude with the cervical fifth of the tooth to be restored. Under these conditions, a veneered gold casting must be considered.

If a porcelain jacket crown, which has fit, occlusion, contour, and harmonious shading, is to be constructed, there must be a concept and skills that can be developed only through long hours of practice. Ceramic technique is highly personalized, and experience or a desire for perfection, and an intimate knowledge of the working properties of the materials involved, are expected. To grasp all the significant details of this subject, the student (dentist or technician) must discipline himself in considerable arduous preparatory study. Otherwise the result can be disappointing failure.[2]

Some of the finest examples of dental art are seen in porcelain jacket crowns, and the greatest possible professional gratification to be derived from clinical restorative dentistry can come from the construction and seating of such restorations. If the operator is proficient in preparing a tooth for a porcelain jacket crown and is capable of its fabrication, or has access to the services of a dependable technician, then *porcelain is the material of choice* for both anterior and posterior teeth.[3, 4]

PREPARATION

A balanced preparation is one which is distributed on the tooth so that the space between the mesial and distal walls and the approximating teeth will be equal, as nearly as possible.[1, 5, 6, 7] Balance will distribute forces, reduce torque, and minimize breakage and unseating.

The length of the prepared tooth stump must be at least two-thirds of the longest inciso-cervical measurement of the restoration. To give general support during incising and at the mesial and distal incisal angles, the incisal edge of the preparation should be parallel with the incisal edge of the finished crown (Fig. 336).

The preparation of an anterior tooth can be accomplished by

(1) reduction of the mesial and distal surfaces without forming a shoulder;

(2) reduction of the incisal edge (steps 1 and 2 may be reversed);

(3) reduction of the lingual surface, one-half at a time (the first cut to be used as a guide for the remaining half);

(4) reduction of the labial surface;

(5) rounding the angles to produce a continuous cervical finishing line at the gingival crest;

(6) fitting the copper band;

(7) further reduction of the tooth and preparation of the shoulder; and

(8) rounding all angles except at the shoulder. (See Figs. 337 and 338.)

Axial Preparation Before Shoulder.   The mesial and distal slices are made using a disk in a straight handpiece, with the impregnated surface of

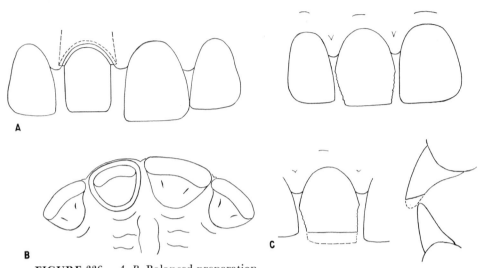

FIGURE 336. *A, B,* Balanced preparation.
C, Incisal reduced for thickness of material and for resistance to thrusts from opposing teeth.

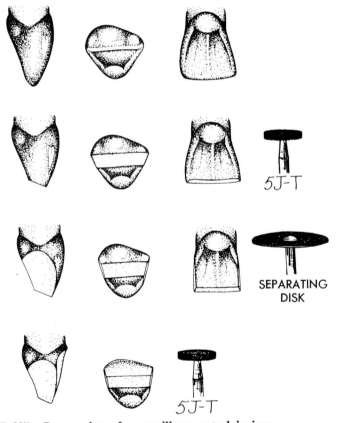

FIGURE 337. Preparation of a maxillary central incisor.
Top to bottom: Uncut tooth; reduction of incisal edge (this can precede or follow proximal slices); proximal slices made; labial surface cut.

the disk toward the pulp. The cut should be made through the tooth structure to the gingival line, and, without forming a cervical shoulder, should
converge slightly both incisally and lingually.

The incisal edge can be reduced with a wheel stone of appropriate
size, and usually this same stone may be used to reduce the labial surface.
The clearance at the incisal edge should be 1.5 mm. plus, at right angles
to the line of force from the opposing teeth, and uniform from mesial to
distal. It is not important that the incisal reduction be at right angles to
the long axis of the tooth.

The lingual surface should be prepared with a round-edge wheel
stone. The natural contour must be approximated, with 1.0 mm. clearance
at all points or paths of contact. The labial reduction, conforming to or
slightly increasing the convex tooth contour in the incisal half, must be
deep enough so the outline of the underlying tooth structure cannot be
seen or so that cement will not adversely alter the shade of the crown. The
incisal edge and angles must be observed for assurance that this has been
done.

The four angles are rounded so that the temporary cervical margin is
at and copies the contour of the gingival crest. Thus far the same rotating
cutting instruments and instrumentation have been used as were specified
for the veneered crown preparation.

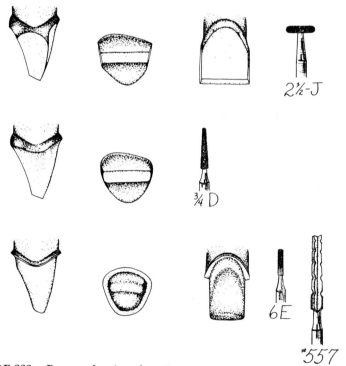

2½-J

¾ D

6E

#557

FIGURE 338. Preparation (continued).
Top to bottom: Lingual surface reduced; corners rounded, band fitted at this time;
shoulder cut.

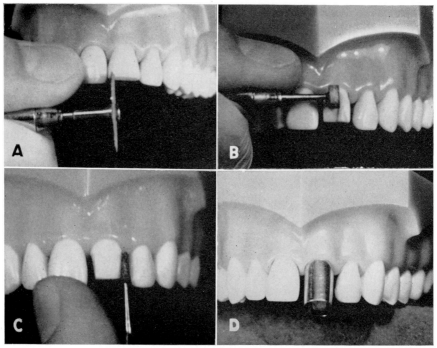

FIGURE 339. Preparing tooth for fitting band. *B,* Labial surface reduced one-half at a time with wheel stone flat surface parallel to long axis. *C,* Corners rounded with long taper stone and reduced labial surfaces smoothed.

Reduction of teeth for jacket crowns can be partially done with accelerated speeds. The preparation can be made with a chamfered cervical, using the same stones or burs designated for the veneered crown. However, the shoulder should be completed and positioned more deliberately and by the methods to be discussed in this chapter. If a copper band is to be used, it should be adapted prior to cutting the shoulder.

Copper Band Fitted (If Needed). Before the tooth is further reduced and the shoulder cut, a copper band can be fitted and contoured with the least difficulty (Fig. 339). For rubber impression materials, the band must clear the tooth by 0.3 mm. at all points. For modeling compound, it should be of such size that, when slipped over the preparation, the cervical portion will be flared a very little and will extend slightly less than 1.0 mm. into the gingival crevice. For either kind of impression, it should be adapted to the outline of the gingival margin.

Forming the Shoulder. Using a cylindrical or taper stone, the tooth structure around the cervical half of the tooth should now be reduced further to outline the shoulder and angle the walls to converge 5 to 7 degrees toward the incisal (Fig. 340). The shoulder, 0.7 mm. wide, can be cut with a No. 557 or an end-cutting bur, or with a cylindrical diamond, and finished with hand instruments to smooth the enamel and dentin. It should simulate the curves of the gingival line and extend into the crevice 0.5 mm., or one-half the depth of the crevice. The shoulder should incline into the crevice from 5 to 10 degrees, forming an angle of approximately 80 degrees apically toward the long axis of the tooth. (See Fig. 341.)

All axio-proximal line angles and mesio- and disto-incisal point angles must be rounded so that they will not act as cleavage points to induce fracture of the crown (Fig. 341), but the taper should not be increased. If the surface of the preparation is smooth, it will be easier to secure an unblemished impression.

NUTTALL'S METHOD.   Nuttall[8] uses a somewhat different but logical technique in the preparation for a jacket crown, reducing the labial, mesial, distal, and incisal, and forming the shoulder on these segments of the cervical. He says:

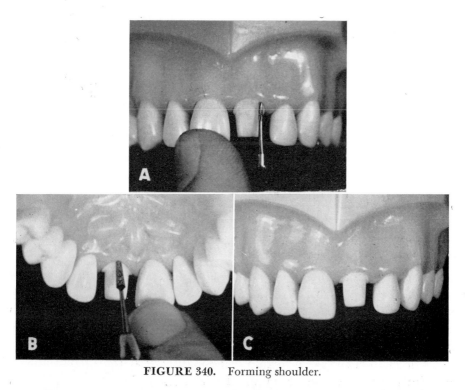

FIGURE 340.   Forming shoulder.

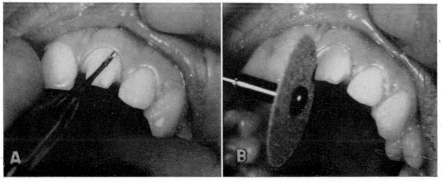

FIGURE 341.   Smoothing preparation and rounding angles.

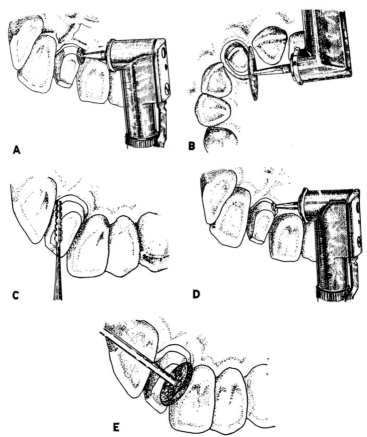

FIGURE 342.   Preparation of the lingual shoulder on a maxillary central incisor. (Courtesy of Dr. E. B. Nuttall, School of Dentistry, University of Maryland.)

"The steps in a routine preparation for the complete porcelain veneer crown may be satisfactorily executed by the average willing operator. However, producing the lingual shoulder often presents difficulties in its clinical management which may be overcome by employing the following approach to the problem [Fig. 342].

"The enamel should be reduced mesio-distally at the lingual gingival area with a 4 mm. diameter mounted wheel (#34 Starlite) with abrasive on all surfaces. The initial reduction must establish a shoulder the same thickness of the instrument and extending into the gingival crevice. [See Fig. 342*A*.]

"A 9 mm. diameter 'safe-on-inside' wheel (#39 S I Starlite) can be used to round the lingual proximal angles and to extend the shoulder in an interproximal direction. [See Fig. 342*B*.]

"The lingual and proximal shoulders can be connected with a #700 tapering crosscut fissure bur. [See Fig. 342*C*.]

"The shoulder finishing instrument (#45 Starlite) should have abrasive only on the periphery and be used to finish the lingual shoulder. [See Fig. 342*D*.]

"The lingual enamel must be removed now with a round edge mounted wheel of suitable diameter (#32 R Starlite). [See Fig. 342*E*.]

"RATIONALE.   The procedure of lingual preparation is frequently approached incorrectly, the enamel being completely removed before the shoulder is prepared, and since dentine does not resist the axial penetration of rotary instruments, this usually results in a lingual shoulder which is too wide.

"In the procedure suggested and illustrated, the enamel in the cingulum area prevents the extension of the preparation in an axial direction. Thus a shoulder of uniform width may be completed to the desired depth."

The technique devised by Nuttall is simple, rapid, and safe. It can be used readily by the novice if he will have the instruments available in the order of use.

Modifications.   On an upper lateral or a lower incisor, because of the constricted neck in relation to the width of the pulp, a No. 556 or 56 bur should be used to make a narrower shoulder. Ideally, the shoulder should be the same width on both the mesial and distal surfaces, but it may be necessary to make one side wider and one narrower in order that the prepared tooth stump will more closely approximate the center of the space to give balanced support to the crown.

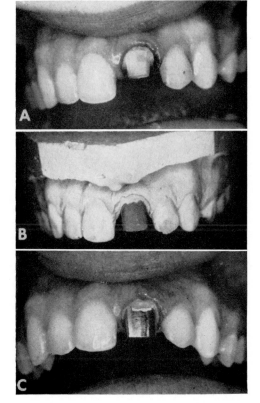

FIGURE 343.   *A,* Tooth stump too short and too conical to support jacket crown. Two porcelain crowns built for this tooth had fractured; one resin crown came off.

B, Cast ferrule designed to restore tooth to correct prepared form.

C, Completed preparation.

Preparation on Pulpless Tooth

When an anterior tooth has been fractured or mutilated by caries, or is pulpless, it must be restored to prepared form with a cast core supported by a post in the root canal (Figs. 344 and 345) or by pins extending into the dentin, or it may be rebuilt with resin, considered by some to have advantages esthetically. When a metal core is used,[9] the depth of reduction on the labial surface should be greater, so that the extra thickness of the

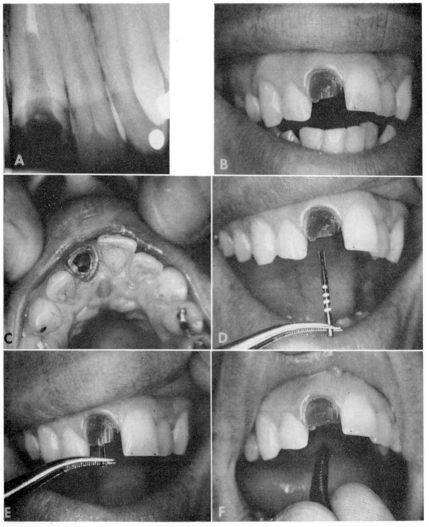

FIGURE 344.   *A,* Radiograph of maxillary central incisor. Canal has been enlarged to receive post.

B, C, Darkened tooth has been semiprepared. Shoulder not extended into crevice.

D, E, Post cut to length, serrated, and tried in canal. Extends beyond incisal edge to give area for pliers to grasp it when pattern is removed.

F, Placing cone of wax into canal.

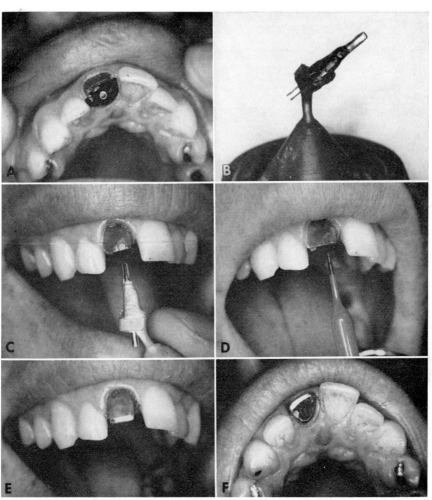

FIGURE 345. *A,* Wax and post in canal ready to carve pattern.
B, Pattern sprued.
C, Casting being fitted.
D, Placing cement in canal. Casting must be seated with light mallet pressure.
E, F, Casting cemented. Preparation completed.

crown will completely hide the prepared tooth stump. If additional tooth reduction and crown bulk are not possible, an opaque liner that will mask the prepared tooth can be used in constructing the crown.

THE DIE AND WORKING CAST

The gingival tissue must be displaced laterally with alum yarn before a polysulfide rubber impression is taken. The preparation segment of the impression is poured with stone which is allowed to set for 1 hour. It is

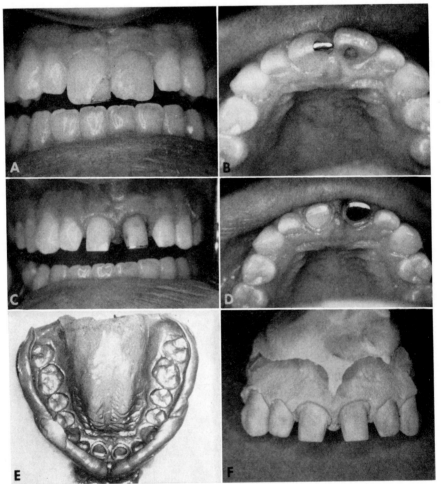

FIGURE 346. *A, B,* Adolescent patient. Left maxillary central pulpless. Right central has receded pulp, due to blow, fracture, and restoration.

C, D, Teeth prepared. Pulpless tooth restored to prepared form with cemented cast core. Incisal angle of right central recontoured with cement.

E, Complete arch polysulfide rubber impression.

F, Cast of prepared area.

removed and sectioned and the replica of the prepared tooth is trimmed to die form (Figs. 346 and 347).

An elastic impression exactly duplicates the prepared area and the tooth contour beyond it. In jacket crown construction, the undercut which extends cervically beyond the shoulder causes considerable inconvenience in the removal of a platinum matrix. A technique devised to overcome this has the undercut waxed out approximately 3.0 mm. apically from the margin of the shoulder, the wax diverging from 3 to 5 degrees. A suitable copper band (that is, one that will have 0.3 to 0.5 mm. clearance at all points) is closed on one end with modeling compound, the interior is coated with

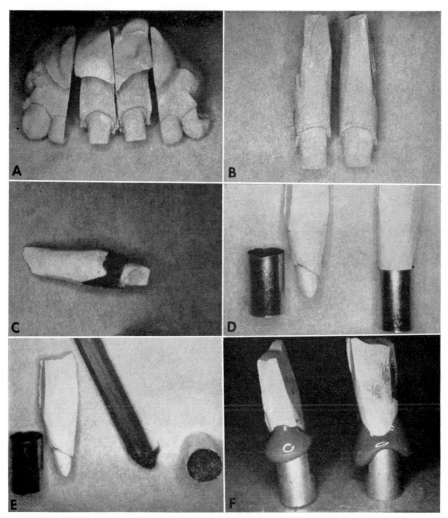

FIGURE 347. *A, B,* Cast sectioned for stone dies.
C, One stone die showing cervical contour undercut waxed out.
D, E, Fitting and preparing copper bands for impressions of stone dies.
F, Elastic impressions of stone dies.

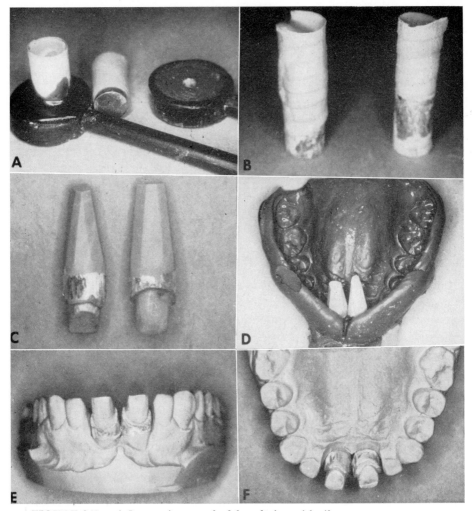

FIGURE 348. *A,* Impression attached for plating with silver.
B, Roots poured.
C, Dies.
D, Placed in same impression from which stone dies were poured.
E, F, Working cast was not articulated because matured crowns were fitted in mouth.

the appropriate rubber cement, and a polysulfide rubber impression is taken of the stone die, which no longer has a cervical undercut. The impression is silver-plated (see Chapter 11) and a stone core is poured and trimmed (Fig. 348).

The silver-plated die is seated in the original rubber base impression and luted to it with baseplate wax, and an intact full arch working cast is poured in stone and allowed to set for 1 hour. The gingival area around the die is cut away to a depth of 3.0 to 4.0 mm. on all sides. If the root of the silver-plated die was lubricated with petrolatum, it can be removed from the cast.

The working and opposing casts should be mounted on an articulator capable of being guided in protrusive or lateral excursions by the approximating and posterior teeth. If only a single anterior crown is being built, and if the matured porcelain form can be taken to the tooth to adjust occlusion, it is possible to dispense with the articulator.

TEMPORARY PROTECTION

Careful protection of the tooth can contribute much to jacket crown success.[10] If the gingival tissue is pushed aside from the shoulder only enough so that later the field may be dry during cementation, normalcy will recur almost immediately and the probability of gingival recession will be minimized. Temporary crowns should have the strength to withstand ordinary chewing and dislodging motions, and should be adjusted to the occlusion to forestall any change in tooth position. All rough edges and sharp points must be removed after fitting.

Self-curing resin should be used for the temporary crown. It can be fabricated on a cast over a simulated preparation, rather than on the tooth. While the effect of the heat generated during curing of the resin will be avoided, there are the disadvantages of poor fit and time used in adjustment. The preparation on the cast may be lubricated or covered with tin foil and the crown form trimmed to fit the shoulder. Incisal and cervical shades should be selected, mixed, and distributed inside a crown form or an alginate impression, which must be seated in alignment, and the resin allowed to polymerize. The contacts of a crown form should be perforated with a No. 6 bur so that the temporary cover will be wide enough to maintain the space. Before cementing with zinc oxide and eugenol over a lubricated stump, it should be machined internally to seat, trimmed at the cervical, and adjusted to the occlusion.

Many operators fabricate the temporary crown on the prepared tooth. If the tooth to be restored is mutilated, it is recontoured with wax on the diagnostic cast and an alginate impression is made. Then, with resin in the tooth being rebuilt, the impression is seated in the mouth over a lubricated stump. Soft tissue is protected by petroleum jelly. When the resin has begun to stiffen, the impression is removed and while still slightly flexible, the temporary crown is taken off and trimmed. It is seated with a zinc oxide and petrolatum or eugenol luting material on the stump, which has been lubricated, and the crown is polished.

Resiliency of the resin will allow removal, whenever expedient, without destroying the crown. While shading will not be satisfying, almost all patients are disposed to accept this situation for short periods. Better shade distribution is possible when the temporary crown is built on a prepared cast.

For shade selection and distribution, see Chapter 21, Esthetic Criteria in a Porcelain Restoration.

THE MATRIX

The matrix, which should be made of 0.001 inch dead-soft platinum foil, is the foundation for the construction of the crown. Platinum will not discolor porcelain and it seems to have an affinity for porcelain. It can be adapted to many shapes without destroying its continuity of surface. The one drawback is that it has an annoying attraction for most contaminating elements or substances. It should be kept in an envelope or clean box, away from all metal grindings. Porcelain has an equal affinity for contaminants, especially those harbored on the platinum foil. Green discoloration around the gingival of a fired jacket crown usually is caused by the die, but internal porosity is due to a number of contaminating influences on the platinum.[11]

A platinum matrix should not be softened or cleaned by heating in the cone of a Bunsen burner flame, but should be kept in the area of combustion. It may be annealed or heated in the furnace to a temperature 25 to 50 degrees higher than the fusing point of the porcelain to be used. This is especially important before vacuum firing, when the matrix must be degassed at 2450° F. if high-fusing porcelain is being used.

Matrix with Proximal Joint

The proximal joint concept is a product of evolution, but it appears that the reasons for placement here were founded on Pettrow's[11] research on functional breakage. When the tinner's joint is placed on the lingual surface of a maxillary anterior die, there will be a line of cleavage in the lingual surface of the porcelain crown. Since this surface receives the thrust from the opposing teeth, the possibility of fracture is increased. One of the fundamentals of jacket crown construction is that bulk adds strength. Generally one of the proximal quadrants of a jacket has its greatest thickness; therefore, if the folded joint of the matrix is moved to either the mesial or distal surface, depending on which has the greater mass, the crown will be stronger.

Technique—Proximal Joint. Before the matrix is formed, the die must be scrubbed with chloroform to remove the oils or other contaminants from the impression. A rectangular piece of platinum (Fig. 349A), approximately 5.0 mm. wider than the greatest inciso-cervical measurement of the preparation, is used. It is applied to whichever proximal surface will be thinner in the finished crown. It is held in position and pushed around the die with the thumb and first finger (Fig. 349B), then held tight with the thumb and finger of the other hand (Fig. 349C). The platinum is adapted to the shoulder with a wedge-shaped orangewood stick or a metal burnisher (Fig. 349D). The protruding ends of the platinum are grasped with cotton pliers (Fig. 349E) and pulled close against the proximal surface of the die. While the platinum is being held in position with the fingers, the flaps are trimmed to 1.5 mm. in width (Fig. 349F). On this same side, the platinum at the incisal edge is cut away at a 45 degree angle; on the opposite proximal surface, it is slit or cut from the top to the edge of the die (Fig. 349G). The two incisal tabs are shortened in length to approximately 1.0 mm. (Fig. 349H).

A tinner's joint is formed with the bend placed at the midline of the platinum extension (Fig. 350A). No attempt is made to shorten either side. The added 0.001 inch of platinum on this surface will not materially lessen the strength of the porcelain crown. After the tinner's joint has been made, the labio-incisal flap is folded over the lingual (Fig. 350B), then the

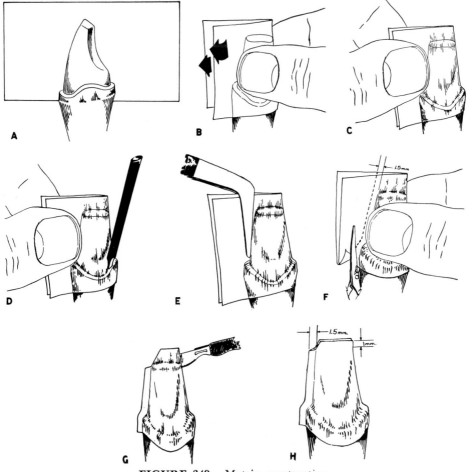

FIGURE 349. Matrix construction.

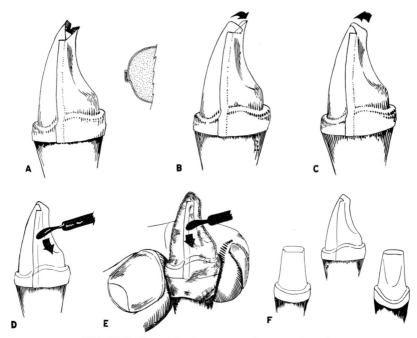

FIGURE 350.   Matrix construction (continued).

lingual flap is folded over the incisal edge toward the labial surface (Fig. 350*C*).

The platinum is burnished from incisal to cervical and all wrinkles are eliminated. (See Fig. 350*D*.) The burnishing is continued over the shoulder and down onto the apron, which should be about 3.0 mm. in width. Before swaging, the matrix is removed and the collar is trimmed to approximately 2.5 mm. in its shortest dimension and made square with the long axis of the matrix so that it can be seated and will stand without toppling. The die and the matrix are placed in the swage and the matrix is adapted to the surface of the die. After swaging it is removed with sticky wax, and the sticky wax is melted off with a torch flame, because the oxidizing areas can be controlled more thoroughly than with a Bunsen burner flame. The matrix is heated to a cherry red for the purpose of rendering it less brittle and removing any impurities.

The matrix is replaced on the die and burnished while being wrapped with, and held in position by, twisted gauze. (See Fig. 350*E*.) It is examined for wrinkles (Fig. 350*F*), and if any are found, they must be removed as nearly as possible by burnishing, since they function as cleavage lines and thus weaken the crown. The excess platinum of the tinner's joint over the shoulder can be either stoned away or left because on this surface the cement is not apt to dissolve. This indentation will not serve as a line of cleavage.

Before reseating the die and matrix, all areas of the working cast that may contact the porcelain during building the crown are painted with a solution of chloroform and clear acrylic powder. This seals the surface of the stone so that water from the porcelain mixture will not be drawn off into the cast.

BUILDING AND FIRING THE CROWN

It should be stated again that dental ceramics must be an expression of the individual. There is no substitute for enforced experience, a desire for perfection, and an encompassing knowledge of the equipment and materials to be used, but the technique and art can be learned by anyone who is willing to expend the effort.

Before constructing a jacket crown of fused porcelain, the dentist or technician should remember these two points:

1. "There are no short cuts in ceramics except not to do it."[12]

2. The firing of porcelain is accumulative; it is a combination of temperature plus time that equals maturity.

Assuming that the die, or reproduction of the prepared tooth, is exact, there are three factors which must be combined in their application and use to create a porcelain jacket crown: the platinum matrix, the furnace, and the porcelain.

The platinum must be adapted to the die intimately, *without wrinkles,* and with minimal thickness in the area of the tinner's joint. The eccentricities of the furnace must be recognized, the firing chamber must be clean, uncontaminated, and capable of being closed to contain the heat, and the pyrometer must be adjusted within the range of acceptable accuracy. Distilled water must be used with the porcelain powder to form the paste from which the jacket will be built to oversize form for firing.

Mixing the Powder.   The proportions of gingival and incisal powders should be placed on separate glass slabs. The powders (for example, two parts No. 6, one part No. 4, and six parts No. 8) must be incorporated thoroughly before the addition of distilled water. Heavy spatulation with a metal instrument must be avoided, or the porcelain will be contaminated by metallic particles. Porcelain is an abrasive, and minute bits of the metal will be transferred to the powder if pressure from the spatula is accompanied by movement (Fig. 351). When a heavy cream consistency has been reached, the mix should be vibrated while remaining on the slab. The porcelain can be mixed and kept in a mound with the spatula. It must remain moist during the working period and be covered between firings. Dry porcelain powder cannot be worked; therefore, before each build-up, water should be added and the mix vibrated. This will cause the escape of entrapped air and will aid condensation. Moist porcelain powder will build with more ease and will be freer of bubbles if applied

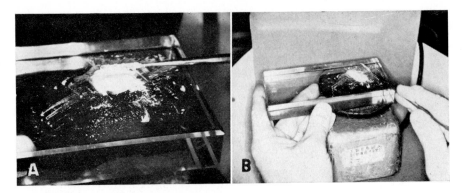

FIGURE 351. Mixing.
A, Mixing measured portions of porcelain powder and water.
B, Vibrating mix.

to the matrix with a spatula or bladed instrument rather than a brush. Excess beyond the angle of the shoulder can be trimmed away.

CERVICAL CONTACT TECHNIQUE

The First Firing or Foundation.   During firing, porcelain will shrink toward its area of greatest bulk and toward the surface to which it is attached. The first bake in making a jacket crown can establish the cervical fit if the porcelain is contoured to place the bulk in the cervical fourth and to appose the marginal area. The first application of porcelain should be very thin over the incisal half or two-thirds of the matrix and over-built in the cervical fifth or fourth. Porcelain of the gingival shade should be used. (See Fig. 352.)

Condensation is gained through light vibration from a serrated instrument and by absorbing the surface moisture with clean gauze. Vibration should be restrained so that the porcelain will not roll or flow out of position, and blotting should take place immediately upon evidence of any moisture on the surface. When moisture no longer comes to the surface, it can be assumed that condensation is sufficient, although it cannot be complete because of the shape of the particles.[13, 14]

Air-Fired 2400° Porcelain.   The "green" porcelain crown should be placed on top of the furnace, or in the preheating chamber, for a minimal time of 10 minutes, and dried completely and slowly so that no cracking will occur. The temperature at which the porcelain is inserted into the furnace is not critical, but in order that there will be no possibility that steam formation will cause an explosion within the crown, it should be placed in front of the open muffle at approximately 1200° F., or lower, and moved into position, ½ inch each move, over a 3 to 5 minute period.

The accepted firing rate of all dental porcelain is sustained by increasing the temperature 100 degrees per minute. Practice or experience with the furnace available will determine how the transformer should be manipulated. The initial firing of high-fusing porcelain should be carried to 2350° F., with no holding period. When 2350° F. is reached, the firing tray should be removed and covered with a beaker or glass until the crown is cool enough to handle. It is returned to the die, again wrapped in gauze, and the platinum apron is burnished from the shoulder toward the apex of the root. It is removed and replaced a number of times to be certain that there is no binding. A crack in the porcelain caused by undersize of the crown due to shrinkage poses no problem.

The Second Firing. The die is placed in the working cast and held so that the lingual of the crown may be supported by one finger covered by a clean gauze, and the crown is built to the incisal height with gingival porcelain. Porcelain is added to the labial surface and the cast is vibrated with a serrated spatula which is moved in one direction only. (Flow of the porcelain can thus be better controlled.) Moisture appearing on the surface is blotted with the gauze. Anatomic contour at this time is not essential.

The lingual of the crown is built in the same way, the porcelain being applied with a sliding motion of the spatula and by vibrating and blotting.

With guidance from the color distribution chart, gingival porcelain is trimmed off the labio-incisal and proximal surfaces at an angle. This is replaced and the contour of the crown restored with the incisal shade. Incisal porcelain is more difficult to handle because of the coarser particle

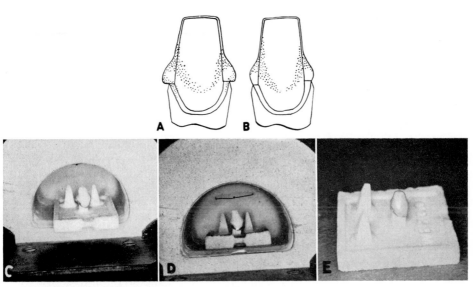

FIGURE 352. First bake.

A, Cross section of first application of porcelain.

B, Cross section of first application after firing.

C, First application drying in muffle opening.

D, In muffle; note relation to thermocouple.

E, After firing.

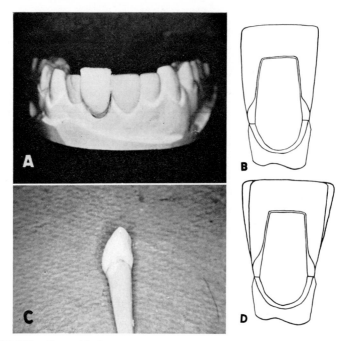

FIGURE 353. Second bake.
A, Die and crown in working cast; incisal has been built longer than approximating teeth to compensate for shrinkage.
B, Cross section of first and second applications of porcelain.
C, Die removed, ready to increase bulk at contacts.
D, Cross section before second firing, showing added porcelain at contact areas.

size needed to produce translucence. It should be flowed on with a brush and built up from 1.0 to 1.5 mm. longer than the finished crown (Fig. 353).

The crown should receive final condensation by burnishing or "whipping" with a large sable's-hair brush. Then the proximal surfaces should be dampened with the die in the cast, and the die and crown removed. The cervical portions must be trimmed to approximate contour but slightly beyond the margin of the shoulder. From 0.5 to 1.0 mm. of porcelain (either gingival or incisal, or both, depending on the color pattern) should be added to each proximal surface.

Following the same technique described previously, the crown is dried on top of the furnace or in the preheating chamber and placed in the furnace. It need not be directly under the thermocouple, but it should not be close to the furnace door. The furnace temperature should be advanced at approximately 100 degrees per minute to 2400° F., with no holding time. The crown is then removed and allowed to cool under a glass beaker.

Contouring. A Busch Silent stone is used to remove the excess at the incisal and to contour the crown. However, at the gingival margin, a concave carborundum or a flexible diamond disk may be used. The crown should be placed on the die and the excess on the proximal surfaces observed (Fig. 354), so that when these surfaces are contoured, equal pressure will be established mesially and distally on the approximating teeth. This will add to the safety and comfort of the cemented crown. Contacts must have strength comparable to that in other sections of the mouth.

The occlusion must be adjusted at this time. If articulated casts have been used, this can be done in the laboratory, or the crown may be taken to the mouth. When a crown is to be adjusted in the mouth, the apron of the platinum matrix must be trimmed to a width of 0.4 mm.

The Third Firing.   The crown is brushed thoroughly with detergent and water, and washed. Any elusive black specks at the surface can be effectively removed by boiling in nitric acid, but those which are embedded must be ground out. The crown is dried and the surface rubbed with dry porcelain powder; if a small bubble or irregularity developed in the surface of the crown during the second firing, or if it becomes necessary to add to the contour, the mix of porcelain should be 75 per cent of 2400° porcelain and 25 per cent of low-fusing, or 1875°,* porcelain. It is then returned to the furnace and carried to 2400° F. and held at this temperature from 2 to 6 minutes. During the holding period, the crown should be examined at least once for luster and surface texture. It is removed from the furnace and covered to cool slowly.

Fitting.   The finished crown should be tried on the tooth before the matrix is removed so that contacts and occlusion may be checked (Fig. 355).

---

* Steele's Apco, The Columbus Dental Mfg. Co., Columbus, Ohio.

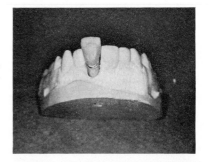

FIGURE 354.   Contouring. Crown after second firing. Contacts, length, occlusion, and contour must be checked and corrected.

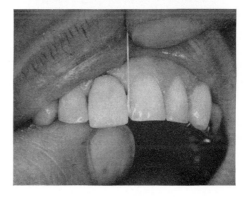

FIGURE   355.   Testing   contact strength when fitting and contouring crown.

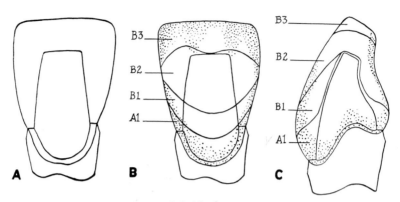

FIGURE 356. *A,* Cross section of finished crown.

B, C, Cross sections showing layers of porcelain: A1, initial application, gingival; B1, second application, gingival; B2, first application, incisal; B3, second application, incisal or incisal mixed with a translucent porcelain.

If any adjustment is made, the ground surface should be covered with an overglaze. If a contact area is slightly lacking in convexity or strength of pressure, this too may be corrected by use of an overglaze, which should be mixed thicker and added in greater bulk.

The matrix can be removed with a pair of straight-beak tweezers by grasping the platinum apron and rolling it toward the center of the crown. Removal of the platinum can be facilitated by the presence of water. The action here has never been explained, but the clinical phenomenon exists. If the matrix was made quite smooth before the crown was built, it should be removed with little effort.

If the shoulder of the preparation has been made 0.5 to 0.8 mm. in width on the labial surface and if the inciso-cervical contour of the tooth has been followed in the preparation, the porcelain should be thick enough to disguise or hide the prepared tooth stump and the underlying cement completely.

If, for some reason, the preparation could not be deep enough, or if the tooth is pulpless and has become quite dark, prior to building up the crown a layer of opaque porcelain should have been applied by brush to the matrix and fired to a low maturity at 2350° F. (Figs. 356 and 357).

CERVICAL DITCHING TECHNIQUE

A clinical case will be used to illustrate this technique for jacket crown construction. The teeth were prepared, extending the shoulders into the gingival crevices approximately 0.4 mm. A working cast with removable silver-plated dies was made and a platinum matrix was formed on each die. (See Figs. 346, 347, and 348.) The technique to be described is for Trubyte 2100° vacuum-fired porcelain, which is built over an opaque.

However, the building sequence has an unlimited application and is probably used more than any other.

Application of the Opaque

The opaque is mixed to a thin, creamy consistency by spatulating and vibrating to help eliminate any air bubbles. It is applied to the matrix

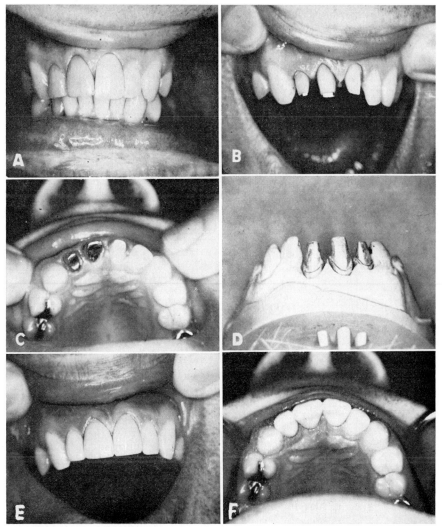

FIGURE 357. Construction of three porcelain jacket crowns on a pulpless lateral and central and a vital central.

A, Discolored maxillary right central and lateral incisors.

B, C, Three teeth prepared. Pulpless teeth built up to prepared form by cast cores, with posts extending into root canals.

D, Working cast. Dies are silver-plated with stone roots. Roots were coated with petrolatum before cast was poured.

E, F, Crowns after cementation.

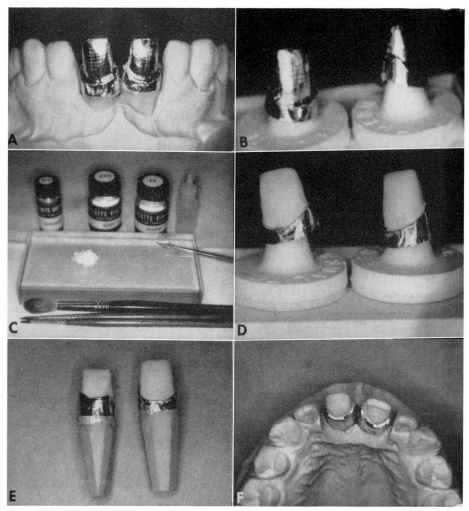

FIGURE 358. *A,* Platinum matrices formed. They were made with proximal joints, were burnished, swaged, and reburnished, then removed with a covering of chilled sticky wax.

B, Matrices on firing trays. To be placed in furnace for degassing and burning off of other impurities.

C, Armamentarium for applying opaque.

D, Opaque applied.

E, F, Opaque fired. Opaque was necessary because of darkened pulpless tooth.

with a spatula, and by alternately vibrating and drying is built up evenly over the matrix surface, except on the shoulder, to a thickness of approximately 0.4 mm. The opaque is dried in front of the open muffle or in the drying chamber of the furnace. When the muffle registers 1600° F., it is placed in the furnace, the vacuum is started immediately, and the temperature is increased 100 degrees per minute until 2100° F. has been reached (Fig. 358).

The tray is removed and placed under a cover to cool. The matrix with the fired opaque is placed on the die and the shoulder is readapted.

Building the Crown

First Firing. Body and incisal porcelain are mixed to a thick, creamy consistency on separate slabs (Fig. 359). The crown is built up to contour with the body porcelain, applying the porcelain with a spatula. The die is vibrated with a serrated instrument, and the moisture that comes to the surface is absorbed with a clean gauze pad (Fig. 360). Porcelain is added, vibrated, and dehydrated until the crown is overcontoured. This is all done with the die in the working cast. The proximal and incisal excess is trimmed, leaving some porcelain overlapping the approximating teeth, and the surface is burnished and smoothed with a large brush, using a whipping motion. The incisal edge and the labial surface are carved away to provide space for the incisal color.

This is added and condensed by vibrating, dehydrating, burnishing, and brushing. It is built about 1.0 mm. overlength. The crown is removed and the grooves formed by the overlapping proximal porcelain are filled with body and incisal so that the crown has extra contour in all dimensions. The lingual is roughly carved to form, but with excess thickness. The die is removed from the working cast, and the cervical porcelain is carved away to form a V-shaped ditch exposing the platinum shoulder of the matrix (Fig. 361). It is dried and placed in the furnace at 1600° F., the vacuum is turned on, and the temperature is increased 100 degrees per minute until 2050° F. has been reached. It is covered while cooling.[8, 15, 16, 17]

Second Firing. The adaptation of the matrix to the shoulder is checked on the die and improved if necessary. When placed in the working cast, the mesio-distal measurement of the crown is sometimes too wide. If so, the contacts must be reduced by grinding with a Busch Silent stone or a Dedeco rubber porcelain wheel so that the die, with the crown in

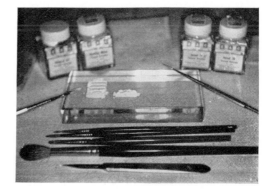

FIGURE 359. Equipment for building porcelain crown.

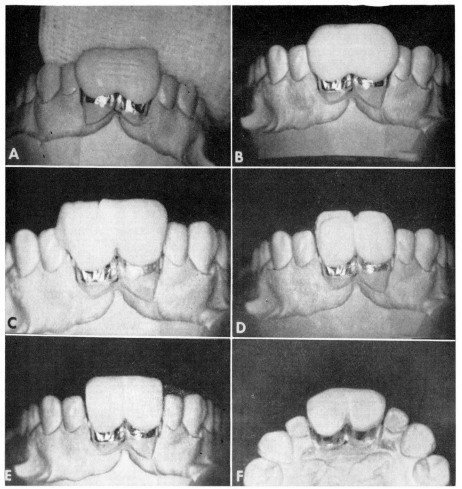

FIGURE 360. *A,* Gauze is held against the lingual surface of the dies and body porcelain is built on the labial surface in a solid mass. Approximating teeth have been coated with lacquer to prevent absorption of moisture from porcelain. Cast was vibrated with serrated instrument and moisture absorbed by gauze as soon as it came to surface.

B, Mass of porcelain condensed by vibrating, absorbing moisture, and brushing.

C, Lingual porcelain added.

D, Body porcelain trimmed and incisal porcelain added.

E, F, All porcelain condensed and matrices cleaned.

place, will seat in the working cast with equal pressure mesially and distally (Fig. 362).

The ditch at the cervical is filled with body-colored porcelain and considerably overcontoured. Porcelain is added wherever shrinkage from the first firing has minimized the contour. The firing cycle is repeated, the temperature being taken to 2100° F., and after cooling the crown is roughly shaped, using stones and rubber porcelain grinding wheels. If the cervical ditch is undercontoured, porcelain is added and the firing cycle is repeated. The crown may receive its final shaping on the working cast.

Preferably it will be taken to the mouth in the low maturity stage so that occlusion and contacts may be re-established, and contour and minute anatomic irregularities checked. Contacts must be very carefully tested and at the mouth-checking stage should seem to be tight. Occlusion must be meticulously developed. Staining should be done at this stage.

Final Firing. Final firing or glazing is done in atmosphere, because if done in vacuum, a pitted surface generally will result. Pitting or bubble formation caused by contamination of the matrix or porcelain is magnified by vacuum firing. The crown is preheated, placed in the furnace at

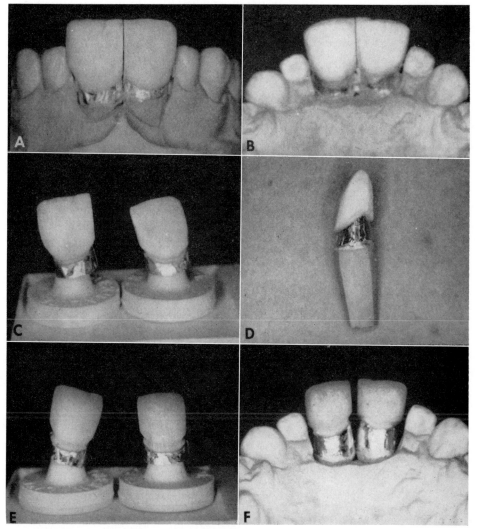

FIGURE 361.   *A, B,* Mass sectioned into two crowns.

C, D, Cervical porcelain carved away to form ditch. Shrinkage will be toward incisal and will not disturb fit of matrix.

E, F, Crowns after first firing.

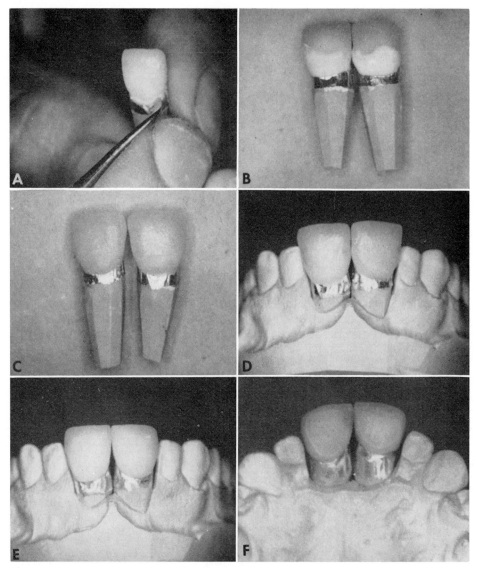

FIGURE 362.   *A*, Readapting matrix to shoulder of die.
B, Ditches filled after crowns were contoured.
C, After second firing.
D, Contacts adjusted; dies seated.
E, *F*, Crowns contoured ready for third firing.

1850° F., carried up to 2100° F. in 3 minutes, and held for 3 minutes (Fig. 363).

The surface texture of the patient's natural teeth should have been observed and the glaze on the crown must be in harmony. This can be developed through variation in the terminal temperature of the glaze firing, which may range from 2000° F. to 2100° F., or by varying the holding time between 2 and 6 minutes.

It must be repeated that before removing the matrix, the crown should be taken to the mouth to check contacts and occlusion; these will almost always be correct if it was tried in the mouth before glazing. If there is a prematurity or if a contact is lacking in pressure, the stoned or under-contoured proximal area can be built up with a special "add-on" porcelain. This is dried, placed in the furnace at 1300° F. and taken to 1775° F. in 5 minutes, and held for 2 minutes. To correct a minute discrepancy, a thick coating of Steele's Super Glaze may be applied and fired at 1945° F.,

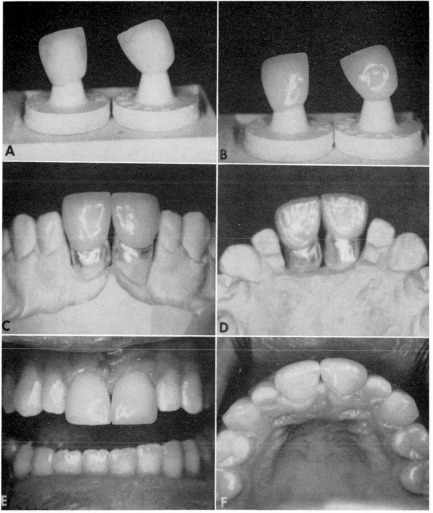

FIGURE 363. *A,* Crowns have been checked for contacts and occlusion, contoured, and cleaned. Ready for glaze firing. Matrices were trimmed to facilitate seating crowns on teeth.

B, Crowns glazed.

C, D, Crowns on working cast.

E, F, Crowns cemented.

making the surface quite smooth and giving the contact the desired strength. The matrix is removed.

When a crown is fabricated in a laboratory, the technician must be instructed to return it with the matrix in place. Otherwise no alterations are possible.

CEMENTATION

It is helpful to have at hand an assortment of zinc phosphate, silico-phosphate, and resin cements so that there will be many shades from which to select the one, or the combination, which will enhance the coloring or harmony of the finished restoration.[8]

For a porcelain crown, the choice of a zinc phosphate cement can be made from trial mixes of powder and glycerin and water after the matrix has been removed. Silicate or resin cement may be selected from a prepared shade guide.

The crown must be cleaned and dried and the tooth isolated and dried. The cements should be mixed not only for strength but also for ease of extrusion. An excess of cement should be placed inside the crown and over the shoulder of the prepared tooth. When it has been seated, the crown should be held in position by the operator. After the hardened excess of cement has been removed, the gingival crevice should be examined for fragments.

The patient must be instructed with regard to the normal care of the restoration and *his* part of the responsibility for the success of the case. The value of hygiene, gingival massage, and periodic examination to ascertain changes in occlusion must be emphasized. The patient should be admonished to avoid biting on thread or pipe stems, or other hard objects that might create a point contact.

BREAKAGE

When a porcelain jacket crown breaks in the mouth,[11] it breaks from the inside out as a result of reciprocal pressures. Sharp line angles or corners cause more breakage than any other factor, owing to increased stress concentration in those areas. Moon-shaped breaks on the labial surface occur because of insufficient length in the prepared tooth. To afford support for the jacket, the abutment preparation at its longest portion should be close to two-thirds of the length of the finished restoration from shoulder to incisal. It must be remembered that an uninterrupted surface has a strength peculiar unto itself; interrupted, it becomes weakened. Therefore, before the platinum matrix is removed for cementation of the crown, all adjustments should be made and the crown reglazed to re-established surface continuity. Even so, equilibration in the future may induce frail areas.

REFERENCES

1. Brecker, S. C.: The Porcelain Jacket Crown. St. Louis, The C. V. Mosby Company, 1951.
2. Theofilis, B. G.: The porcelain jacket crown. Senior thesis, Indiana Univ. School Den., June 1955.
3. Bartels, J. C.: Full porcelain veneer crowns. J. Pros. Den., 7:533, July 1957.
4. Bastian, C. C.: Porcelain jacket crown. D. Clin. North America, March 1959, p. 133.
5. Rieser, J., and Aaronson, W.: Different technic of anterior porcelain jacket crown preparation. J.A.D.A., 56:559, April 1958.
6. Fairley, J. M., and Deubert, L. W.: Preparation of maxillary central incisor for a porcelain jacket restoration. Brit. D. J., 104:208, March 18, 1958.
7. Bartels, J. C.: Preparation of the anterior teeth for porcelain jacket crowns. J. South. California D. A., 30:199, June 1962.
8. Nuttall, E. B.: Personal communication.
9. Mumford, G.: Recent studies in porcelain and porcelain jacket crown construction. Paper read before the Partial Prosthodontics Section, American Dental Association meeting, Philadelphia, Oct. 1961.
10. Malson, T. S.: Protection for jacket crown preparations. Ohio D. J., 33:139, June 1959.
11. Pettrow, J. N.: Practical factors in building and firing characteristics of dental porcelain. J. Pros. Den., 11:334, March–April 1961.
12. Pettrow, J. N.: Personal communication.
13. Baker, C. R.: Condensation of dental porcelain. J. Pros. Den., 10:1094, Nov.–Dec. 1960.
14. Vines, R. F., and Semmelman, J. O.: Densification of dental porcelain. J. D. Res., 36:950, Dec. 1957.
15. Dunton, H.: Personal communication.
16. Jones, R. J.: Personal communication.
17. Moskey, M. S.: Personal communication.

Bartels, J. C.: Porcelain as an esthetic restorative material. D. Clin. North America, Nov. 1963, p. 831.

Bastian, C. C.: Restoration of lower anterior teeth. J. Pros. Den., 6:684, Sept. 1956.

Blancheri, R. L.: Optical illusions and cosmetic grinding. Rev. Association Den. Mexicana, 8:103, 1950.

Blazoudakis, C.: Personal communication.

Clark, E. B.: The color problem in dentistry. D. Digest, 37:499, 571, 646, 732, 815, 1931.

Felcher, F. R.: The Art of Porcelain in Dentistry. St. Louis, The C. V. Mosby Company, 1932.

Hobo, S.: A study of the fit of porcelain inlays using different technics. Master's thesis, Indiana Univ. School Den., 1964.

Manners, P.: Removal of jacket crowns. J. Pros. Den., 7:814, Nov. 1957.

Miller, C. J.: Inlays, Crowns and Bridges. Philadelphia, W. B. Saunders Company, 1962.

Nuttall, E. B.: Factors influencing success of porcelain jacket restorations. J. Pros. Den., 11:743, July–Aug. 1961.

Sacchi, H., and Paffenbarger, G. C.: A simple technic for making dental porcelain jacket crowns. J.A.D.A., 54:366, March 1957.

Yock, D. H.: Porcelain jacket veneer crown preparation. Iowa D. J., 43:267, Oct. 1957.

25

THE CONSTRUCTION OF CROWNS
AND BRIDGES WITH RESIN VENEERS

For more than two decades, resins have been used to restore individual teeth and to veneer crowns and bridges. As with many materials and processes achieving wide popularity almost instantaneously, there have been widespread abuses in application and expectations, extravagant claims for adaptability and for improved physical properties, and just as frequently unwarranted and unjust criticisms. Because of its successes and in spite of its failures, acrylic resin remains a part of the armamentarium of the dental profession.

In addition to acrylic resin, others are also available for veneering purposes. These include acrylic copolymers, vinyl, and epoxy resins. Each type has certain advantages and disadvantages in terms of the inherent physical properties. However, none has been shown to be markedly superior and all have the general characteristics that will be described here.[1, 2]

Physical Properties of Acrylic Resin

Acrylic resin is translucent in varying degrees, sometimes a desirable trait in a tooth-colored restoration. This translucent quality gives it a natural look in the mouth because it is capable of assuming shade values from the approximating teeth. The esthetic appearance of a veneered restoration may be influenced considerably by the underlying metal, but this can be controlled in some measure by using opaquing or masking materials or if the veneer is 1.0 mm. or more thick and helps to serve as its own mask. Properly manipulated, most of the resin materials procurable today are

430

reasonably color-stable. Resin will flow and alter its shape when subjected to even relatively light loads over long periods of time, and it undergoes elastic deformation under intermittent stresses that may be too light to cause permanent change.[3] Therefore, a resin veneer must be protected from occlusal forces by a thickness of gold, which is visible in many cases.

Acrylic resin does not bond to the metallic portion of the restoration.[4] It must depend on some type of mechanical lock. This inherent weakness, coupled with a high coefficient of thermal expansion in resin as compared with gold, may allow a space to form at the interface between the gold and the veneer, even though the veneer is protected by metal from the forces of occlusion. Debris from the oral cavity probably can penetrate under the veneer and discolor it, or induce tarnish and corrosion of the underlying metal, either of which could cause discoloration of the veneer.[5] Adequate retention and protection, and technique in packing and curing, will minimize such a space, although it can never be eliminated completely. The veneer is easy to apply, or to remove for remaking if the shade is unsatisfactory.

Since pure gold is a relatively inert material, gold-plating the area to be veneered will lessen the chance of tarnish of the underlying metal. Gold-plating may be done by the usual electrical process or by flash-plating.*

Clinical experience has shown that an acrylic resin veneer may be abraded severely during tooth brushing. This problem probably cannot be resolved altogether with the resins presently available, but by using a semi-soft brush and a tooth paste containing no coarse abrasives, and with patient education in regard to proper brushing technique, labial and buccal abrasion will be less pronounced.[5, 6] A resin veneer will wear rapidly under the cast retentive clasp arm of a partial denture, or under a heavy occlusal or incisal load if the opposing arches are subjected to normal wear and closure.[3]

There is very little or no difference in the preparation[7] of a tooth for a crown to be veneered with resin and one to be veneered with porcelain, except in length. For a resin veneer crown the prepared tooth, under ideal conditions, can be left 0.5 to 0.8 mm. longer than when a bonded porcelain veneer crown will be used (Fig. 364).

The Die

Any acceptable method of obtaining the dies and working casts may be used for constructing resin veneer crowns and bridges, but there are obvious advantages in using an indirect technique. Metalized dies are excellent; stone dies and intact working casts, poured in one impression, give splendid results.

---

* Gold Plating Solution, The L. D. Caulk Company, Milford, Del.

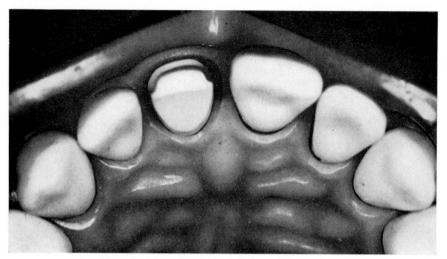

FIGURE 364.   Width and lingual extension of shoulder.

The Shade

The shade should be selected using a New Hue,* Biotone,* or Myerson† shade guide. The choice will depend on the acrylic resin to be used, or on the shade of the tooth, and possibly on the resin favored by the technician.

A shade distribution chart, made with care, should be sent to the laboratory.

THE RESIN VENEER CROWN

The Wax Pattern

It is advisable that the pattern be carved to anatomic form (Fig. 365) before an attempt is made to shape the area to be veneered, because correct contour cannot be visualized when dealing with only a portion of a tooth. After form, contact, and occlusion have been attained, the veneer outline should be drawn on the wax pattern with a sharp instrument. Then the wax in the area of the veneer may be removed completely to the labial surface of the die, and a single layer of 28-gauge sheet wax adapted to the die surface and sealed to the pattern; or a uniform layer of the original wax, about 0.5 mm. thick, may be left (Fig. 366). The latter method is preferable, since carving wax resists deformation during handling more effectively than the softer sheet wax.

---

* The Dentists' Supply Company, York, Penna.
† Tooth Corp., Cambridge, Mass.

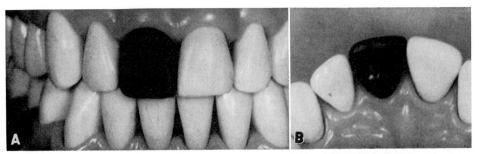

FIGURE 365. Wax pattern from labial (*A*) and incisal (*B*).

FIGURE 366. Labial of pattern reduced.

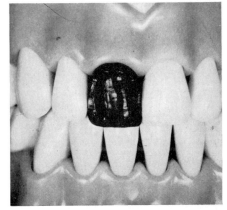

The occlusal and cervical peripheral wax around the area to be veneered is not cut down as far as the gold casting will be reduced. This excess wax will allow molten metal to be fed into the thin labial portion of the casting from a surrounding area of considerably heavier bulk, and will assure a complete casting in the thin section, which will back the veneer. An accessory wax sprue rod, or vent, joining the labial surface of the pattern and the sprue former, may be helpful in securing a complete casting. The proximal outlines should be established in the wax, since the proximal retentive loops will make it impossible to alter the outline here after the casting has been made.

Retention. Retentive wire loops, 27-gauge or 28-gauge, incorporated in the proximal of the pattern, will offer maximal retention for the veneer.[5] They can be purchased or they may be formed from wire of proper size and physical properties. The wire must be nonoxidizing in order to form a union with the casting, soft enough so that adjustments can be made after the casting has been completed, and have a fusing range high enough for gold to be cast to it without changing its physical properties.* The loops should be staplelike in shape, about 1.0 mm. in diameter and 1.5 mm. in

---

* Zephyr wire, The J. M. Ney Company, Hartford, Conn.; Pliant wire, J. F. Jelenko & Co., Inc., New Rochelle, N. Y.

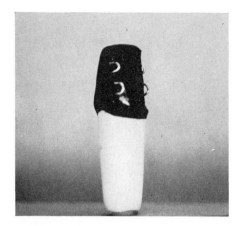

FIGURE 367.   Retentive loops.

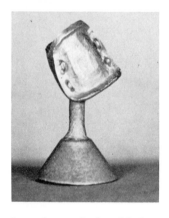

FIGURE 368.   The casting.

length, and should be placed approximately 0.7 to 1.0 mm. inside the peripheral margin of the veneer area, perpendicular to the surface of the wax at that point (Fig. 367).

If the loops are warmed very slightly in a flame while being held by tweezers, the wire can be forced into the wax far enough to be held securely. Then a small instrument should be heated and placed in contact with the wire loop. Enough heat will be conducted from the instrument to melt the wax around the points of the wire, making it a simple matter to guide the loop to place. At no time should the hot instrument come into contact with the wax.

The wire should extend into the pattern about 0.5 mm., leaving an exposed loop 1.0 mm. high and 1.0 mm. wide. The number of loops will depend on the length of the tooth involved; in most instances two loops can be inserted on each side. The wire must not be placed so far incisally on an anterior crown that it will show through the thin resin in that area.

Plastic beads may be added to the surface to be veneered. They will form irregular nodules to supplement the loop and undercut retention and further reduce the amount of percolation. Beads should not supply the only retention for the veneer.

The Casting

Because a veneered gold crown has almost-parallel walls and a small inside diameter, an investment and casting technique capable of maximal expansion must be used. Inlay Cristobalite and Control Powder, used with an asbestos liner and a burnout temperature of 1250° F., is satisfactory. A hard crown and bridge or partial denture gold should be used (Fig. 368).

The final peripheral outline of the casting can be established by further reduction of the incisal protection and the cervical collar of gold, using a No. 557 or 558 steel bur. To augment the retention afforded by the wire loops and to make certain that the bulk of resin in these areas will provide the required color in the veneer, undercuts must be placed incisally and cervically (Fig. 369), using a No. 33½ or 34 inverted cone, No. ½ round, and No. 14 wheel burs. The thickness of metal remaining between the opposing teeth and the resin veneer must be checked after the undercuts have been made. The minimum should be 1.0 mm. If the unit is a part of a bridge or splint, it should be soldered, and then the surface to be veneered should be cleaned and smoothed with a metal bur.

If it is possible that the tips of the loops will be visible through the resin, they may be bent toward the midline of the restoration (Fig. 370),

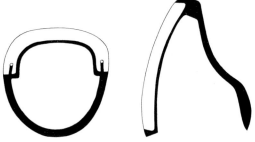
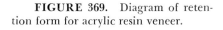

FIGURE 369. Diagram of retention form for acrylic resin veneer.

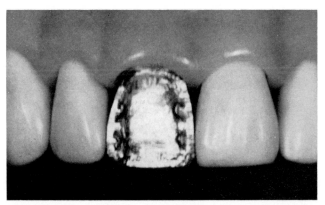

FIGURE 370. Peripheral outline established in casting. Loops bent toward center of crown.

thereby bringing a greater thickness of the veneering material over the wires. Bending is necessary in the majority of cases and will not appreciably affect the retentive qualities of the loops. If the veneered area is to be plated, it must be done at this time, after which the restoration can be polished and scrubbed clean.[8]

The Mold

The contour for the finished veneer, with the exact form and surface markings desired, must be produced in tooth-colored wax. The restoration should be invested in a small amount of stone, labial or buccal surface up, with the stone approaching but not in contact with the wax veneer. No undercuts on the metallic portion may be left unfilled by stone, because they would cause fracture of the second half of the mold when the flask was opened, or, even worse, might effect deformation of the casting. If the restoration is complicated, of five, six, or more units, those not to be veneered may be wrapped in a thin layer of wet asbestos to make subsequent removal from the stone easier. However, all areas to be veneered must be supported by hard stone to ensure adequate resistance to the high pressures to which these sections are subjected during packing.

After the first layer of stone has set, it must be trimmed circumferentially to within approximately 2.0 mm. of the restoration and then invested in plaster or stone in the bottom half of the flask. This double-investing technique makes it possible to remove the crown or bridge from the bulk of the investing stone without danger of damage to the restoration. The surface of the investing stone in the first half of the flask should be lubricated with petroleum jelly and the excess carefully wiped away without obliterating any detail of the wax veneer.

The second half of the mold must be poured with well-spatulated, bubble-free stone, without trapping air bubbles over the wax pattern. When it has set, the mold should be warmed in a water bath to prevent the wax from sticking to the mold, the flask opened, and the surface examined for imperfections (Fig. 371). If there are no bubbles or voids in the counterdie, the wax can be flushed from the mold by a stream of boiling water and all traces of the wax residue removed with a solvent such as chloroform. The case may be veneered with resin when the mold has cooled to room temperature.

Veneering Resins

There are many tooth-colored acrylic resins available to the dental profession. The majority are satisfactory; choice depends solely on personal preference. There are several opaque or masking materials also, but the resin ones appear to be the most successful. The paint and lacquer opaques seem to act as contaminating agents or to produce discoloration of the veneer. A resin masking material has the advantage of becoming an integral, inseparable part of the veneer during the process of polymerization, permitting masking in the retentive areas of the casting without loss of retention. The autopolymerizing or self-curing resin restorative materials are not suitable for veneers, being very difficult to handle and not as color-stable as heat-cured resins.

Masking. It is not always necessary to use a masking material. If the veneer is sufficiently thick, the color, especially the darker shades, should not be influenced by the underlying metal. However, masking probably will improve the shade of a veneer if it is no thicker than 1.0 mm.

The medium chosen should be approximately the same color or should be blended to complement the shade selected for the finished veneer. If a close match is impossible, a darker opaque will be better than a lighter one, separate colors being used for masking the cervical and incisal sections. A thin, uniform coating, just thick enough to obliterate the color of the metal, should be applied, with no build-up of masking material around the peripheral margin of the veneer. As soon as the masking layer has set, the main body of the veneer may be applied.

The Veneer—Gingival. The gingival portion of the veneer should be prepared first, placing the resin powder or blended powders of the pre-selected shade in a small, covered mixing jar. Only enough monomer should be added to wet all particles of the powder. The powder and liquid must be mixed slightly to obtain uniform color, the jar covered tightly to prevent evaporation of the liquid, and then set aside until the resin has reached a doughy consistency. Several sheets of cellophane should be placed in a bowl of water so that a fresh piece will be at hand each time the flask is to be closed.

Gingival resin, roughly equal to the bulk of the veneer, should be placed over the metal and shaped to approximate form with a stainless steel spatula. After a damp sheet of cellophane has been placed between the two halves of the flask, the mold must be closed with a bench press, then opened

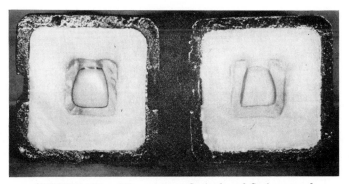

FIGURE 371. Wax pattern flasked and flask opened.

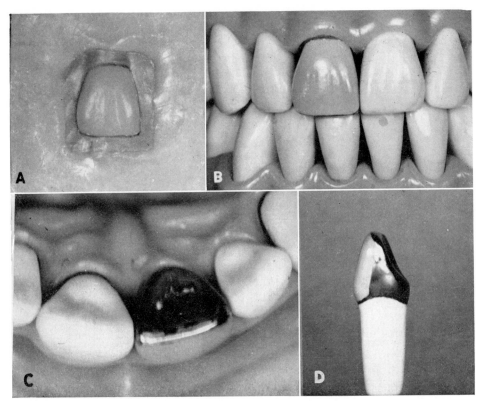

FIGURE 372. The processed and finished crown.
A, Crown in flask.
B, C, D, Finished crown.

and the veneer examined for contour and surface detail. A lack of material, flow, or details would indicate the need for more resin, in which case a small amount is added, a fresh damp sheet of cellophane is placed for separation, and the flask is again closed in a press. Trial packing must be repeated until all contours and surface details are registered and the resin has a firm consistency.

The Veneer—Incisal. As soon as the flask is opened, the incisal area must be trimmed with a sharp instrument to remove the bulk to be replaced by the incisal shade; that which remains may be reshaped with a flat instrument. The incisal powder, mixed in a Dappen dish, will have a sandlike consistency when all particles have been wet by monomer. After it has been carried to place and patted to form, a moist sheet of cellophane is placed over the first half of the flask and the top portion is positioned without pressure and kept there for approximately 5 minutes. This will assure blending of the two shades without displacing the gingival portion. The flask should be opened to check the shade distribution. If the incisal has reached a doughy consistency, it is ready for the application of packing pressure. If more incisal must be added or an excess removed, corrections are made before the flask is closed under pressure. The flask must be opened for a final check, all excess trimmed from the periphery of the veneer, and a new sheet of cellophane inserted between the halves before the flask can be closed for processing.

Processing and Finishing

Processing should be completed by immersing the flask and press in a room-temperature water bath and raising the temperature of the water to 212° F. over a period of 30 minutes. Then the case must be boiled for an additional 30 minutes, after which press and flask should be removed from the boiling water and allowed to bench-cool to room temperature. (See Fig. 372.) Only then should the flask be opened and the restoration carefully removed from the investing stone so that the margins will not be damaged or the restoration distorted. If the packing was done meticulously and all excess removed before the final closure of the flask, there will be only a little additional flash of resin at the margins of the veneer. This can be removed with a sharp knife or a fissure bur, and the areas polished. The cellophane used between the two halves of the flask will give the veneer a surface texture that should not be disturbed while polishing the margins.

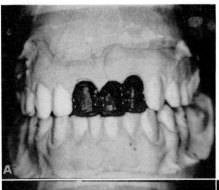

FIGURE 373.   Construction of a resin veneered bridge.

A, Three wax patterns with retentive loops. They were cast individually.

B, Soldered bridge.

C, Waxed labial veneers.

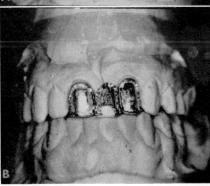
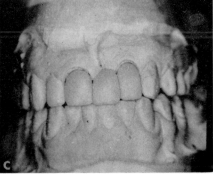

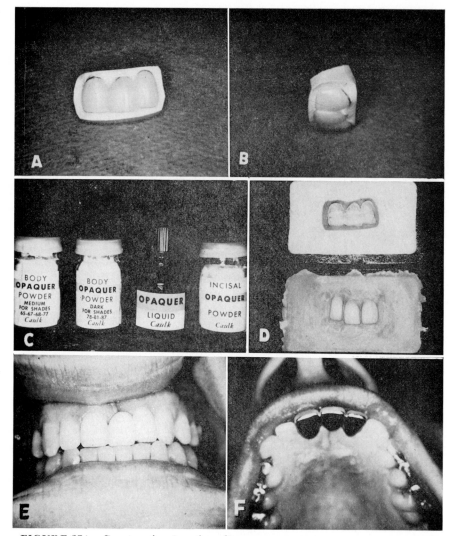

FIGURE 374. Construction (continued).
A, Bridge invested, ready for flasking.
B, Side view, showing investment extended just to height of contour.
C, Opaque.
D, Flask separated, wax eliminated, opaque applied.
E, F, Bridge seated.

The finished restoration should be stored in water until it can be cemented. This will permit the veneer to attain equilibrium with water and thus be dimensionally stable when it is placed in the mouth and subject to sorption of fluids. (See Figs. 373, 374, and 375.)

The proponents of dry-heat and vacuum-curing of resin veneers claim that with these techniques a harder material results, which is more resistant to abrasion and shade change and is not irritating to tissue in a static situation. Several workers in dental materials have been unable to substantiate these empirical findings in the research laboratory. However, it is possible that some phase of curing technique or environment was not followed or reproduced.[9, 10, 11, 12]

Resin veneer crowns may be cemented by the technique elected by the operator. If resin cement is used, the veneer should be protected from contact with the cervical excess of cement.

BRIDGES VENEERED WITH RESIN

Resin veneers are attached to bridge retainers and pontics by the same mechanical devices as with crowns, although pontics may be hollow, with the resin built around crossed wires or rods and into very irregular spaces.

It is the considered observation of the authors that the ridge-contacting areas of pontics, since the relationship is static, should not be veneered with resin because of tissue irritation. However, Eich[13] and others infer that this does not occur to a greater degree with resin than with porcelain or metal.

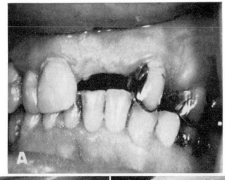

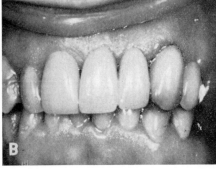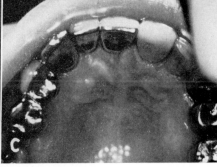

FIGURE 375. Six-unit bridge.

A, Mouth presented with maxillary left central and lateral incisors and first bicuspid missing.

B, C, Bridge seated. Coping and resin jacket crown on right central incisor; resin veneered gold crown on left cuspid; partial veneer crown on left second bicuspid. Pontic facings are Steele's.

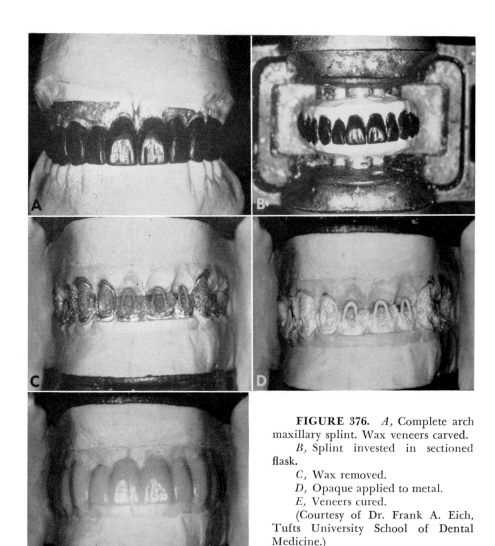

FIGURE 376.   *A,* Complete arch maxillary splint. Wax veneers carved.

B, Splint invested in sectioned flask.

C, Wax removed.

D, Opaque applied to metal.

E, Veneers cured.

(Courtesy of Dr. Frank A. Eich, Tufts University School of Dental Medicine.)

In the event that this procedure becomes necessary, ridge contact must be reduced to the minimum.

Where both retainers and pontics are to be veneered with resin, shading will be more uniform if all veneers are approximately the same thickness. This is especially true in an anterior fixed prosthesis. When pontics are posterior to the cuspid, it becomes progressively less important.[14]

When veneering long prostheses or splints, a sectional flask should be used, in order that the counterdie may be divided and opened and closed laterally on hinges (Fig. 376).

Packing, trial packing, and curing follow the routine for the single-unit crown.

REFERENCES

1. Kafalias, M. C., Swartz, M. L., and Phillips, R. W.: Physical properties of selected dental resins, Part I. J. Pros. Den., *13*:1087, 1963.
2. FitzRoy, D. C., Swartz, M. L., and Phillips, R. W.: Physical properties of selected dental resins, Part II. J. Pros. Den., *13*:1108, Nov.–Dec. 1963.
3. Peyton, F. A., and Craig, R. G.: Current evaluation of plastics in crown and bridge prosthesis. J. Pros. Den., *13*:743, July–Aug. 1963.
4. Swartz, M. L., and Phillips, R. W.: A study of adaptation of veneers to cast gold crowns. J. Pros. Den., 7:817, Nov. 1957.
5. Skinner, E. W., and Phillips, R. W.: The Science of Dental Materials. 5th ed. Philadelphia, W. B. Saunders Company, 1960.
6. Coy, H. D.: An evaluation of acrylic resin as a restorative material. J.A.D.A., *48*:266, March 1954.
7. Davis, M. C., and Klein, G.: Combination gold and acrylic restorations. J. Pros. Den., *4*:510, July 1954.
8. Cohn, L. A.: The acrylic-faced cast gold crown. J. Pros. Den., *1*:112, Jan.–March 1951.
9. Vieira, D. F., and Phillips, R. W.: Influence of certain variables on the abrasion of acrylic resin veneering materials. J. Pros. Den., *12*:720, July–Aug. 1962.
10. Pincus, C. L.: New concepts in mold techniques and high temperature processing of acrylic resins for maximum esthetics. Technical procedure. J. South. California D. A., *24*:26, Feb. 1956.
11. Ryge, G., and Foley, D. E.: Effect of dry heat processing on the physical properties of acrylic crowns. J.A.D.A., *66*:672, May 1963.
12. Hedegard, B.: Evaluation of materials for anterior bridges with special reference to acrylic resins. Internat. D. J., *12*:33, March 1962.
13. Eich, F. A.: Personal communication.
14. Yock, D. H.: Indications for the use of plastic resins in crown and bridge prosthesis. J.A.D.A., *46*:505, May 1953.

26

THE RESIN JACKET CROWN

It must be noted that the novice or student can learn readily to construct a jacket crown of resin that fits and is esthetically and biologically acceptable. Using products now available, a thoroughly cured resin crown seems to have satisfactory color stability, and wear on the contact areas of an anterior jacket does not constitute a hazard to arch length or embrasure form.[1, 2] It is true that a resin crown will abrade on the labial and linguo-incisal, but it is not a restoration to be looked on with scorn or to be seated apologetically. It will give long service and, in almost all instances, will be in harmony with the approximating teeth.

A more adverse reaction from occlusal pressure and abrasion will be found on posterior resin crowns. Pressure will be generated in many directions during mastication, tending to break adhesion of cement, or after an extended period of wear, to split the crown. Therefore, resin jacket crowns should be limited to maxillary incisors and cuspids where there is at least a normal overjet in the maxillo-mandibular relationship.

PREPARATION

The preparation to receive a resin jacket crown is identical to that for a porcelain jacket, with one exception. Areas of contact in centric occlusion and eccentric excursions should be cut 0.25 mm. deeper than for porcelain, to provide for wear and to minimize flexing of the crown.

Color Selection. See Chapter 24, The Porcelain Jacket Crown, and Chapter 25, The Construction of Crowns and Bridges with Resin Veneers.

Dies and Working Casts. See Chapter 10, The Working Cast, and Chapter 11, Individual Dies Constructed from Tube Impressions.

444

THE MATRIX

A matrix should be formed from 0.001 platinum foil, even though the crown is to be made of resin. Platinum is easier to handle than tin foil. and it may be swaged to the die and adapted to the shoulder of the preparation if the pattern is taken to the mouth. Since it is tougher and will have fewer wrinkles on the surface, platinum foil can be removed from a resin crown with less effort and less chance that any particles of metal will be retained in the resin, especially at the incisal.

The instruments needed for forming a matrix are scissors, cotton pliers of stainless steel or some noncorrosive metal, an orangewood stick pointed on one end and flattened on the other, a burnisher shaped like a nailhead

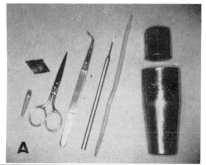

FIGURE 377. *A,* Instruments used in forming a platinum matrix: die and platinum, scissors, pliers, burnisher, orangewood stick, swage.

B, Platinum foil and diagram for cutting.

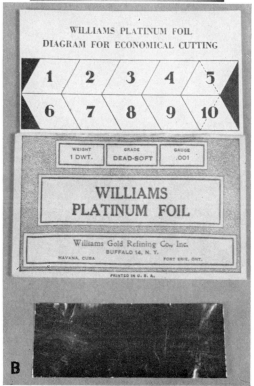

on one end and with near-parallel sides on the other, soldering tweezers, a mallet, a swage, and a small, fine-grit wheel stone (Fig. 377).

The matrix may be made using a proximal joint, but if it is necessary to conserve platinum foil and to secure the greatest number of matrices from the rectangular sheet supplied by any manufacturer, the piece to be used for the individual matrix should be cut in diamond form instead of rectangular and the joint shifted to the lingual surface. Usually a marked cardboard guide is included by the manufacturer in the envelope with the platinum.

Matrix with Lingual Joint

The foil must be placed on the labial of the die so that it covers both

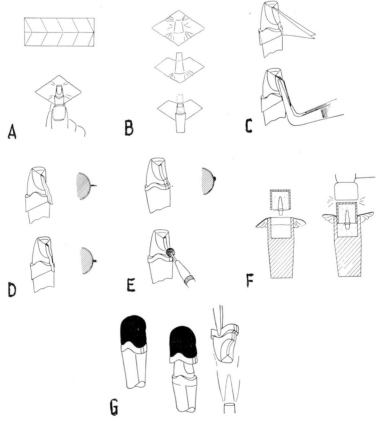

FIGURE 378.   Construction of platinum matrix.
A, Diamond of platinum pushed against die.
B, Flap cut and burnished over linguo-incisal.
C, Ends pulled tight on lingual surface.
D, Flaps trimmed and folded to start tinner's joint.
E, Fold continued to left, completing tinner's joint; excess platinum taken off shoulder
F, Matrix swaged on die for closest possible adaptation.
G, Matrix covered with sticky wax, removed, and wax melted off.

the shoulder and the incisal edge, and should be held in position by the first finger while the die is grasped by the thumb and second and third fingers. The ends are pulled together around and at the center of the lingual surface. Holding the matrix in this position and using the flattened end of the orangewood stick, the platinum is burnished to conform to the labial and proximal surfaces and shoulder of the die. The platinum is then grasped with the cotton pliers and closed tight against the lingual surface so that the excess and the two ends project from, and at right angles to, the lingual surface. The platinum is cut at the corners from the topmost labial edge to the incisal of the die. The lingual is opened and a triangular piece is removed on each side, making the second cuts continuous with the incisal edge and at right angles to the first. The labio-incisal extension is cut off, leaving about 3.0 mm. to be folded lingually over the incisal and onto the lingual surface. The lingual flaps are closed again and the folds drawn tight with the cotton pliers. The flaps are trimmed so that the lingual extension of each is 1.5 mm. Either the right or left flap is narrowed by one-half and both are readapted to the lingual surface. The longer flap is folded over the shorter, the bend being made at the margin of the shorter flap (Fig. 378).

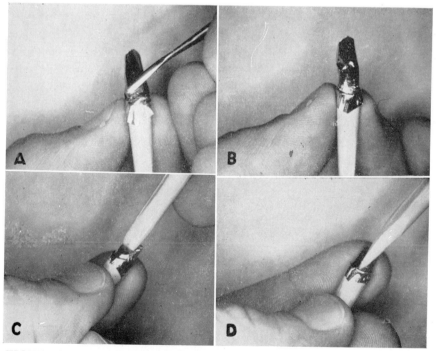

FIGURE 379.   Instrumentation in burnishing matrix.
A, Platinum being burnished to labial surface and shoulder.
B, Labial burnished ready to cut incisal flap.
C, Burnishing tinner's joint.
D, Burnishing shoulder.

Folding is continued in the same direction, to form a tinner's joint. The folded lingual surface and shoulder must be burnished with the orange-wood stick (Fig. 379). The matrix is covered with sticky wax and removed. The irregular apron is trimmed evenly so that 2.0 mm. of platinum foil will extend cervically at all points beyond the shoulder, to stiffen the matrix during manipulation and waxing. The wax is melted off and the platinum is annealed at the same time. The matrix is replaced on the die, burnished with the stick, and using a swage, the matrix is given the closest possible adaptation to the die. This is essential in the construction of any jacket crown. Again the matrix should be covered with sticky wax and removed. After the wax has been melted off, the matrix is placed on the die, wrapped in gauze, and burnished inciso-cervically to remove or smooth any minute wrinkles. It is returned to the working cast after the stone around the shoulder of the die is trimmed away so that the platinum will not be distorted.

A small, fine-grit wheel stone can be used on the shoulder area of the matrix to remove three of the four layers of platinum in the tinner's joint.

THE WAX PATTERN—DIRECT WAXING

Ivory-colored or tooth-tint wax should be used for the pattern to avoid the possibility of later contamination of the investment and resin with blue, purple, or green pigment. The wax pattern, a replica of the finished crown, should be taken to the mouth and checked for contour, alignment, contact, and occlusion (Fig. 380). It will be necessary to shorten the apron of the matrix so that the pattern can be seated on the prepared tooth. On the die, a V-shaped portion of wax can be removed from the cervical, uncovering the platinum over the shoulder. The pattern is returned to the tooth and the exposed platinum is adapted to the preparation. With the pattern re-

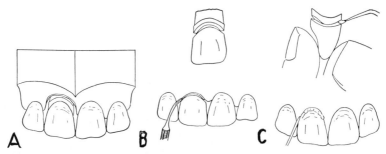

FIGURE 380.   Checking wax pattern for resin crown on tooth.
A, Completed wax pattern on working cast.
B, Cervical of matrix uncovered; platinum being burnished to shoulder of prepared tooth.
C, Crevice is filled with wax outside the mouth and carving is completed on tooth.

moved, the crevice is filled with wax and carved to contour on the tooth, or on the die if its accuracy was verified.

A completely indirect technique, if satisfactory for other types of construction, is suitable for building a resin jacket crown. Contact areas on the approximating teeth of the stone cast may be scraped slightly to assure a tight contact; then the crown can be adjusted prior to cementation.

LABORATORY PROCEDURE FOR CONSTRUCTION OF A RESIN JACKET CROWN

The first technique to be described was developed by M. S. Moskey,[3, 4] who designed a three-piece flask to allow complete labial and lingual color control during packing (Fig. 381). This had not been possible before, because either the lingual or the labial surface was concealed. However, with this method the center section of the flask, in which the pattern will be invested, is an open frame permitting the gingival, middle third, and incisal mixes to be applied as precisely as if the case were mounted on an open cast. The outside sections of the flask, acting as lingual and labial counterdies to register and mold the material to the desired form, are used for compression.

Flasking the Pattern—The Three-Piece Flask. The wax crown should be invested in the Moskey flask in the following manner (Fig. 382). After mixing stone to a thick, creamy consistency, the wax pattern should be removed from the die, the core filled with stone, and set aside. Only mild vibration can be used if air bubbles are to be avoided. The center section of the flask must be filled with the mixed stone and the wax pattern placed in the center, with the incisal edge tipping lingually. The investment must be smoothed so that the labial surface of the pattern is entirely exposed. (See Fig. 382B.)

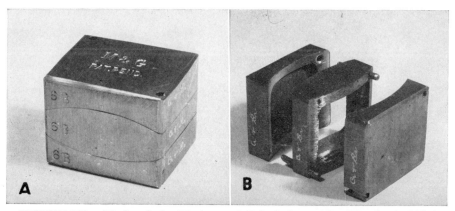

FIGURE 381.   Moskey flask. (Moskey and Geiss Laboratories, Cleveland, Ohio.)

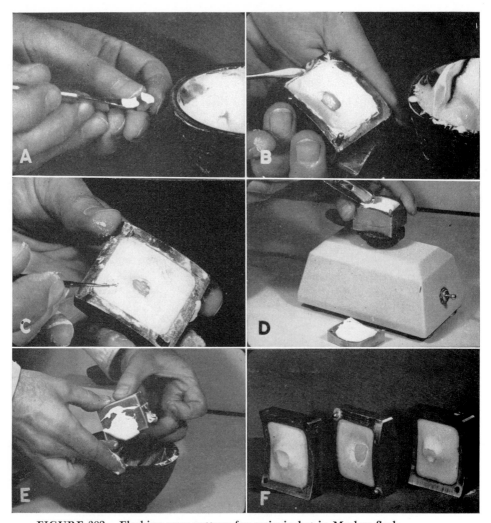

FIGURE 382.   Flasking wax pattern for resin jacket in Moskey flask.

A, Pattern being filled with stone.

B, Pattern is placed in stone in center of middle section of flask, labial surface up.

C, Lingual of pattern must be uncovered before stone sets; carving must not be mutilated.

D, E, Flasking completed.

F, Flask opened.

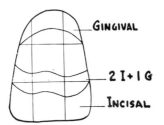

FIGURE 383.   Color distribution chart.

Before the investment has set, the lingual surface of the pattern must be uncovered, leaving only the mesial, distal, and incisal surfaces and the gingival apron covered with investment. Cleaning and smoothing the investment should be done so that no scratches will be made on the wax pattern. After the investment has set, separating medium must be painted on each side.

A little bubble-free investment is painted on the lingual and labial surfaces of the pattern. Then each outside section of the flask must be filled with investment and closed gently against the central part. It is placed in a hand press to expel the excess stone and to assure closure while the stone is setting.

The two ends are separated from the center section of the flask, the wax is flushed away with boiling water, and any feather edges of stone that may have formed around the pattern are cut off and washed away with cold water. The flask must cool completely before packing is begun.

It is recommended that the walls and exposed edges be covered with thin tin foil or painted with sodium silicate (water glass) before packing. Tin foil is better because with it the resin can be cured in contact with metal only. Curing against metal produces a superior surface and eliminates the possibility of crazing in the resin.[5]

Packing—The Three-Piece Flask. The selected shades (Fig. 383) of gingival and incisal resin powders are mixed in two Dappen dishes, and the gingival color is the first to be saturated with monomer (Fig. 384). It should stand for about 3 minutes before mixing the incisal. The incisal color should be of a thinner consistency than the gingival when it is applied; therefore it must be mixed later. When the gingival mixture has reached the dough stage, it is ready to pack. Several sheets of cellophane should be placed in a bowl of water so that a new piece can be used each time the flask is closed.

After placing a wet sheet of cellophane on the lingual surface of the exposed jacket in the middle section of the flask, the gingival color should be placed on the labial surface with a small spatula, tapering it toward the incisal and stopping about 1.0 mm. short of the incisal edge. The remaining space must be filled with the incisal color. There is no need to overbuild the labial, since the lingual side is to be packed also, and pressure will be applied from there.

Using finger pressure only, a moist piece of cellophane should be placed on the labial section of the flask before it is positioned against the middle part. The lingual surface is packed in the same manner as the labial except that more material must be added to obtain bulk for compression. Cellophane must be used between the lingual surface and the outside section when they are assembled in a hand press for test packing.

Following the test packing, the center section may be held up to the light to check the translucence of the incisal edge and the distribution of

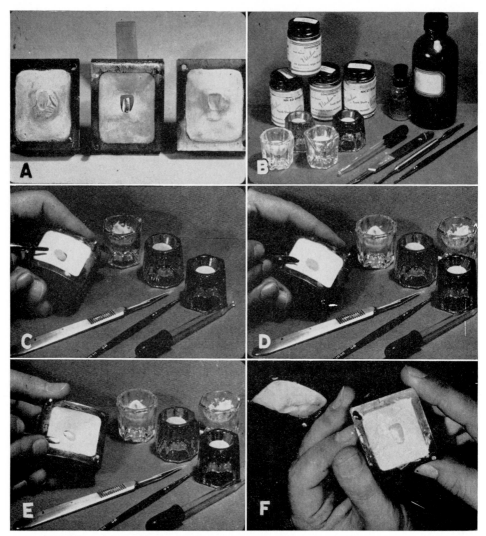

FIGURE 384. Packing resin jacket crown in three-piece flask.

A, Flask open, wax eliminated, ready for packing.

B, One brand of acrylic resin for jacket crowns and equipment for mixing and packing; to prevent evaporation, covered jars may be used instead of Dappen dishes.

C, Packing gingival shade on labial surface.

D, Incisal shade placed on labial surface.

E, Lingual ready to pack; shade distribution about the same as on labial; labial third of flask is in position with cellophane covering resin.

F, Placing sheet of moistened cellophane before closing flask.

shades. At this stage, any characterizations that were charted (such as check lines, stains, and calcified areas) may be added. The stains must be mixed in separate Dappen dishes and saturated with monomer (Fig. 385). Flaps can be cut on the labial surface of the crown with a razor blade or a very sharp knife, and with a clean spatula the desired stains can be added beneath the flaps. The flaps must be cautiously closed and the labial surface smoothed.

A thin piece of tin foil should be adapted to the lingual and labial outside sections of the flask before it is closed for the final time. The press-enclosed flask is placed in a container of room-temperature water, which should be brought to 212° F. in not less than 30 minutes. Boiling is continued for 30 minutes, after which the flask is bench-cooled to room temperature.

Flasking—The Two-Section Flask. The acrylic resin jacket crown may be invested, packed, and processed in a two-section flask also. A small amount of die stone is mixed with a mechanical spatulator and vacuumed to remove the air bubbles. The inside of the crown is filled and the pattern is positioned, lingual side down, in a small mass of stone placed on a glass slab or other suitable surface. The stone is carried to a point lingual to the labial line angles on the proximal and incisal surfaces so that the polished flash line will not be visible. No matter how well polished, this line can be detected if it is to the labial of the interproximal shadow. At the cervical, the investment is carried flush with the apron of the platinum matrix. After the stone has set completely, the mass is trimmed so that it is no more than 3.0 mm. thick at any point. This procedure allows greater control of flask-

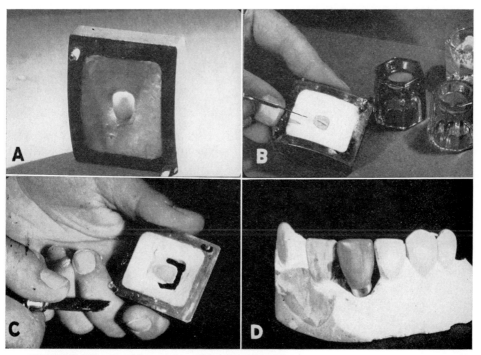

FIGURE 385. Packing and staining (continued).
A, Checking packed resin for shade distribution.
B, Staining labial to produce hairline check.
C, Removing cured crown.
D, Finished crown on working cast; note staining.

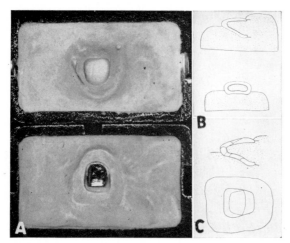

FIGURE 386. Packing in two-piece flask.

A, Pattern invested in flask; wax washed away.

B, Cross section of flasked pattern.

C, Increments of resin are added to blend gingival and incisal shades.

ing materials and prevents the pattern from settling too far into the flask (Fig. 386).

Using a fresh mix of stone, the pattern is set in the bottom section of the flask, slightly above the level of the edge of the flask. After the hardened stone has been smoothed, the surface is lubricated with petroleum jelly and the second half is poured. Any excess separating medium or air bubbles trapped on or near the pattern will produce defects on the surface of the crown.

Packing—The Two-Section Flask. When the stone in the top half of the flask has set, it is warmed in hot water, opened before the wax has melted, and all wax is flushed away with a stream of clean, boiling water. When the case may be comfortably held in the bare hands, the portion of the mold in the bottom section of the flask is coated with a single layer of a foil substitute, such as Al-Cote.* If this should be done while the case is hot, the foil substitute will peel from the surface of the stone after it dries.

When the acrylic resin has reached a relatively thick doughlike state, the mold is packed completely with the selected gingival shade, trial packing being employed and more material being added if necessary. Except that attention must be given to forcing resin into the lingual portion of the mold, the technique of packing and processing is exactly the same as for the resin veneer crown which is discussed in Chapter 25.

Deflasking and Polishing. After the flask has air-cooled to room temperature, it is taken from the press and opened. The stone is removed from around the restoration with a sharp knife until it may be easily freed from the flask. Resin is not a strong material and could be damaged by prying. Any stone remaining on the surface of the resin can be flaked off with a sharp instrument.

---

* The L. D. Caulk Company, Milford, Del.

The stone inside the crown may be partially eliminated with a small round bur inserted into the mid-portion of the material, and the remainder may be chipped away by using a small pointed instrument.

The platinum is loosened by grasping the apron of the matrix at the lap joint with tweezers and pulling toward the center of the crown. Then, with a twisting motion, the matrix can be wound onto the beaks of the instrument and freed. If the matrix was adapted to the die without wrinkles,

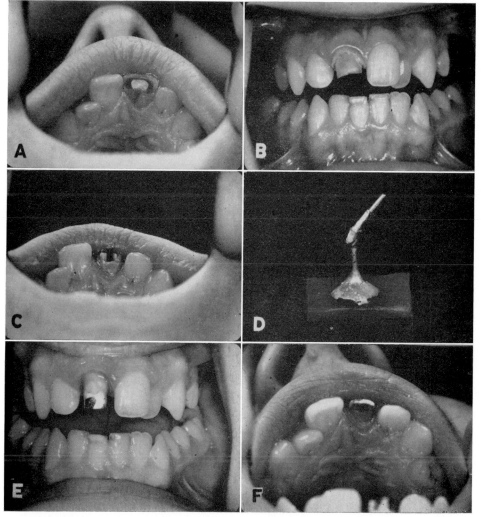

FIGURE 387.   Sequence of steps in constructing a resin jacket crown for a pulpless maxillary central incisor using amalgam die, wax transfer, and plaster impression.

A, Fractured central following endodontic therapy.

B, Shoulder partly formed in preparation of tooth.

C, Post of high-fusing clasp wire fitted into root canal and extending out to what will be the incisal edge of prepared tooth.

D, Cast core.

E, *F*, Finished preparation with cast core cemented.

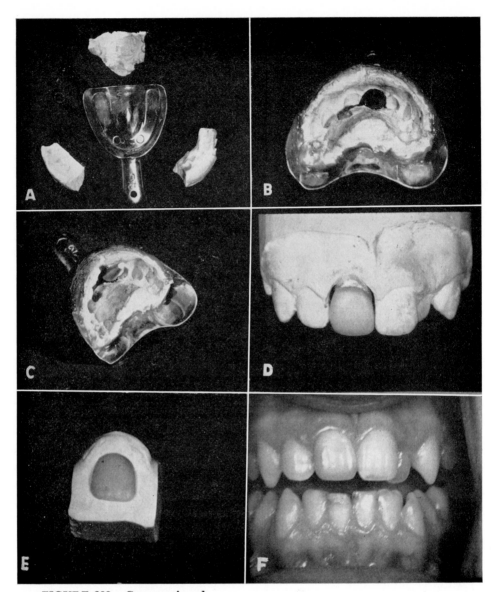

FIGURE 388. Case continued.
A, B, C, Plaster impression with amalgam die seated, ready to pour working cast.
D, Working cast and wax pattern.
E, First step in flasking pattern.
F, Finished crown on tooth.

the foil will separate intact by this one operation. However, any bits of remaining platinum may be obliterated with a round bur.

The flash is cut from the crown with either small fissure burs or suitable carborundum stones. To protect the margin, flash at the cervical should be removed with the crown in place on the die. The crown can be polished with fine pumice in a rubber cup or on a small felt wheel. Wet whiting on a felt wheel, or a prepared resin polishing agent on a small dry rag wheel, will produce a luster on the surface. To avoid abrading the resin, it is better to use a handpiece, rather than the greater speed of a lathe, for polishing.

CEMENTATION

Before a resin crown is seated permanently, it should be tried on the tooth and examined for color, shape, position, occlusion, contact points,

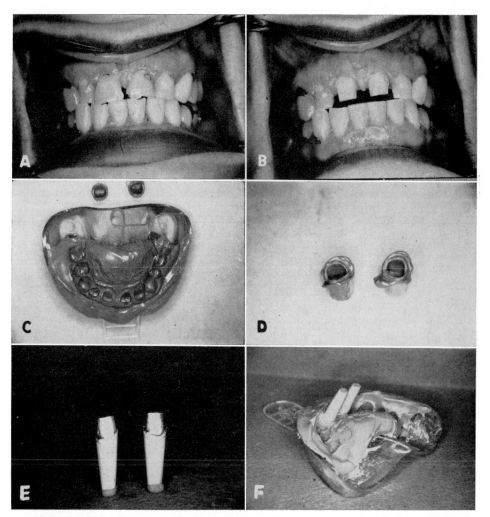

FIGURE 389.   Sequence of steps in constructing two crowns for vital maxillary central incisors using silver-plated dies and a polysulfide rubber impression.

A, Central incisors before preparation.

B, After preparation; this is an end-to-end occlusion, making it necessary to have greater incisal clearance.

C, Polysulfide rubber impression for working cast was stored in a humidifier until dies were completed.

D, Polysulfide rubber impressions for metalized dies.

E, Dies.

F, Dies in impression ready for boxing.

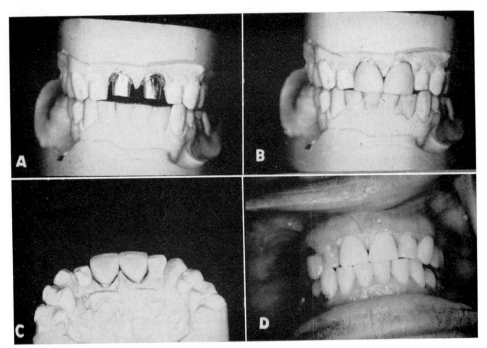

FIGURE 390.   Case continued.
A, Working and opposing casts before mounting.
B, *C*, Wax patterns.
D, Completed crowns.

soft-tissue relationship, and fit. Zinc phosphate cement is preferred and may be selected after making test mixtures of the powders with water and glycerin. The cement should be mixed at a ratio that will assure maximal physical properties, but should not be so thick that undue pressure will be necessary when the crown is cemented.

REFERENCES

1. Chevalier, P. L.: Personal communication.
2. Pincus, C. L.: Esthetic variations in jacket crowns and bridge restoration involving periodontal and other deformities. Its application to oral rehabilitation. New York J. Den., *24*:132, March 1954 (Abstract).
3. Theofilis, B. G.: The porcelain jacket crown. Senior thesis, Indiana Univ. School Den., June 1955.
4. Moskey, M. S.: Personal communication.
5. Fairhurst, C. W., and Ryge, G.: Effect of tin-foil substitutes on the strength of denture base resins. J. Pros. Den., *5*:508, July 1955.

Swartz, M. L., Phillips, R. W., Day, R., and Johnston, J. F.: A laboratory and clinical investigation of certain resin restorative and cementing materials. Part I. In vitro tests on adhesive characteristics. Part II. A twenty-eight month clinical evaluation of a resin cement. J. Pros. Den., *5*:698, Sept.–Oct. 1955.

27

BRIDGE PATTERNS

There is a divergence of opinion among dentists concerning the use of complete coverage of the abutment tooth. It is the contention of some men that the dentist is not fully aware of his responsibility, or, if he is aware of it, that he does not meet his responsibility if any surface of the abutment is permitted to remain uncovered so that it may be susceptible later to a carious lesion.

The authors do not subscribe to this philosophy. A noteworthy number of bridges, held in place by inlays, pinlays, or partial veneer crowns, have served for such long periods that the occluding surfaces have been worn to a point necessitating replacement of the original bridges. Many teeth that have been prepared for partial veneer crowns and other types of retainers not covering all of the enamel surfaces have resisted caries so effectively that they are now supporting the third bridge.

It is true that there are numerous situations in which caries, movement of teeth, a short clinical crown, or the need for maximal retention makes a full veneer gold crown the retainer of choice. Periodic clinic surveys* have disclosed that full veneer or veneered gold crowns constitute between 55 and 60 per cent of all retainers used. These, it must be remembered, were placed in mouths that cannot be considered exactly typical of those to be found in practices in which fixed partial denture construction may be one of the major efforts. Oral hygiene concepts and routine clinical care render mouths of patients in private practice far more receptive to the construction of bridges.

In the following review of bridge patterns, it will be observed that a variety of retainers have been suggested. Selection was governed by *tooth form, tooth position, space length, occlusion,* and *caries* (either existing or previously treated).

---

* Indiana University School of Dentistry

MAXILLARY PATTERNS

Absence of a **single central incisor** is one of the patterns seen most frequently, doubtless because of the embarrassment which it causes the patient (Fig. 391). In private practice, barring accident, this plight generally can be alleviated by inserting a temporary partial denture at the time of extraction, which is preferable to the immediate construction of a fixed prosthesis. This will help to mold the gingival tissue and will maintain the approximating and opposing teeth in their natural positions, provided that it is not worn indefinitely.

Unless the teeth are exceedingly thin and unless the proximal surfaces or incisal angles are restored or carious, a pinledge retainer may be used on each abutment. If the distal surfaces are carious or have small restorations, such areas can be filled with gold foil, or possibly with resin or silicate cement, and the pinledge still may be used. Caries on the mesial surfaces presents somewhat greater difficulties, but again gold foil may be used to rebuild the teeth to normal form, after which they can be treated as sound.

There is no valid argument against using partial veneer crowns with this central incisor pontic except that in many cases it is useless to destroy so much tooth surface. The pinledge retainer is less conspicuous than the partial veneer crown, although the special types of partial veneer preparations advocated by Vedder,[1] Grubb,[2] and Willey[3] work beautifully.

The pinledge can be used on either a long or a short tooth, but some bulk labio-lingually in the incisal half is a requisite. Now and then a modification that does not bring the preparation onto the incisal fourth of the lingual surface can be used. While the pins will be more centralized in their locations, if they are given maximal length and are cast, stability will not be jeopardized.

The veneered gold crown must be used, of course, when the caries index is high. Inlays seldom, if ever, provide satisfactory retention in this space. A broken-stress bridge or a cantilever pontic is contraindicated.

A missing **single lateral incisor** (Fig. 392) can produce a sizable problem for the student of crown and bridge prosthodontics.[4, 5] Very often a lateral incisor is replaced by cantilevering the pontic from a partial veneer crown retainer on the cuspid, with no rest at the mesial of the pontic. Some students, and some practitioners as well, believe that the teacher is being merely theoretical when he insists that this practice is detrimental to the tissue surrounding the single abutment, or when he asserts that alignment cannot be sustained throughout the lifetime of the bridge. Rotation to the labial is bound to occur and the mesio-lingual margin of the lateral pontic will overlap the disto-labial line angle of the central incisor. This is unsightly. Even more serious is the change which the anterior movement of the cuspid will bring about in the contact relationships of all posterior teeth in the quadrant.

When the space is narrow, when the forces from the opposing teeth are weak, or when the cuspid root is long and the alveolar recession is slight, there may be some justification for the two-unit bridge. However, a disto-lingual inlay in the central incisor, with a rest extending from the mesial of the lateral pontic into a recess previously prepared in this inlay, is favored in the event that two soldered retainers cannot be used.

The pinledge is indicated on each abutment unless caries, tooth position, or pulp size prohibits its use. A partial veneer crown is acceptable, unless, as in the central incisor pattern, the caries index, shortness of the teeth, or leverages demand that the veneered gold crown be used.

A bridge replacing **both central incisors** (Fig. 393) will require more support than can be secured ordinarily from the lateral incisors, which usually have short and frail roots. Splinting the lateral incisors and cuspids as multiple abutments, and using partial veneer or veneered gold crowns as retainers will insure gratifying results for the longest period.

When the lever arm is short and the clinical crowns are relatively short and stubby, four pinledge retainers can be used. Cast pins will furnish ample resistance to displacement. The partial veneer preparation cannot be adapted readily to such tooth form. Proximal caries which weakens an incisal angle, or a high caries index, would point to the veneered crown.[1]

Figure 391.   Figure 392.

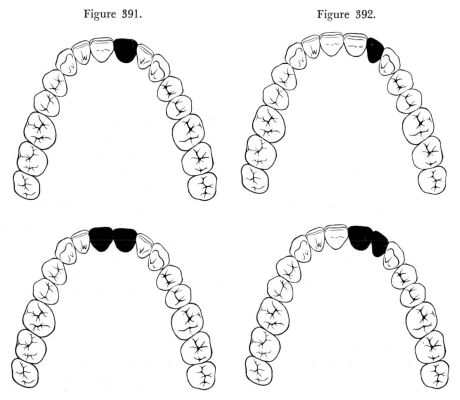

Figure 393.   Figure 394.

The replacement of the **approximating central and lateral incisors** (Fig. 394) usually will involve only two abutment teeth, namely, the remaining central incisor and the cuspid approximating the space. Considerable success has been experienced with this type of bridge, using a partial veneer crown on the cuspid and a pinledge or partial veneer retainer on the central.

If the alveolus around the central incisor has receded markedly, the lateral incisor should be included. While a lone lateral incisor is not a strong tooth and does not afford maximal retention, when it is splinted to the central incisor, the ensuing two-rooted multiple abutment will provide resistance to rotation and displacement greater than the sum of the two. When the lateral incisor is badly aligned and three abutments are needed, the prosthesis may be attached to the central incisor, cuspid, and first bicuspid, with a partial veneer or veneered crown on the central.

Building a bridge to replace the **central incisor on one side of the median line and the lateral incisor in the adjacent quadrant** (Fig. 395) is an entirely different matter from the one just discussed. The cuspid and central incisor will have an equal amount of periodontal membrane area, but, because of distribution the support will not be comparable to that derived from the two abutments in the preceding pattern. The proximity of the central incisor to the cuspid would allow a cantilever central pontic to exert too much leverage on the central incisor; consequently, the remaining lateral incisor must be used as a terminal abutment. The option between pinledge, partial veneer, or veneered gold crown retainers will be decided by proximal caries, incisal angles, tooth form, long-axis relationship, and incidence of caries.

In a case where **both lateral incisors** are missing (Fig. 396), two three-unit bridges should be constructed, rather than one of six units, although the continuous replacement might be in order if recession has added as much as 25 per cent to the crown length of the central incisors. Pinledges, partial veneer, or veneered gold crowns could be used for the longer bridge. Condition and form of the abutments will dictate the choice.

When the **two centrals and one lateral incisor** have been lost (Fig. 397), removal of the remaining lateral and construction of a six-unit bridge are sometimes proposed. Unless this action is warranted by resorption of the alveolus, the lateral incisor should be retained. Its extraction will elongate the lever arm, and often the first bicuspids must be included as abutments. The teeth should be prepared for partial veneer or veneered crowns, depending on the restorations, caries index, or the length of the clinical crowns.

Replacing **one central and two lateral incisors** (Fig. 398) is not an exacting task unless the remaining central has drifted out of position. If there is harmony in the long-axis relationship, this bridge can be constructed by using partial veneer or veneered crowns on the cuspids and remaining central incisor. If the teeth are short, with contact areas very close to the gingival line, the retention of the partial veneer preparations must be increased with two extra pinholes in each lingual surface.

When replacing **four incisors** (Fig. 399), it has been the custom to use only the cuspids as abutments. Many bridges so constructed have failed, and faulty preparations or fit of castings cannot be held accountable for all these failures. The lever arm extends too far beyond the line of rotation. Retention and balance must be obtained through posterior extension. The cuspids and the first bicuspids, with partial veneer or veneered crowns as the retainers, will have compensating resistance to incising and rotating thrusts, and the life of the prosthesis will be prolonged. In a few cases, when the lever arm was very long, the second bicuspids have been included also. When the cuspids are of average length and the bicuspids are short, a combination of retainers may be indicated, partial veneer crowns being used on the cuspids and veneered gold crowns on the bicuspids.

Replacement of a **single cuspid** (Fig. 400) may become necessary for one of several reasons. With the increase in orthodontic treatment, cuspids are being extracted because of impaction or malposition. They are also lost through mishap or extensive caries, or they may be congenitally missing.

In a young patient the alveolar process will be pliable and the cusps of all teeth will retain much of the angulation present at the time of erup-

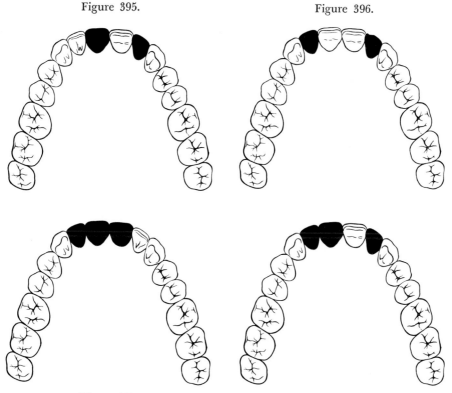

Figure 395.

Figure 396.

Figure 397.

Figure 398.

tion. A bridge constructed here must have more abutments than will be needed in the mouth of the adult, where the alveolus will be rigid and clinical crowns will be shortened by abrasion.

If a bridge is built for an adolescent, using only the first bicuspid and lateral incisor as abutments, the unit usually will move labially and forward into such a position that the mesio-lingual portion of the lateral will overlap the disto-labial line angle of the central incisor. This in turn causes loss or alteration of contact between the first and second bicuspids and the first molar. Even in a young adult, three abutments must be used to prevent such movement. Some authorities approve the use of the two bicuspids and the lateral incisor. Others feel that the central and lateral incisors and the first bicuspid will maintain the pontic in correct position more competently. Notwithstanding some difference of opinion, there is general agreement on the number of abutments.

To reach a decision, tooth form and occlusion must be studied. If the bicuspids are short occluso-cervically, they will serve poorly; if the central and lateral incisors are thin labio-lingually, with an excessive vertical overlap, their use may be contraindicated. If anterior retainers can be made that will be pleasing in appearance, the central and lateral incisors and the first bicuspid are preferred.

When the caries index is low, pinledge retainers on the central and lateral and a partial veneer crown on the first bicuspid will hold the bridge. However, if diagnostic casts and mouth examination reveal that considerable torque will be manifested in lateral excursions, partial veneer or veneered crowns should be used on the central and lateral incisors. Veneered crowns are obligatory if the caries index is high or if the teeth to be used as abutments are badly mutilated. If the first and second bicuspids and the lateral incisor are used, partial veneer or veneered crowns would be advisable.

In older patients, when abrasion has reduced the oblique forces from lateral excursions, the first bicuspid and lateral incisor may be ample for support. A few bridges replacing the cuspid have been retained for long periods by using an MO inlay in the first bicuspid and a pinledge on the lateral incisor, but the majority have been built with two partial veneer or veneered crowns.

When **both cuspids** are missing (Fig. 401), two fixed prostheses should be made, rather than an unbroken bridge from first bicuspid to first bicuspid.

The stringent measures proposed in the replacement of the cuspid are imperative because of the tremendous forces that bear on this tooth. Being situated at the corner of the arch, it receives anterior thrusts from the posterior teeth during mastication, and lateral force from the incising and protrusive movements of the opposing teeth. These are transferred to the cemented retainers and to the abutments.

Fortunately the absence of the **cuspid and approximating lateral incisor** (Fig. 402) occurs infrequently. While Ante's law can be satisfied in the replacement of these two teeth, resistance to the lever arm is not readily obtained. No less than three abutments should be used. If three will suffice, the two bicuspids and the central incisor are recommended. When the crown-root ratio, the contour of the arch, or the occlusion is abnormal, the second central incisor should be used, also. Partial veneer or veneered crowns must be used as the retainers.

A bridge to replace a **first bicuspid** (Fig. 403) must be constructed for many people. Sometimes, when the occlusion is receptive, an MO inlay in the second bicuspid and a pinledge on the cuspid will retain this prosthesis. The primary objectives, along with esthetic considerations, should be protection of the abutment teeth and retention. These can be assured by using a partial veneer or veneered crown on each abutment tooth.

In replacing the **cuspid and first bicuspid** (Fig. 404), the opposing forces are more powerful than those against the cuspid and the lateral. As a rule, the first molar, second bicuspid, and lateral and central incisors must be used as abutments. Even if the teeth are short, partial veneer crowns can be used unless the caries index makes veneered or full veneer gold crowns mandatory.

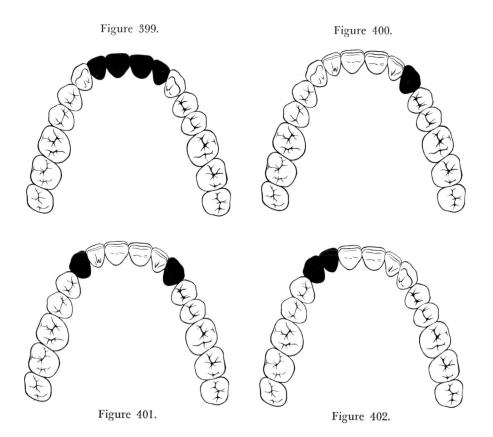

Figure 399.

Figure 400.

Figure 401.

Figure 402.

Figure 403.

Figure 404.

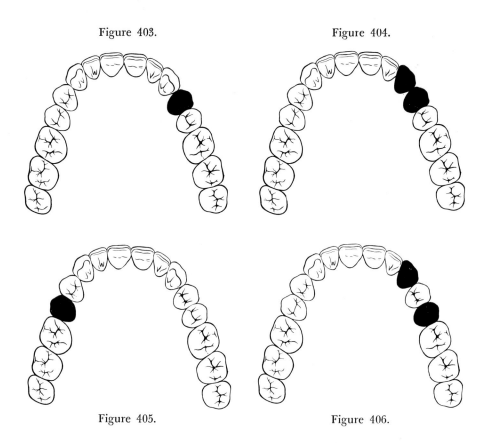

Figure 405.

Figure 406.

Inlays may be used to replace the **second bicuspid** (Fig. 405) unless one (or more) of the specific contraindications for inlays exists; then retainers must be partial veneer or veneered or full veneer gold crowns.

When the **cuspid and second bicuspid** are missing (Fig. 406), the bony structure around the first bicuspid and lateral incisor must be examined critically. If the occlusion is normal and the crown-root ratio of the first bicuspid is no worse than one-to-one, three abutments will be sufficient. The lateral incisor, first bicuspid, and first molar retainers may be partial veneer or veneered or full veneer gold crowns, subject to tooth form, long-axis relationship, and caries index. If the alveolus encircling the lateral incisor and first bicuspid is reduced, but still may be considered safe, the central incisor should be added. Partial veneer or veneered crowns may be used on the central and lateral incisors and first bicuspid, with a full veneer gold crown as the retainer on the molar.

When **both central incisors and one first bicuspid** are missing (Fig. 407), it is to be hoped that a survey of the diagnostic cast will show that the long-axis relationship of the two cuspids, two laterals, and second bicuspid is harmonious. The most desirable method of restoration will be an extension of the pattern advised for the two central incisors, using partial veneer or veneered gold crowns as retainers on the five abutments. Occasionally the terminal cuspid can be excluded.

When the **lateral incisor and first bicuspid** have been lost (Fig. 408), usually the second bicuspid and cuspid will withstand migration or destructive stimulation; but if the alveolar process around the cuspid has receded more than one-third, the central incisor should be used as the terminal abutment. Partial veneer or veneered crowns will be required for retainers.

When the **first bicuspid and central incisor in the same quadrant** are to be replaced (Fig. 409), two three-unit bridges should be built, because there is no purpose in complicating construction by having to parallel four abutments. Nevertheless, if the alveolar process has receded and the abutments must be splinted, the same abutments, namely, the second bicuspid, cuspid, and lateral and central incisors, can be prepared for either partial veneer or veneered crowns.

A bridge replacing the **approximating bicuspids** (Fig. 410) is quite successful, as a rule, using a full veneer gold crown on the first molar and a partial veneer on the cuspid. In case the anterior abutment cannot be prepared for this retainer, a veneered crown must be used.

When the **approximating bicuspids and a lateral incisor** have been lost (Fig. 411), the normal periodontal membrane area of the first molar

Figure 407.　　　　　　　　　　　　Figure 408.

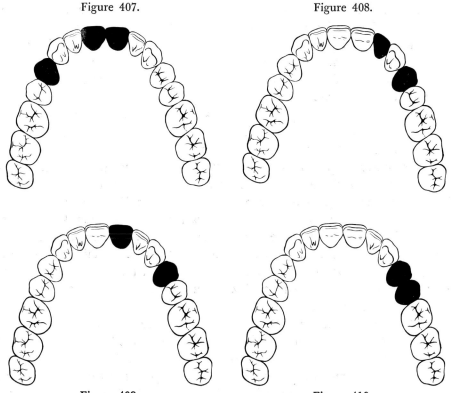

Figure 409.　　　　　　　　　　　　Figure 410.

and cuspid will exceed that of the missing teeth. The occlusion of the lateral pontic will demonstrate whether the central incisor must enter into the plan of treatment. If the relationship is benign and the crown-root ratio of the cuspid is favorable, the lateral pontic can be cantilevered without adversely affecting the cuspid.

However, if these three teeth are missing, there will of necessity be some resorption of the alveolus around the cuspid. Construction must be guided by the amount remaining and its capacity to resist the forces against the abutment teeth. The first molar and the cuspid should be capable of holding this bridge, using a full veneer gold crown on the molar and a partial veneer on the cuspid. The acceptability of the partial veneer crown will depend on tooth form and caries index.

Two bridges should be constructed for replacing **two bicuspids and the central incisor in the same quadrant** (Fig. 412) for the same reasons discussed under the first bicuspid and the central incisor patterns.

Is it possible that the **four incisors and a first bicuspid** can be lost (Fig. 413), leaving an isolated cuspid with a suitable crown-root ratio? Ordinarily the answer would be No. However, extraction of the cuspid would be no solution. If the crown-root ratio is close to one-to-one and not further complicated by an active atrophy, and if clinically the cuspid is not mobile, it should be used as a "pier," with the first molar and second bicuspid on the same side of the median line, and the cuspid and first bicuspid on the other, being used as the terminal multiple abutments.

The degree of the lower cuspid "lift" and the possibility of balancing the occlusion on each side of the isolated cuspid should be calculated. Every effort should be made to promote a wide distribution of the load, to protect the cuspid and ensure its long life. Some enlargement or thickening of the periodontal membrane may be expected and need not be viewed with alarm, provided that there is no discomfort.

In a mouth where recession is minimal, the cuspid and first bicuspid on one side are prepared for abutments; on the opposite side, the cuspid and second bicuspid. Partial veneer or veneered crowns are constructed for the retainers, contingent on the condition of the individual tooth.

When the **four incisors and the four bicuspids** must be replaced (Fig. 414), a removable bridge merits consideration. Support and retention may be found on the cuspids and the first molars. Usually the cuspids must be reshaped with partial veneer or veneered crowns and the molars must be recontoured or realigned with full veneer gold crowns to supply rest seats and undercuts.

Except when the alveolus has receded around one of the cuspids, a fixed partial denture is more utilitarian and comfortable. This prosthesis should be retained by partial veneer or veneered and full veneer gold crowns.

If there are missing the **two bicuspids and the lateral and central incisors in one quadrant** (Fig. 415), a fixed prosthesis should be constructed if half of the alveolar process remains around the cuspid. Even if a bicuspid or molar is missing on the opposite side, a removable partial denture would not take precedence over two bridges. In the latter situation, retainers for the longer bridge would be a full veneer gold crown on the first molar and veneered or partial veneer crowns on the cuspid and on the central and lateral incisors across the median line.

When a bridge is being constructed to replace a **first molar** (Fig. 416), the second molar abutment should be crowned and the second bicuspid prepared to receive a partial veneer or veneered crown, because the occluding surface of the first molar pontic would be so much larger than the occlusal seat of a second molar inlay retainer. An inlay-supported bridge would be feasible only under ideal circumstances and if precisely constructed.

When the **approximating first molar and second bicuspid** have been lost (Fig. 417), the second molar retainer should be a full veneer gold crown. Coronal length and the caries index will control the first bicuspid retainer, either a partial veneer or veneered crown. If this space appears bilaterally (Fig. 418), bridges should be constructed unless the alveolar process has receded so far that bracing would be helpful, in which case a removable prosthesis must be considered.

Figure 411.   Figure 412.

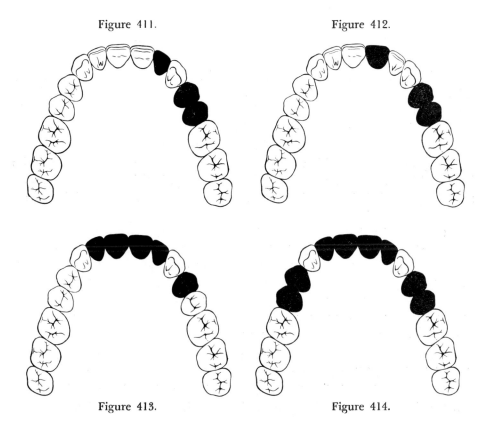

Figure 413.   Figure 414.

Figure 415.

Figure 416.

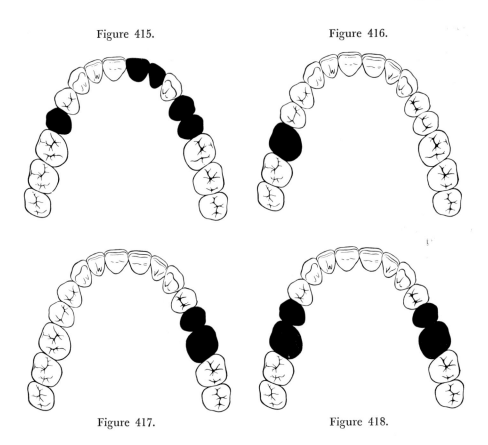

Figure 417.

Figure 418.

When the **first molar and first bicuspid on the same side** are missing, (Fig. 419), three teeth should be used as abutments because there would be excessive leverage on the second bicuspid from a cantilever first bicuspid pontic. A full veneer gold crown retainer is indicated for the second molar. If the cuspid and second bicuspid are short, a veneered crown may be necessary on the bicuspid, with pin retention on the cuspid. If the caries index is high, veneered crowns will be mandatory. If this pattern is bilateral (Fig. 420), and if it is possible to insert bridges, a removable partial denture is contraindicated.

Occasionally there will be missing the **two bicuspids and central incisor on one side and the lateral incisor, second bicuspid, and first molar on the opposite side of the median line** (Fig. 421). A removable prosthesis is contraindicated unless the supporting structure of the remaining teeth has receded grossly. Even then the central and lateral incisors should be replaced by an immovable bridge, and a removable bridge should be constructed to replace the molar and bicuspids.

If 50 per cent or more of the alveolus remains, three separate fixed units should be built. This treatment plan enlists the first molar and cuspid as abutments for the missing first and second bicuspids; the lateral, central, and cuspid for the anterior prosthesis; and the first bicuspid and second molar for the third bridge. Because of the great number of teeth missing, partial veneer, veneered, and full veneer gold crowns should be used for retainers.

If a mouth is presented with the **four incisors lost and the second bicuspid missing on one side and the second bicuspid and first molar missing on the other** (Fig. 422), a removable partial denture might be contemplated if the anterior ridge has resorbed abnormally. It is practicable to construct a continuous bridge using the first molar, first bicuspid, cuspid, cuspid, first bicuspid, and second molar as abutments, and veneered and full veneer gold crowns as retainers. There will be no more mouth preparation in making a bridge than would be needed for the stabilization of a removable prosthesis, and esthetically the bridge probably will be superior.

To replace a **second molar** (Fig. 423), full veneer gold crown retainers should be placed on the third and first molars. When the third molar is useless as an abutment, it should be extracted. A fixed prosthesis can be constructed, using the first molar and second bicuspid as abutments, with a cantilever second molar pontic.[4] Such a pontic must be smaller and have harmonious occlusion in all excursions. Its primary function is to keep the opposing tooth in position, not to furnish additional surface for mastication.

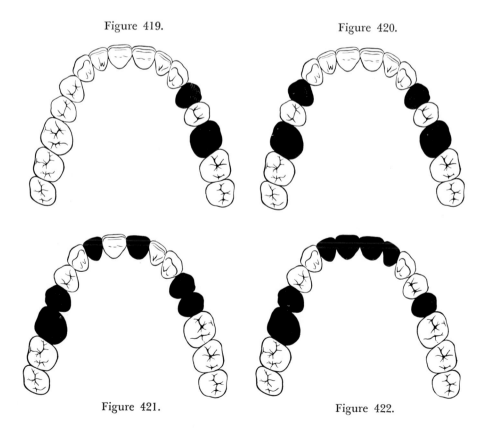

Figure 419.   Figure 420.

Figure 421.   Figure 422.

Figure 423.   Figure 424.

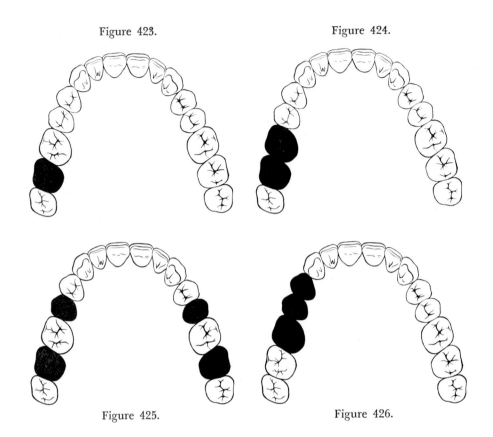

Figure 425.   Figure 426.

On a few occasions when the **approximating first and second molars** (Fig. 424) have been lost and the third molar has remained in position, it has been used as an abutment for a fixed prosthesis. Such treatment seldom can be sanctioned unless in position, crown, and root form the third molar closely resembles the second molar. Otherwise it should be removed and the area restored with a Class II partial denture.

When a **second bicuspid and second molar** are missing (Fig. 425), probably the third molar has been or should be extracted. In the rare event that it qualifies as an abutment, the third molar, first molar, and first bicuspid must be used for stability, with full veneer and veneered gold crowns as retainers. If the first bicuspid is long and substantial, it can be prepared for a partial veneer crown. In a majority of cases, the third molar should be extracted and a bridge constructed having a cantilever second molar pontic. Usually the cuspid will not be included as a third abutment.

If this condition occurs bilaterally, the third molars should not be retained. Bridges should be constructed supplying the second bicuspids, with full veneer gold crown retainers on the first molars and partial veneer or veneered crowns on the first bicuspids. The second molars can then be attached to a Class I removable prosthesis.

When the **approximating first molar, second bicuspid, and first**

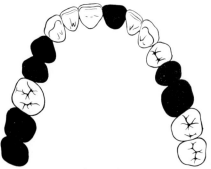

Figure 427.

bicuspid have been lost (Fig. 426), a bridge from second molar to cuspid may not fulfill all requirements. However, if the occlusion is favorable, if the musculature of the face is not extremely powerful, and if the second molar and cuspid to be used as abutments are rugged, in good alignment, and well supported, a bridge can be made that will be comfortable and efficient for a worth-while period.

Although the span is long, the lever arm will be negative. The pontics must be modified drastically through increased embrasure size, exaggerated spillways, and a decreased bucco-lingual measurement. Alveolar response will be favorable if equilibration is maintained. Some bridges of this type have ben retained by a full veneer gold crown on the second molar and a partial veneer on the cuspid, but often a veneered crown can be used to advantage on the cuspid.

When there are missing the **third molar, second molar, second bicuspid, and first bicuspid on the right side, and the central incisor, second bicuspid, and first molar on the left side** (Fig. 427), two bridges and a Class II, Modification I, partial denture should be built. One bridge will supply the right bicuspids, using the first molar and cuspid as abutments; the other, the left central incisor, with the approximating central and lateral as the abutment teeth. The molar retainer should be a full veneer gold crown. The others will be dictated by mouth conditions. After the left first bicuspid and second molar have been prepared or recontoured for retention and support, the left second bicuspid and first molar and right second molar spaces should be filled by the removable partial denture.

MANDIBULAR PATTERNS

Lower incisors are not easily prepared for partial veneer or veneered gold crowns. These teeth are small and the preparations must be delicately done; but when veneered crowns for these teeth are well made, the effect is pleasing.

Figure 428.   Figure 429.

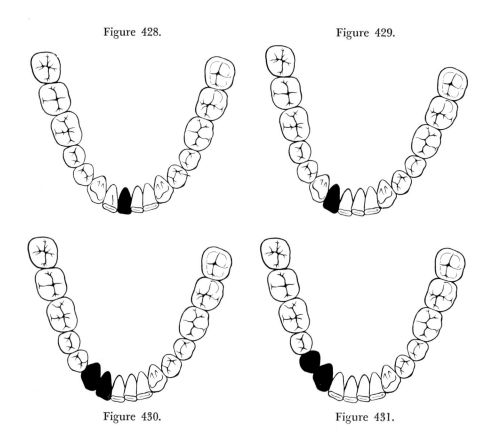

Figure 430.   Figure 431.

Replacement of a **single central incisor** by a bridge (Fig. 428) can be complicated by proximal caries, rotation, or angulation of designated abutments, an end-to-end occlusion, or frail crown form. If the alveolus on the adjacent central has resorbed more than one-fourth in linear measurement, three abutments should be used. The MacBoyle or veneered crown retainer will overcome either proximal caries or rotation; caries-free teeth in regular alignment will accept the pinledge.

A mandibular cantilever **single lateral incisor** pontic (Fig. 429) has even less merit than the maxillary cantilever lateral. The adjacent cuspid and central incisor must be used, and if one central incisor will not be adequate, the two centrals must be splinted. There are times when the life of the remaining incisors can be prolonged by a continuous splint running from cuspid to cuspid, adding one tooth and rigidly joining the five remaining. Caries, alignment, and patient acceptance of metal display will guide the dentist in choosing between pinledge, MacBoyle, or veneered crown retainers.

Replacing a **single cuspid** can pose many problems, especially when it has been extracted because of an eccentric position. This space will be reduced through the contact area but be normal or near-normal in width at the cervical, and any pontic built for it will have to be narrow. The approximating bicuspid and lateral incisor seldom will have compatible long axes, and often it will be necessary to extract one of these teeth before a suitable bridge can be built.

If the lateral incisor is removed (Fig. 430), the first bicuspid and two central incisors should be able to carry the prosthesis; if the first bicuspid is lost (Fig. 431), the central and lateral incisors and the second bicuspid probably will suffice. A survey of the alignment of the abutment teeth will show which tooth should be sacrificed. According to tooth condition, the retainers would be pinledges and a partial veneer or veneered crown, or veneered crowns throughout.

When **both lateral incisors** have been lost (Fig. 432), the alveolar process must be measured. If they have been removed because of lingual or labial malpositions, enough bony tissue should remain to give support to the centrals; but if they were extracted for any other reason, it might be better to remove the centrals also, and construct four pontics between the cuspid abutments. If the centrals can be retained, a continuous unit still is desirable, using partial veneer crowns on the cuspids and MacBoyles or pinledge retainers on the centrals. When the pulps have receded and the caries index is high, all abutments can be prepared for veneered crowns.

A bridge replacing **both central incisors** (Fig. 433) ordinarily can be

Figure 432.   Figure 433.

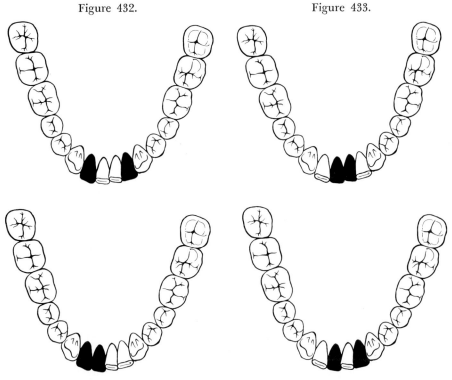

Figure 434.   Figure 435.

Figure 436.   Figure 437.

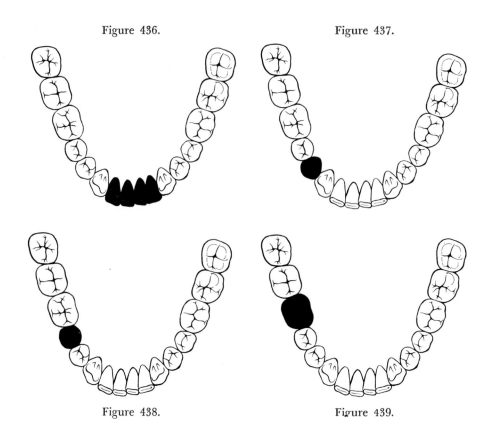

Figure 438.   Figure 439.

capably supported by the mandibular laterals. They are larger than the centrals, with root surface and form a little more adapted to resisting an added load. Pinledges, partial veneers, MacBoyles, or veneered crowns can be used for retainers, and preference is in the order named if there is no caries.

If the **central and lateral incisors in one quadrant** are missing (Fig. 434), three teeth must serve as abutments, namely, the remaining central and lateral, which should receive pinledge retainers (provided caries and alignment permit such preparations), and the cuspid, which may be prepared for either the partial veneer crown or the pinledge.

In the lower arch, replacing a **central incisor on one side of the median line and a lateral incisor on the other** (Fig. 435) calls for a solution similar to that for the same pattern above. The remaining central and lateral incisors and the cuspid will be required for support. Pinledge retainers or MacBoyles on the central and lateral and a partial veneer crown or pinledge on the cuspid will stabilize the prosthesis, although veneered crowns may be used on all abutments. It may be expedient to include the remaining cuspid if it will blend the shading or if realignment will improve esthetic appearance. If the supporting tissue is minimal, it will be advisable to remove the central and lateral and to build a six-unit prosthesis anchored on the cuspids.

If **three incisors** have been lost, it is logical to extract the one that remains (Fig. 436), so that a cuspid-to-cuspid bridge may be built.

A **first bicuspid** (Fig. 437) can be replaced by using partial veneer or veneered crowns as retainers on the cuspid and second bicuspid. The type of construction in which a porcelain veneer is fused to the gold structure may be advocated here.

Inlays will retain a **second bicuspid** pontic (Fig. 438) unless the occlusion, the occluso-cervical measurement of the crowns, or the caries index contraindicates their use. Such a bridge should have a broken-stress joint between the pontic and the first bicuspid inlay. If the first bicuspid has been weakened by caries and a partial veneer or a veneered crown must be employed, a full veneer gold crown should be placed on the first molar and two solder joints should be used.

Frequently the **first molar** (Fig. 439) can be replaced by using inlay retainers. However, if the abutment teeth have drifted so that the occlusion has been disarranged, a full veneer gold crown on the second molar and either a partial veneer or veneered crown on the second bicuspid will be essential.

Figure 440.   Figure 441.

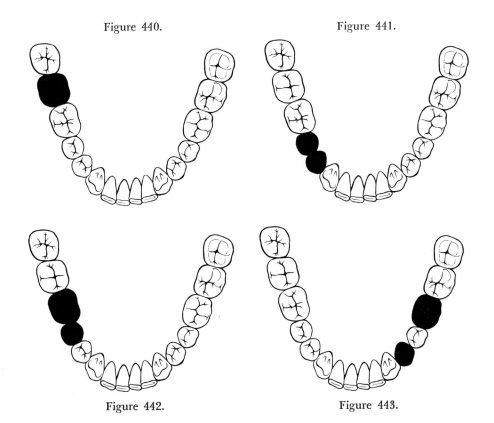

Figure 442.   Figure 443.

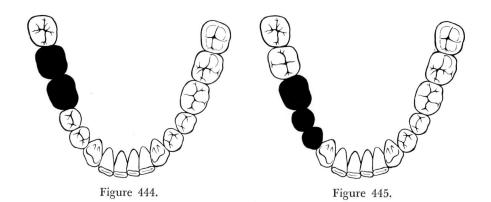

Figure 444.   Figure 445.

When the third and first molars can be used in the replacement of the **second molar** (Fig. 440), the retainers should be full veneer gold crowns. If the clinical crown of the third molar has insufficient length, surgery may be warranted to remove some of the overlying soft tissue. If this is impracticable, the construction of a bridge is contraindicated.

When the **approximating bicuspids** (Fig. 441) have been missing for an extended period of time and the molars have moved forward, with a resultant mesial inclination, often all posterior teeth on that side of the mouth must be rebuilt or reshaped to regain maximal occlusion and function. Even under initial receptive conditions, a full veneer gold crown on the molar and a partial veneer or veneered crown on the cuspid will be the preferred retainers.

When the **second bicuspid and first molar** have been removed (Fig. 442), the first bicuspid is not a good single abutment. It should be splinted to the cuspid. Veneered and full veneer gold crowns will be required to retain this bridge except when the cuspid and first bicuspid are appropriate for partial veneer crowns.

When supplying the **first bicuspid and first molar** (Fig. 443), the second molar, second bicuspid, and cuspid should be used as abutments. A full veneer gold crown and two veneered or partial veneer crowns may be used for retainers.

When the **first and second molars** are missing (Fig. 444) and the third molar is suitable as an abutment, both bicuspids will be indispensable, under most circumstances, to stabilize the anterior end of the bridge. Full veneer and veneered gold crowns must be used as the retainers. If the opposing teeth have extruded, the occlusal plane must be restored or be recontoured to eliminate eccentric interference.

It is hazardous to construct a mandibular bridge that substitutes for **both bicuspids and the first molar** (Fig. 445). The span is too long, even if the opposing teeth have not extruded or can be restored to their former occlusal plane. A noticeable lever arm may be developed, owing to the position of the cuspid. Without losing embrasure space through an increase in size of the solder joints, there might not be strength to withstand breakage or flexing that would destroy cement adhesion.

A removable bridge will be safer. The cuspid should be recontoured with a partial veneer or veneered crown, to support as well as retain the prosthesis, and the second molar should be rebuilt with a full veneer gold crown to afford retention, and depth for an occlusal rest seat. Two approximating teeth on the opposite side should be prepared to receive an embrasure clasp. The masticating efficiency of such a prosthesis will be equal to that of a bridge.

*   *   *   *   *

Innumerable patterns may be encountered. It is felt that the principles of retention and stabilization and the combinations of abutment teeth set forth in this chapter can be applied to restore effectively any single space or combination of spaces.

REFERENCES

1. Vedder, F. B.: Personal communication.
2. Grubb, H. D.: Fixed bridgework. J. Pros. Den., *3*:121, Jan. 1953.
3. Willey, R. E.: Preparation of abutments for veneer retainers. J.A.D.A., *53*:141, Aug. 1956.
4. Ewing, J. E.: Re-evaluation of the cantilever principle. J. Pros. Den., 7:78, Jan. 1957.
5. Moulton, G. H.: Esthetics in anterior fixed bridge prosthodontics. J.A.D.A., *52*:36, Jan. 1956.

Adams, J. D.: Planning posterior bridges. J.A.D.A., *53*:647, Dec. 1956.
Klaffenbach, A. O.: Biomechanical restoration and maintenance of the permanent first molar space. J.A.D.A., *45*:633, Dec. 1952.

28

SPLINTING TEETH

The term "splinting" denotes a rigid or semirigid attachment of one tooth to another, or the comparative immobilization or support of a series of teeth by either a removable or attached appliance. The extent, and perhaps the number, of individual tooth movements usually is restricted because of the union.

Teeth are splinted in the construction of fixed partial prostheses, in preparing mouths to support and retain removable partial prostheses, and for mutual or individual support in periodontally affected mouths. When two or more approximating or separated teeth are joined, forces from mastication, whether against the teeth themselves or transmitted from a prosthesis, will be shared. Splinting is also useful for long range retention following orthodontic treatment.

Splinting is indicated in fixed partial construction when the space is long or when an individual abutment tooth at one or both ends of the space will yield to the torque from the lever arm of the prosthesis. Because of counter balancing, two teeth splinted will provide support, and resistance to forces, greater than the sum of the support or the resistance of the in dividual teeth (Fig. 446).

If splinted teeth are to be used as abutments for either fixed or removable partial prostheses, the occlusion table should be reduced; the embrasures should be kept as large as possible; the solder joints should be as small as is consistent with strength, and round rather than oblong; and the joints should be placed at the normal points of contact between the teeth. Any periodontal involvement should be eradicated. Teeth with short crowns, or those irregularly aligned, are very poor subjects for splinting.

Splinting may be effected by solder joints (Figs. 447 and 448), by precision attachments, or by simultaneous support from extensive clasps or adapted bars that are a part of a removable framework.

When teeth are joined rigidly by solder joints, any force directed against one tooth will be in part transmitted to the one (or the others) to which the recipient is splinted. When two teeth are interlocked by a precision attachment, lateral pressures and any force in line with its path of insertion, except one directed solely to the tooth containing the female attachment, will be shared by the other. Splinting by clasping minimizes any tendency toward lateral movement or rotation by the involved teeth, but they can move into and out of their sockets, one by one, on the application or release of pressure.

When teeth are splinted, there are potential hygienic and periodontal risks. If teeth are short, the solder joint will occupy much of the cervical embrasure, thus reducing the amount of stimulation for the underlying gingival tissue. If in addition the solder joint is wide bucco-lingually, over-protection for the septal gingival tissue is increased. Therefore it is axiomatic in splinting with solder joints that the joint be kept to minimal size, that without obliterating the occlusal embrasure it be placed at the maximal height occlusally (proximally), that it be round for the easiest possible cleansing, and that its structure be such that maximal strength will accrue from minimal size.

Teeth may be splinted in sections when there is a variable long-axis relationship and the sectional splints may be joined and mutually supported by a precision or semiprecision attachment. The precision attachment has some features that contraindicate its use in splinting. First is the amount of tooth structure that must be cut away to receive the female portion. Secondly, if it is to have the greatest effectiveness, the attachment must run the full length of the crown occluso- or linguo-cervically. This effaces the cervical embrasure and seriously encroaches on the lingual space. Hygiene is very

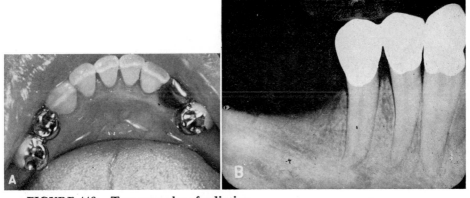

FIGURE 446.   Two examples of splinting.

A, Note occlusal rest seats, small solder joints, and normal embrasures.

B, Second bicuspid radiograph shows evidence of the torque from a poorly designed clasp. The recontoured and splinted tooth became comfortable.

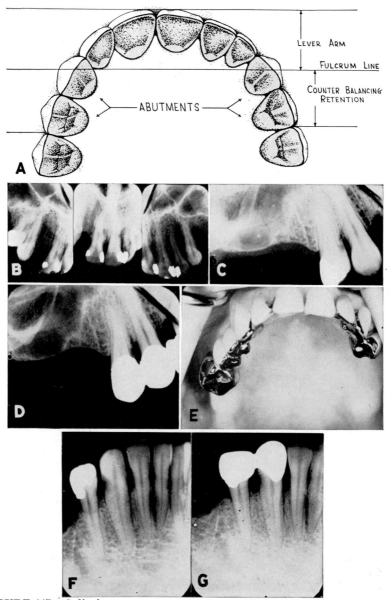

FIGURE 447.   Splinting.

A, Cuspid and bicuspid retainers splinted to form "multiple abutments."

B, C, Good alveolar process and crown-root ratio on cuspid and first bicuspid. Lateral incisor space.

D, Splinted cuspid and bicuspid abutments; cantilever lateral incisor pontic.

E, The three-unit bridge.

F, Reduced support around first bicuspid; too weak for partial denture abutment.

G, Splinted first bicuspid and cuspid; now a strong abutment.

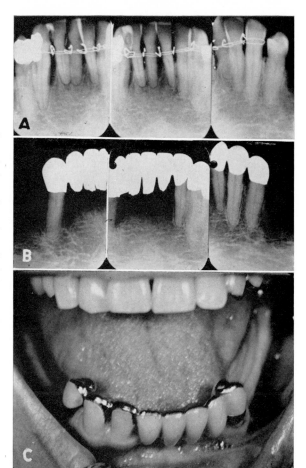

FIGURE 448. Bridge constructed with four abutments.

A, Radiographically, situation not acceptable. Did not respond to periodontal treatment. Three incisors and one cuspid removed.

B, Radiographs showing embrasures.

C, Bridge shown in *B.* The three splinted abutments will stabilize the single bicuspid on the left side of the arch. It has good bony support and will receive bilateral bracing from removable partial denture.

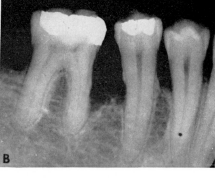

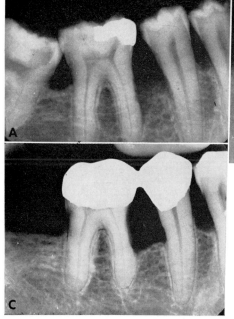

FIGURE 449. *A,* Radiograph showing pocketing around mesial root of mandibular first molar.

B, Second molar lost due to carious exposure. First molar and second bicuspid separated. Pocket advanced.

C, Three years following periodontal surgery, reshaping of alveolar process, and splinting. Molar has served during this time as an abutment for a removable partial denture. Notice reduced masticating area on molar.

483

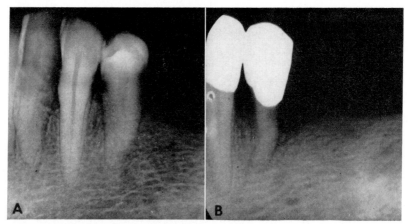

FIGURE 450.   *A,* Radiograph of bicuspid and cuspid to be splinted in the preparation of mouth for removable partial denture.

B, Seventeen months later. Bicuspid must be extracted. Masticating area increased in size and crown-root ratio altered. Marginal ridges too high.

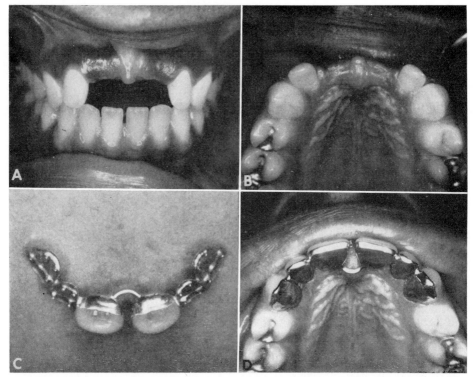

FIGURE 451.   *A, B,* Anterior space too wide for prosthesis to be supported by lateral incisors only.

C, D, Six-unit anterior bridge. Lateral incisors and cuspids splinted on each side, providing counterbalancing retention to offset lever arm and to bring strong cuspid abutments into support of bridge. There will be no labial drifting.

difficult to achieve with the fixea precision attachment splint, and invariably periodontal disturbances will follow its use.

Splinting with clasps is occasionally indicated, but bulk, exaggerated contours, and temporary food retention all tend to make this approach unpopular with the patient if used for an extended period of time. This method is more often employed to provide temporary support during periodontal treatment or as a means of retaining severely affected teeth until it is possible to remove and replace them.

Posterior teeth should be splinted by using full or partial veneer crowns (Fig. 449). Special attention must be given to the preparation of the teeth proximally. These areas must be reduced more than is normal so that the casting will have strength even though lingual and cervical embrasures are enlarged. The approximating occlusal margins of the preparations must also be deepened slightly so that spillways may feed into the lingual embrasure between the splinted teeth. Intercuspal distance sometimes may be constricted bucco-lingually to reduce loads further (Fig. 450).

Anterior teeth are splinted using veneered crowns, partial veneer crowns, and pinledges (Fig. 451). Each has its peculiar set of indications, although these may be interrelated. Veneered crowns are used when teeth must be rebuilt, esthetic appearance heightened, or a tooth clasped or used to house a precision attachment (Fig. 452). Partial veneer crowns will suffice

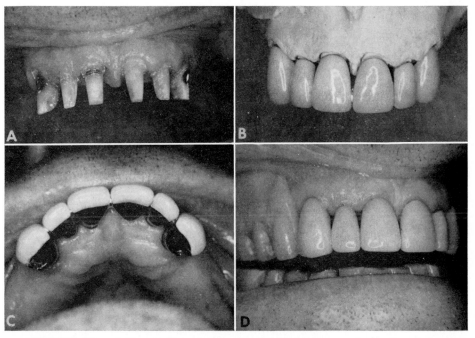

FIGURE 452.   *A,* Six maxillary anterior teeth following removal of splint previously.

   B, C, Six-unit splint. Cuspids house precision attachments.

   D, Splint and partial denture in mouth.

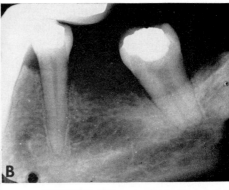

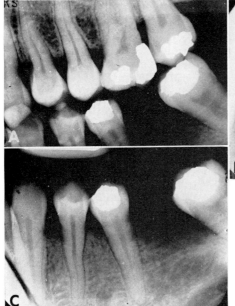

FIGURE 453. *A,* Occluding teeth; mandibular first molar missing, with second molar inclined mesially. Maxillary first molar extruded on distal.

B, Considerable loss of supporting alveolar bone around molar.

C, Bicuspids, if splinted, would provide excellent support for bridge and against lateral forces on molar. Periodontal surgery would give bicuspids sufficient crown length for splinting.

to support a partial denture or an abutment tooth. Much of the time pinledges are used to build lingual surfaces into occlusion or when teeth are periodontally affected.

Many times, of necessity, teeth must be splinted (Fig. 453). When selecting cases where it is to be done, certain requirements must be fulfilled or success may be uncertain.

REFERENCES

Glickman, I., Stein, R. S., and Smulow, I. B.: Effect of increased functional forces upon the periodontium of splinted and non-splinted teeth. J. Periodont., *32:*290, Oct. 1961.

Hudson, W. C.: Provisional coverage and splinting procedures in crown and bridge ceramics and rehabilitation. D. Practitioner & D. Record, *8:*198, March 1958.

Karlstrom, S.: The Pontostructor Method. Stockholm, A. B. Nordiska Bokhandelns, 1955.

Morris, M. L.: The diagnosis, prognosis and treatment of the loose tooth. Oral Surg., Oral Med. & Oral Path., *6:*957, 1037, Aug.–Sept. 1953.

Sanell, C., and Feldman, A. J.: Horizontal pin splint for lower anterior teeth. J. Pros. Den., *12:*138, Jan.–Feb. 1962.

Shooshan, E. D.: Pin-ledge casting technique—its application in periodontal splinting. D. Clin. North America, March 1960, p. 189.

Weinberg, L. A.: Force distribution in splinted anterior teeth. Oral Surg., Oral Med. & Oral Path., *10:*484, May 1957.

Weinberg, L. A.: Force distribution in splinted posterior teeth. Oral Surg., Oral Med. & Oral Path., *10:*1268, Dec. 1957.

Winslow, M. B.: Fixed splint and bridge assembly. J.A.D.A., *51:*47, July 1955.

29

THE CONSTRUCTION OF CROWNS AND BRIDGES IN THE PREPARATION OF PARTIALLY EDENTULOUS MOUTHS FOR CLASP-RETAINED REMOVABLE PROSTHESES

In the rebuilding of a partially edentulous mouth, the philosophy should be one of rendering a real oral health service, not one of merely "filling the space."[1] A fixed partial denture is the restoration of choice when existing conditions and space length will permit (Fig. 454). In many instances, however, a removable prothesis must be employed for a portion or all of the replacement (Fig. 455).[2, 3]

Restoration, preservation, and prevention are all of vital concern. Esthetic appearance, mastication, phonetic ability, and comfort should be restored, at the same time preserving teeth, alveolar process, gingival tissue, tooth position, occlusion, and oral and systemic health. Finally, any further loss of teeth and injury to supporting tissues must be prevented by bringing the forces acting on the removable partial denture within the limits of tissue tolerance.[4, 5]

The most important step in achieving these objectives is adequate preparation of the mouth before construction of a prosthesis. Mouth preparation can be defined as the series of operations necessary to enable a mouth to accept and support a partial denture for the maximal period of time and with minimal adverse reaction on the remaining natural teeth and supporting tissues.[6, 7, 8]

487

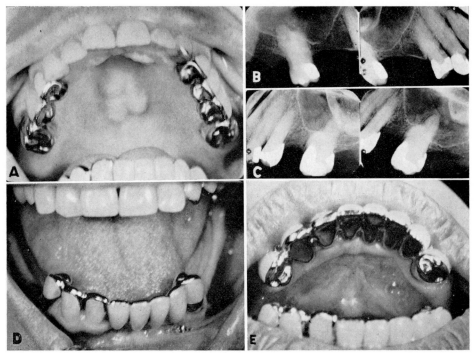

FIGURE 454. *A*, Maxillary arch in which two bridges have been placed. Such spaces are restored frequently with one removable partial denture. While this could be done, it would require rebuilding each of the abutment teeth for support and retention, and would require bars (major connectors) crossing the palate anteriorly and posteriorly to the torus. The plane of occlusion was made acceptable to the construction of the mandibular prosthesis.

B, C, The radiographs substantiate the treatment plan. There are properly distributed healthy abutment teeth to support fixed replacements.

D, E, A bridge was placed in the anterior of the mandibular arch of this mouth. Four teeth are supporting four pontics. The bony process was good, and the first bicuspid, cuspid, and lateral incisor on the right will give the needed support to the left first bicuspid. Also, through the splinting action of the bridge, the bicuspids will be much stronger in their role of abutments for the Class I partial denture. The elimination of the anterior modification space simplifies construction of the removable prosthesis.

A clasp-retained prosthesis can contribute much to oral health, provided that the mouth is correctly prepared for its retention and support and for positioning of its parts. Otherwise it can be an instrument of destruction.

Restorative dentistry, which plays a major part in mouth preparation, includes rebuilding individual teeth with crowns, inlays, or other restorations; splinting teeth by connecting adjacent restorations with a solder joint; and placement of fixed prostheses before the removable partial denture is constructed. Often it is advisable to restore an anterior space with a bridge before building the removable prosthesis, to avoid restrictions in selecting the most desirable path of insertion, and to make construction more simple, design more efficient, and maintenance and repair easier.[9, 10]

Existing conditions in each individual case, such as extent of caries,

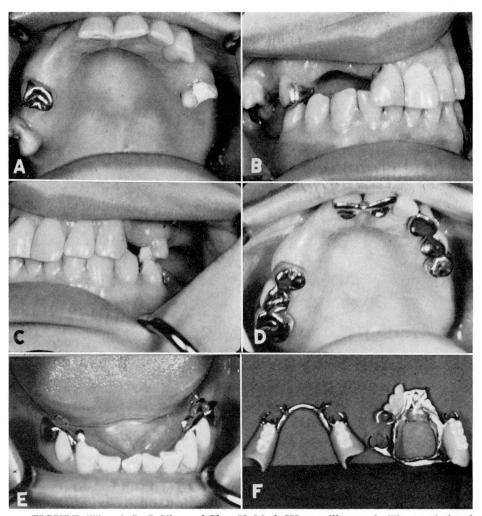

FIGURE 455.   *A, B, C,* Views of Class II, Mod. III, maxillary arch. The two isolated bicuspids were vital and well supported. The molar was inclined buccally so far that clasping was contraindicated without major recontouring.

D, The preparation of the arch for a removable prosthesis included two fixed restorations and one splint. This stabilized all abutment teeth, eliminated two modification spaces, and changed the classification to Class II, Mod. I. The forms of the molar and the bicuspids were made suitable for clasping and support, and the incisors were splinted and recontoured to give support and to receive force parallel to their long axes.

E, The opposing arch was prepared by splinting the bicuspids on each side with a crown and a partial veneer crown. Note the occlusal rest seats for the clasps on the distals of the second bicuspids and for the secondary retainers on the mesials of the first bicuspids. Guiding planes were made also on the distal surfaces of the second bicuspids and at the mesio-lingual line angles of the first bicuspids.

F, The prostheses built for this mouth. The mandibular has two retainers and four rests; the maxillary, three retainers and four rests.

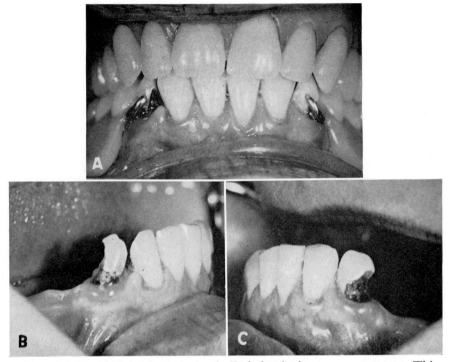

FIGURE 456. Carious abutment teeth. Endodontic therapy was necessary. This was followed by building the teeth to prepared form with cast cores retained by posts in the root canals.

caries index, quantity and quality of remaining supporting tissue, and tooth contours, will dictate the amount and kind of restorative dentistry.

Carious teeth must be restored and caries controlled by whatever procedures are feasible. A high caries index will make it necessary to cover the abutment teeth with crowns (Figs. 456 and 457). Splinting may be essential to distribute the forces that will be brought to bear on the remaining teeth. This is a service often indicated but seldom delivered, yet it is one of the best methods available for distributing forces over a wider area (Fig. 458). (See Chapter 28, Splinting Teeth.)

Although many phases of dentistry may be pursued in properly preparing a partially edentulous mouth, it is the purpose of this chapter to discuss what is probably the most neglected phase of treatment in all dentistry, the construction of crowns and bridges that *fulfill* the specific requirements of support, retention, and ideal design for partial dentures and removable bridges.[11,12,13]

These requirements encompass (1) the establishment of abutment tooth contour that will remove any interference with the rigid portion of the partial denture framework and reciprocal clasp arms during insertion or removal (Fig. 459); (2) protection of the abutment tooth against caries; (3) restoration of a favorable occlusal plane and harmonious occlusion; and

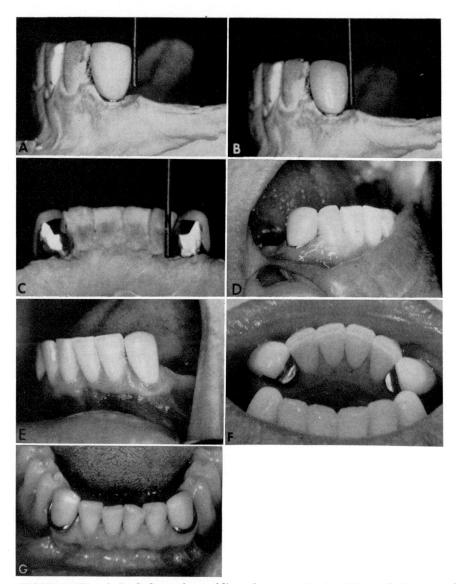

FIGURE 457. *A, B, C,* Surveying guiding planes on distal and lingual of crown: *A,* before glazing; *B, C,* after glazing.

D, E, The crowns built to reconstruct and recontour abutments shown in preceding figure. The frameworks are cast gold; the veneers are porcelain bonded to the castings. Retentive undercuts of the desired depth, and specifically positioned at the mesio-cervical, were located with a surveyor and ground into the porcelain. Guiding planes, partly on gold and partly on the veneer, were placed at the distal. An overglaze was used.

F, The type of lingual contour in the castings. The prosthesis will be supported, the gingival tissue protected, and the force directed along the long axes of the abutments.

G, Partial denture in position.

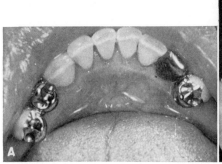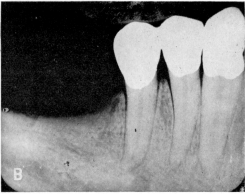

FIGURE 458. Examples of splinting.

A, Note occlusal rest seats, small solder joints, and normal embrasures.

B, Second bicuspid radiograph shows evidence of the torque from a poorly designed clasp. The recontoured and splinted tooth became comfortable.

(4) elimination of modification areas that might complicate design, tolerance, and maintenance.

INDICATIONS

Crowns or bridges (or both) for the support and retention of removable partial prostheses are indicated

(1) when abutment teeth are carious or the caries index is high;

(2) when crown form must be changed on either normal or tipped teeth to accommodate a benign clasp design (see Fig. 460);

(3) when splinting is necessary because of alveolar recession or root form;

(4) to restore occlusion or to correct the occlusal plane when teeth have extruded, and thus regain occlusal harmony in the finished partial denture;

(5) to allow more freedom in selecting the path of insertion when an anterior modification space exists;

(6) to splint a bicuspid that is standing alone so that it may resist torque or leverage; and

(7) for esthetic reasons. (See Figs. 461 and 462.)

PRELIMINARY DESIGN AND TREATMENT PLANNING

Before the preparations are started, the diagnostic cast should be surveyed, a preliminary design made for the cast metal framework, and the path of insertion established. At the same time the amount of recontouring of teeth to be used for retention or support of the prosthesis should be diagrammed. If one (or more) of the abutment teeth does not require recontouring, the path of insertion should be selected with this in mind. Reduction of the abutments can be guided by the space measurements when the analyzing rod is in contact with the height-of-contour line.

The crown surfaces that are to be contacted by minor connectors and nonretentive sections of clasps must be parallel to each other and to the path of insertion, to form planes that guide the prosthesis along the predetermined path of insertion. They will provide, also, for balanced and equalized retention, strategically located and of the accepted, but not excessive, depth for the designated clasp design. This can be accomplished by using a surveyor while carving the wax pattern. Thus it will be possible to procure bracing and reciprocation. Since secondary retainers should never be placed on inclined planes, the cingulum areas of anterior teeth must be elevated to create ledges (see Fig. 457C), which will direct the forces parallel to the long axes of the roots.

TOOTH PREPARATION

In the preparation of a tooth to be clasped or to support a secondary retainer, there must be more reduction of the marginal ridge so that an occlusal rest seat in the finished crown may have enough depth (Fig. 463). Rest seats are located in the marginal ridge areas of the occlusal surfaces and over the crests of the alveolar ridges. Rest seats should be spoon-shaped (see Fig. 458A), slanting slightly toward the center of the teeth, and must be a minimum of 1.5 mm. deep, 2.0 mm. wide, and 2.5 mm. long.[14]

The axial preparation of a tooth to be reshaped must be done so that the right contour for clasping can be built into the completed restoration.

The gingival margin of the crown, whenever possible, must be extended into the sulcus. When one (or more) of the surfaces of the tooth is not covered, inhibiting treatments of stannous fluoride should be used.

TAKING THE IMPRESSIONS

An accurate indirect technique is necessary to produce such exact contour in the restoration. After the teeth have been prepared and adequate tissue displacement has been obtained, a full arch polysulfide rubber impression is made. Two casts are poured, one being sectioned for dies and the other left intact, to be used as a working cast (Fig. 464). The working and opposing casts are occluded, using a face-bow and a Kerr Bite Frame or an occlusion rim, so that occlusion and contact may be established on

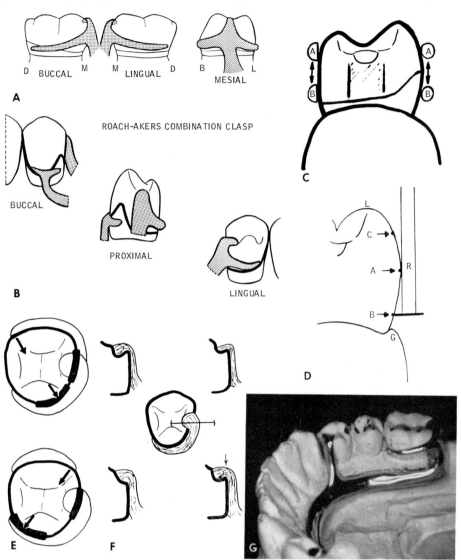

FIGURE 459. *A,* Left, survey line produced on buccal of recontoured tooth brings clasp arm low on tooth and forms a retentive undercut which accepts only the flexible portion of the clasp arm. Center, survey line (or height of contour) on lingual is low. Reciprocal, nonretentive clasp arm can contact and support tooth at all times while retentive arm is flexing and going over height of contour into or out of retentive undercut. Right, clasp close to cervical line and closer to point of rotation in root.

B, Recontouring tooth for Roach-Akers clasp. Buccal shows survey line, or height of contour, developed to produce retentive undercut next to edentulous area. Under force of mastication, retentive tip moves away from tooth. Proximal and lingual views show stabilizing, or nonretentive, clasp arm above a height of contour placed down very near but not on gingival line.

C, Guiding planes on lingual and proximal of recontoured abutment. Occlusal and cervical margins of lingual plane are above and below point where buccal clasp arm begins to flex over height of contour and into undercut. Thus, stabilizing lingual arm supports tooth during seating of prosthesis.

D, Convexity above and below height of contour the same in length and depth.

E, Heavy lines show guiding planes opposite retentive undercuts.

F, Three incorrect and one correct occlusal rests and rest seats. Top left: Seat too

(Legend continued on facing page)

494

the wax patterns. The working cast must be removable so that the patterns can be surveyed. Alginate may be used for the opposing cast impression.

SURVEYING THE WAX PATTERNS

The wax pattern for either a crown or a pontic that will retain or support a removable partial denture must first be carved to have harmonious form and occlusion. Then the working cast is transferred to a surveying table (Fig. 465), where guiding plane areas, to be contacted by a minor connector and a reciprocal clasp arm, will be formed with a warmed analyzing rod. These must be parallel to the path of insertion. The predetermined amount of undercut should be measured and located ideally on the pattern,

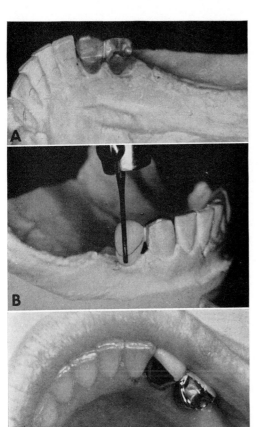

FIGURE 460. *A,* Splinted castings for removable partial denture. Rest seat in bicuspid and shelf on cuspid. Line on cast shows height of proposed lingual plate.

B, Marking survey line and developing height of contour and mesio-buccal retentive undercut on a bonded porcelain veneer.

C, Finished retainer shown in *A.*

angular and rest too thin crossing margin. Will fracture. Top right: Not enough bulk. Will fracture. Bottom left: Too sloping. Tendency to slide will cause clasp arms to exert adverse pressure. Bottom right: Correct as to bulk and contour.

G, Framework on cast. Guiding plane surfaces on distal of molar, lingual of molar, and mesio-lingual of bicuspid. Strut for secondary retainer placed in mesio-lingual embrasure. Lingual clasp arm low on tooth but entirely above height of contour.

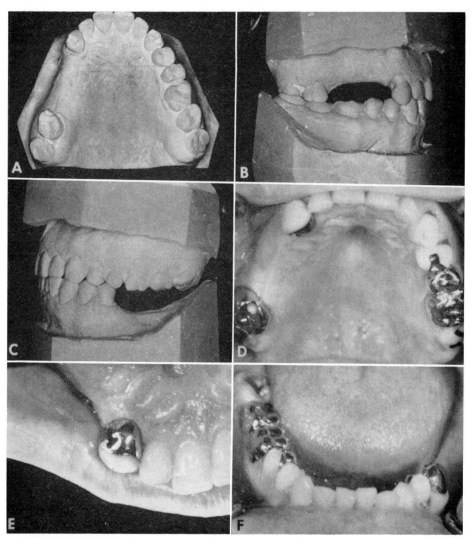

FIGURE 461. *A, B,* Cast of maxillary Class III arch. Cuspid abutment has poor crown-root ratio because of apicoectomy.

C, Class II occluded mandibular arch.

D, Maxillary mouth preparation. Bonded porcelain veneer on cuspid housing precision attachment. Recontoured molar with rest seat and disto-buccal retentive undercut. Recontoured molar and bicuspid on opposite side. Back-to-back clasps will cross occluding surfaces above contacts.

E, Mirror view of cuspid crown.

F, Mandibular mouth preparation. First and second molars to be clasped. Occluding surfaces grooved for crossing clasp. Rest seat in mesio-lingual occlusal of bicuspid. Bicuspid crowned for clasping.

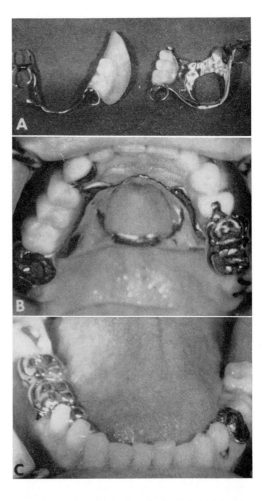

FIGURE 462.   *A,* Removable partial dentures.
B, C, Prostheses in position.

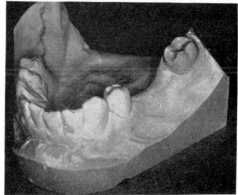

FIGURE 463.   Preparation of molar to make room for adequate rest seat in casting.

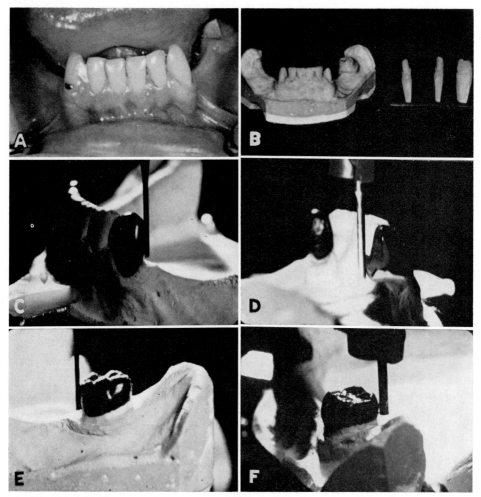

FIGURE 464.   *A,* A Class II, Mod. I, mandibular arch.

B, The working cast and dies for mouth preparation.

C, Placing distal guiding plane on pattern for left cuspid crown; surveyor table is set at correct tilt for predetermined path of insertion.

D, Carving guiding plane on lingual of raised cingulum, mandibular right cuspid.

E, Checking guiding plane, parallel to path of insertion, with warmed analyzing rod of surveying instrument.

F, Checking position and depth of retentive undercut of mandibular molar crown.

eliminating all interfering contours except the measured suprabulge above the undercut. Also, while the cast is on the surveying table, any modifications should be made in the height of contour and the buccal and lingual surfaces that are needed to form supporting areas that will balance and stabilize the tooth during insertion and removal of the partial denture.[15] (See Fig. 464C, D, E, and F.)

After occlusion, contact areas, and contour have been obtained, the wax pattern is returned to the die for correction or completion of the cervical margin, and for polishing. The polished casting is placed on the working cast and checked with the surveyor analyzing rod for exactness of guiding planes, and with an undercut gauge for depth of undercut. It is then cemented on the abutment tooth, completing the restorative phase of mouth preparation. (See Fig. 466.)

Removable partial dentures should not be built around isolated bicuspids or incisors. Such teeth may be splinted with bridges to cuspids anteriorly, molars posteriorly, or to cuspids or other incisors laterally.[6] A bridge built for this purpose gives superb support to the abutment tooth, eliminates an awkward modification space, enhances incising if in the anterior, and provides rest seat, guiding plane, and embrasure areas for secondary retainers and minor connectors.

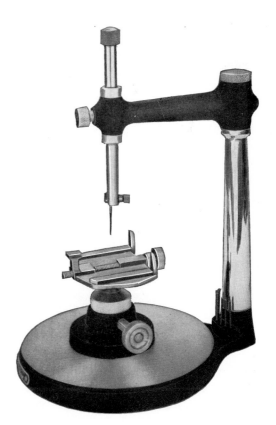

FIGURE 465.   Surveyor (Ney).

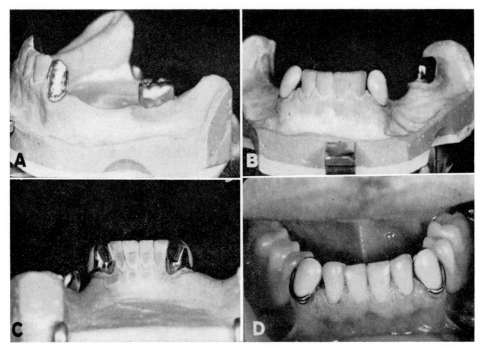

FIGURE 466. *A,* Castings from wax patterns shown in Figure 464; note guiding planes.

B, Veneered cuspid crowns and polished molar crown.

C, Lingual form of cuspid crowns.

D, Class II, Mod. I, mandibular partial denture which occludes with maxillary complete denture.

A crown on an abutment tooth may be undercontoured, with a shelf as a supporting area for clasp arms which restore normal contour to the tooth. Pontics or connectors may be contoured or grooved for clasps which cross the occlusal surface. Preparation of abutment teeth or pontic design must be planned to facilitate such a clasping situation. Cingulums of retainers or pontics may be contoured or recessed to support lingual plates or rests.[16]

A tooth with receded alveolar process may be doubly supported by another bridge abutment and the bilateral bracing from a removable partial denture.

*   *   *   *   *

From the foregoing discussion, it is evident that before a student or dentist is qualified to prepare mouths and to construct biologically acceptable partial dentures, he must have a good foundation in crown and bridge prosthodontics. These two fields of dentistry are inseparable, since the success of the partial denture will depend entirely on the quality of the preparatory crown and bridge work.

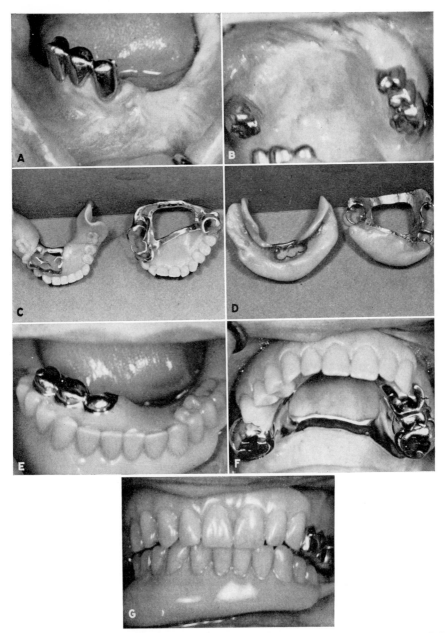

FIGURE 467. Rebuilding a mutilated mouth. Preservation of the seven remaining teeth is essential if the patient masticates and has normal appearance. Portions of both mandibular and maxillary arches shot away. Repaired by bone grafts and plastic surgery.

A, Mandibular cuspid treated endodontically. Crowns extended as far as possible cervically. Guiding planes on buccal surfaces, retention on lingual. Rest seats mesially and distally on splint.

B, Three teeth splinted and contoured for buccal and lingual retention. Clasp arms reciprocate. Mesial and distal occlusal rests. Grooves for crossing occlusion. Right molar contoured for ring clasp and two occlusal rests.

C, D, The mandibular and maxillary prostheses.

E, Mandibular prosthesis in mouth, built around three abutment teeth to restore contour to face.

F, Maxillary prosthesis in mouth. It is supported by four rests, one strut, and scar tissue.

G, Mastication, appearance, and enunciation satisfactory to patient. Without recontoured crowns and splinting, such a case is hopeless.

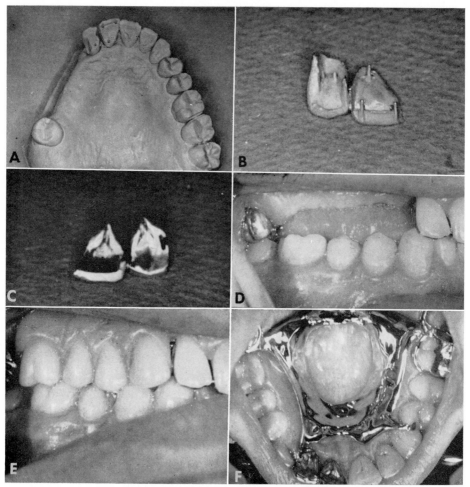

FIGURE 468.   *A,* Cast of maxillary arch. Right molar crowned, with mesial rest seat. Left molars prepared for clasping. Lateral and central incisors prepared for splinting. Lateral will house precision attachment. Same preparation, although less deep, would be required for Sherer rest seat.

B, C, D, Splinted retainer for lateral and central.

E, Partial denture in place. Esthetic appearance acceptable.

F, Mirror view of partial denture. Four points of support and stabilization. Four areas of retention.

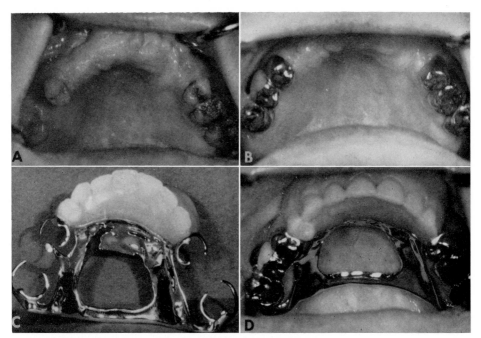

FIGURE 469.   *A,* Class IV maxillary arch resulting from accident.

B, Mouth preparation. Bridge on right splinting molar and bicuspid. Abutments will be clasped and provide support as well as retention. All teeth on left crowned. Retention and support pattern same as on right side.

C, D, Partial denture before seating, and seated. Class IV removable partial denture must have retention as far as possible behind the fulcrum line. Anterior support must be rugged.

REFERENCES

 1. Jordan, L. G.: Designing removable partial dentures with external attachments (clasps). J. Pros. Den., *2*:716, Nov. 1952.
 2. Frechette, A. R.: Partial denture planning with special reference to stress distribution. J. Ontario D. A., *30*:318, Oct. 1953.
 3. Smith, G. P.: Factors affecting the choice of partial prosthesis—fixed or removable. D. Clin. North America, March 1959, p. 3.
 4. Applegate, O. C.: Essentials of Removable Partial Denture Prosthesis. 2nd ed. Philadelphia, W. B. Saunders Company, 1959, p. 182.
 5. Eich, F. A.: Role of removable partial dentures in the destruction of the natural dentition. D. Clin. North America, Nov. 1962, p. 717.
 6. Johnston, J. F., and Bogan, R. L.: Partial denture design and related mouth preparation. Bul. Virginia D. A., *40*:25, March 1963 (Abstract).
 7. Johnston, J. F.: Preparation of mouths for fixed and removable partial dentures. J. Pros. Den., *11*:456, May–June 1961.
 8. Cunningham, D. M.: Mouth preparation for removable appliances. Arizona D. J., *2*:154, Dec. 1956.
 9. Steffel, V. L.: Planning removable partial dentures. J. Pros. Den., *12*:524, May–June 1962.
10. Johnston, J. F.: Preparation of mouths for fixed and removable partial dentures. Alum. Bul. Indiana Univ. School Den., Sept. 1960, p. 4.

11. Towle, H. J., Jr.: Mouth preparation for removable partial dentures. New York J. Den., *31*:119, April 1961.
12. Glann, G. W., and Appleby, R. C.: Mouth preparation for removable partial dentures. J. Pros. Den., *10*:698, July–Aug. 1960.
13. Mills, M. L.: Mouth preparation for the removable partial denture. J.A.D.A., *60*:154, Feb. 1960.
14. Perry, C.: Importance and preparation of the occlusal rest. J. Michigan D. A., *42*:97, March 1960.
15. DeRisi, M. C.: Surveying for removable partial denture prosthesis. J.A.D.A., *63*:603, Nov. 1961.
16. McCracken, W. L.: Partial Denture Construction. 2nd ed. St. Louis, The C. V. Mosby Company, 1964.

Martone, A. L.: A challenge of the partially edentulous mouth. J. Pros. Den., *8*:942, Nov.–Dec. 1958.
McCracken, W. L.: Mouth preparation for partial dentures. Bul. Alabama D. A., *39*:37, Oct. 1955.
McCracken, W. L.: Mouth preparation for partial dentures. J. Pros. Den., *6*:39, Jan. 1956.
Metty, A. C.: Obtaining efficient soft tissue support for the partial denture base. J.A.D.A., *56*:679, May 1958.
Perry, C.: Philosophy of partial denture design. Bul. St. Louis D. Soc., *25*:48, May 1954 (Digest).
Schuyler, C. H.: Analysis of the use and relative value of the precision attachment and the clasp in partial denture planning. J. Pros. Den., *3*:711, Sept. 1953.
Steffel, V. L.: Postgraduate course, Ohio State Univ. School Den., 1953.
Steffel, V. L.: Clasp partial dentures. J.A.D.A., *66*:803, June 1963.
Terkla, L. G., and Laney, W. R.: Partial Dentures. 3rd ed. St. Louis, The C. V. Mosby Company, 1963.

30

ORTHODONTIC POSITIONING OF ABUTMENTS AND ASSOCIATED TEETH

Abutment alignment is one of the most important factors influencing the design, esthetic effect, and longevity of a fixed partial denture. Improved axial directions of the abutment teeth will not only provide a more suitable foundation for the prosthesis—that is, one better able to accept additional forces—but also will make it possible to utilize teeth that otherwise would be unusable as abutments.

Reorientation of abutment teeth will enable the prosthodontist to cope with many uncertainties associated with pathologic axial inclinations of abutments. The purpose of this chapter, therefore, is to demonstrate a few of the more typical problems that may exist because of poor alignment of the abutment teeth, and to suggest methods of treatment. It is not the intent here either to discuss all of the abnormalities that may be present, or to elaborate on the various techniques that may be used to correct them.

Considerations that may be used as the basis for a successful solution for some of these situations will be set forth. Only one technique will be outlined, namely, that of the so-called "working retainer." This appliance is sufficiently versatile to effect a majority of the tooth movements that the prosthodontist may wish to do himself. However, it does have limitations, which must be recognized. These will be mentioned in the section on technical procedures.

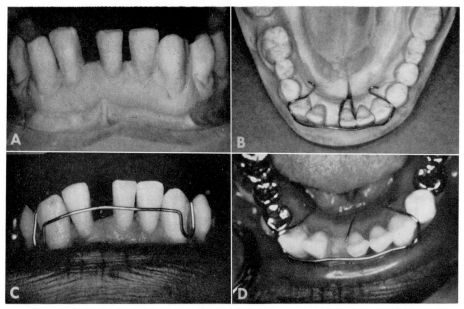

FIGURE 470.   *A,* Cast of mandibular arch.
B, C, D, Incisor abutments were first moved lingually, then laterally (*D*).

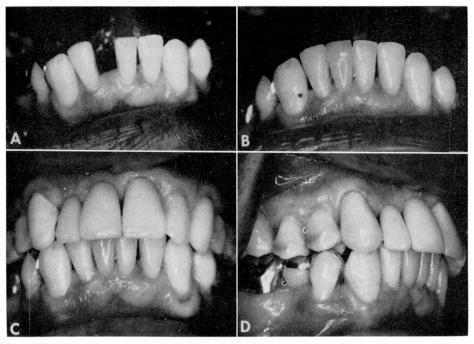

FIGURE 471.   *A,* Repositioned abutments.
B, C, D, Views of mandibular anterior bridge and occluding maxillary bridge.

SOME TYPICAL PROBLEMS

It may be desirable to alter the positions of the abutment teeth for one or more of the following reasons:

1. A lack of contact with adjacent teeth, if uncorrected, can result in a food trap is the retainer is overcontoured in an attempt to make contact.

2. Axial tilting can lead to a crushing of the periodontal membrane under an additional load, with subsequent periodontal and alveolar atrophy.

3. Teeth can display occlusal interference in eccentric excursions. (An example of this is a mandibular second molar tipped forward into a first molar space, the mesial of the tooth rotating to the lingual, the disto-buccal being elevated above the occlusion table, and cuspal interference with the mesio-lingual cusp of the maxillary second molar occurring during lateral excursions.)

4. When there is a rotation effecting disturbances in inclined-plane relationships, it might be difficult to design the preparation of the abutment tooth so that it will meet the demands of both appearance and mechanics.

5. When teeth are tipped labially or lingually, or when anterior teeth

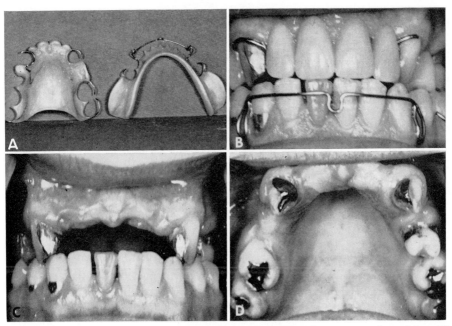

FIGURE 472. *A,* Working retainers that were used to improve tooth position. The maxillary left cuspid clasp is free of acrylic resin over most of its length so that it can be activated to cause labial movement of the tooth. The labial wire on the mandibular anteriors will be used to move the incisors lingually and together.

B, Appliances in the mouth. The mandibular posterior supplied teeth are set high to increase the vertical dimension so that the left cuspid will be free to move into proper position.

C, Left cuspid has moved to position. Teeth have temporary amalgam restorations.

D, Occlusal view of *C.*

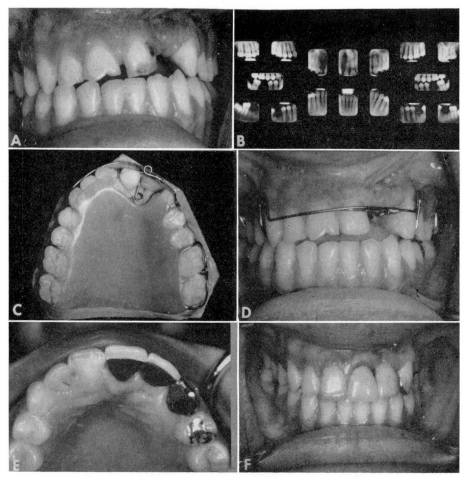

FIGURE 473.   *A, B,* Mouth of adolescent. Lateral incisor missing, owing to repaired cleft. Axial inclination and pulp size of central made preparation impossible.

   C, Appliance to correct inclination of central. Tooth will be tipped instead of being moved bodily, but this will suffice.

   D, Repositioning almost completed.

   E, F, Bridge on realigned abutments.

are flared labially with an unsatisfactory esthetic effect, preparations could result in overreduction.

   This list is incomplete, but these are the problems most frequently encountered.

PHYSIOLOGIC CONSIDERATIONS OF TOOTH MOVEMENT

   The periodontal membrane is composed primarily of collagenous fibers, and the majority of the fibers are oriented obliquely and directed apically as the cementum of the tooth is approached. Orban[1] states that the blood supply for this structure is derived from the blood vessels (1) entering the apical foramen, (2) passing over the alveolar crest from the gingivae, and (3) penetrating the wall of the alveolus, with the major supply coming from the last-mentioned.

The periodontal membrane is more vascular on the side next to the alveolus, and this characteristic is greater in the apical third than in the coronal portion. Bone is a highly vascular tissue, but cementum is an avas-

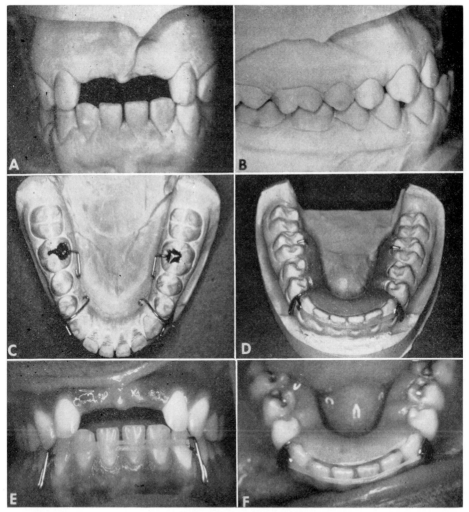

FIGURE 474.   *A, B,* Casts of opposing arches. Observe relationship of incisal edges of mandibular teeth to maxillary ridge. This position and width of space made situation very difficult.

C, D, Appliance to move mandibular incisors lingually. Force exerted lingually by elastic band stretched over labial surfaces. Resin contoured to give freedom of movement and to maintain alignment.

E, F, Appliance at work. Movement short of that desired.

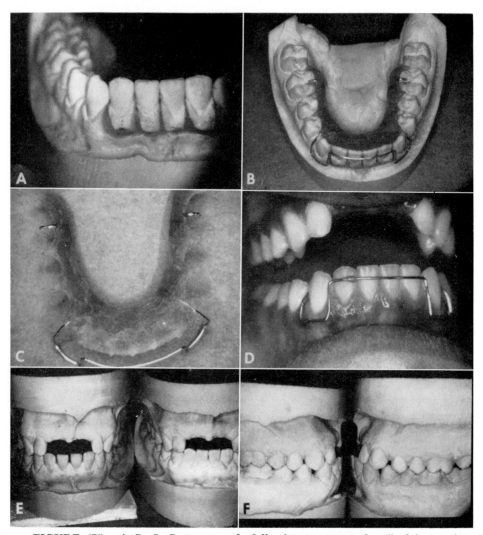

FIGURE 475. *A, B, C,* Cast was made following treatment described in previous figure. It was sectioned, teeth were aligned, and a Hawley retainer made.

D, Second appliance pushed mobile teeth into alignment. Patient was uncomfortable for about two hours.

E, F, Contrasting casts showing realigned mandibular incisors. Occlusion now suitable for maxillary bridge. (See Case History 1 in Chapter 36.)

cular structure. It is quite possible that the resorption differences of bone and cementum are due to these dissimilarities in vascularity and that the more common presence of resorption in the region of the apex may be changes in the periodontal membrane as force is applied to it. As a consequence of such compression, stasis of the blood at the compression site lowers the pH, which in turn causes an increased solubility of the mineral traced to the higher vascularity of the periodontal membrane at this point.

Hemley[2] believes that the actual resorptive mechanism stems from pH

salts of the bone, resulting in resorption. Relief of the stasis allows a resumption of the normal pH, and local calcium is deposited in the formation of new bone.

Oppenheim[3] has found that a force applied to the crown of a tooth produces a tipping movement, the fulcrum of which is located approximately at the beginning of the apical third of the root. The distance of this fulcrum point from the apex is a function of the degree of force applied to the tooth. This creates four areas of activity in the periodontal membrane, two of resorption and two of deposition (Fig. 476).

Reitan[4] has noted a cellular increase in the periodontal membrane within the first to second day of tooth movement in humans, and also an increase, particularly marked around the ninth day, in the osteoid present on the alveolar wall. Under pressure there occurs either direct resorption of bone or hyalinization of the periodontal membrane, with resorption in adjacent areas of the bone. Cellular proliferation is stated to be a response to tension of the fibers of the periodontal membrane.

Owing to the thickening of the periodontal membrane around the tooth during movement, mobility to the extent of approximately 1.0 mm. may ensue. To permit the tissues to reorganize around the root, active treatment is followed by a period of retention[5] in which the teeth are held during undisturbed reparative processes. This is accomplished by having the working appliance adjusted passively to maintain the new positions of the abutment teeth. One alternative would be to prepare the abutment teeth and then to stabilize them with a temporary acrylic resin bridge to be worn during fabrication of the prosthesis.

FIGURE 476.   Diagram showing the areas of pressure (P) and tension (T) along the root of a tooth receiving a buccal tipping force.

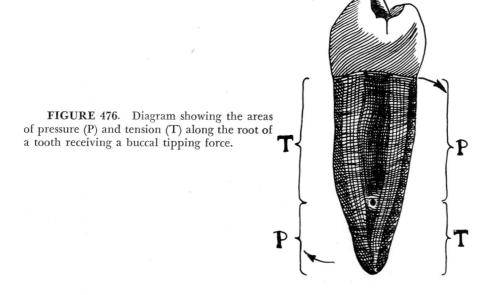

DIAGNOSIS, ANALYSIS, AND TREATMENT PLANNING

"Diagnosis," as used here, refers to the recognition of an existing problem concerning the position of the abutment teeth. The simple recognition of such disturbance is followed by a scrutiny of the abnormality, which is termed "analysis." Information obtained in the analytical process is the basis for the formulation of the treatment plan, which may include repositioning of the abutment teeth.

Abutment position must not be considered a problem separate from the design of the prosthesis. It is one of the factors that dictate this choice and should enter into the treatment planning much the same as does the caries index of the mouth. Malpositions of teeth to be used as abutments are only one phase that must be contemplated in the restoration of a mouth to an optimal level. For instance, a complete denture opposing the arch to be restored would decrease the forces on a bridge and might make it unnecessary to reposition the abutment teeth for better resistance to stresses.

In the analysis, information is gleaned from diagnostic casts, intraoral radiographs, and oral examination. The diagnostic casts, plus the radiographs, will show the axial inclinations of the teeth in a mesio-distal direction. The casts also will divulge facio-lingual axial inclinations, abnormal rotations, and resistance to orthodontic movement of abutment teeth caused by interlocking cuspal relations, unerupted teeth, or ankylosis. Ankylosed teeth cannot be moved, but cuspal interferences may be minimized either by spot grinding of the offending cusps or by the construction of a bite plane against which the lower incisors occlude, thus prohibiting articulation in the posterior segments.

Examination of the mouth will disclose cuspal relations in lateral excursions. If an excessive curve of Spee exists, a view of the interocclusal space in rest position will show whether the excessive vertical overlap is due to infraclusion of the posterior teeth or to supraclusion of the anterior teeth.

Isolation of the reason for the exaggerated vertical overlap will determine the ideal solution. If the interocclusal space is more than 3.0 to 5.0 mm., undereruption of the buccal segments, especially the mandibular bicuspids and maxillary molars, is the probable cause. Sometimes a bite plane, occluding against the lower incisors, will prevent the occlusion of the posterior teeth and allow their eruption, thus reducing the vertical overlap. If the interocclusal space is within the 3.0 to 5.0 mm. range, usually there is an overeruption of the anterior teeth. Such a situation should be handled by an orthodontist, inasmuch as it requires depression of teeth, the most challenging type of movement, and involves procedures not within the scope of the restorative dentist.

After completing the analysis, the design of the appliance is considered.

To the maximal extent permitted by limiting factors, it must correct the problem as it has been visualized. The analytical process should show the directions and the distance desired in tooth movement. The limiting factors include those inherent in the appliance, the patient, and the operator.

It is possible for a tooth to undergo movement in three planes of space simultaneously, as, for example, distally, lingually, and occlusally. The appliance to be described will not perform bodily movement of teeth and will not actively erupt teeth. Tissues may not respond as anticipated, and movement may be extremely difficult if not impossible. In other individuals, eruption is not easily obtained when using bite planes, and the new positions are sometimes unstable. **Lack of skill and comprehension of the potentialities of the appliance definitely can preclude achievement of the result expected.**

APPLIANCE DESIGN

Factors presented by each individual case determine the design of the appliance. It is constructed of an acrylic resin base, the working arms being formed from stainless steel wire varying from 0.025 to 0.030 inch. In general, the smaller wire is used instead of its heavier counterpart, to produce a lighter force which will act for a longer time and through a greater distance.

The passive wire to be activated should be deformed 1.0 mm. in the direction toward which movement is desired (Fig. 477). Therefore, by opening slightly the primary coil (Fig. 477 at *1*), the free arm of this coil, which extends to the secondary coil, is displaced 0.5 mm. An additional 0.5 mm. is then gained by opening the secondary coil (Fig. 477 at *2*). The result is a displacement paralleling the direction sought in the movement (mesial in this instance).

If only the primary coil were opened in this case, the resultant movement would have a labial component that might be undesirable. The degree of displacement of the working arm will vary with the size of the wire

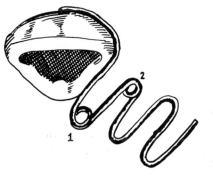

FIGURE 477. Double cantilever spring as used to apply a direct proximal thrust on an incisor. 1, The primary coil; 2, the secondary coil.

being used, usually with a greater displacement being placed in the thinner wires.

Types of tooth movement, and some basic designs that can be realized with the working retainer, are illustrated.

Labio-Lingual Movement of Incisors

Lingual tipping of an incisor can be effected by utilizing a labial arch wire that is deformed to place a force on the labial surface of the tooth to be moved. One design for this arch wire is shown in Figure 478.

The acrylic resin is cut away on the lingual surface of the central to be repositioned, and the pressure is kept on the central incisor by gradually building an inset into the arch passing over it or closing the vertical loops, or both (Fig. 479). This is done by making slight adjustments in the arch wire at two-week intervals. This inset will keep the arch from being in contact on the labial surface of the other incisors and cuspids.

Force is then generated in the loops overlying the cuspids and is transmitted to the central incisor. The wire should rest in contact across the labial surface of the central if there is no need to rotate this tooth. This can be checked by drawing a length of dental floss between the wire and the tooth to test the accuracy of fit.

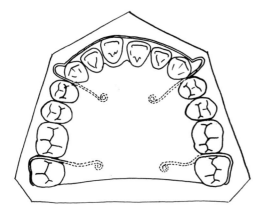

FIGURE 478. Design of appliance to tip an incisor lingually. The acrylic resin, as shown, is relieved on the lingual of the incisor to allow movement.

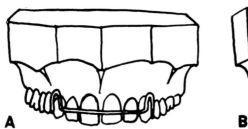
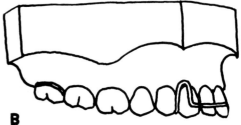

A   B

FIGURE 479. *A,* Labial view of appliance shown in Figure 478.
B, Buccal view of appliance shown in Figure 478; closure of the vertical loops applies a distal thrust to any teeth contacting the labial arch.

Labial tipping of an incisor is achieved by placing a double cantilever spring on the lingual surface, as suggested by Adams[6] and shown in Figure 480. With this type of movement, owing to the slope of the lingual surface, there is a tendency for a force on the lingual of most incisors to unseat the appliance because of a component directed downward; but usually this can be counteracted with wire clasps on the labial surfaces of the cuspids. As a rule, the posterior end must be retained with clasps around a molar on each side.

Mesial and Distal Tipping of Anterior Teeth

This is accomplished with a lever, as shown in Figure 481. The labial arch wire is contoured to curb rotation of the tooth being tipped to the distal. Rotation is also controlled by the judicious relief of the acrylic resin on the mesio-lingual as the tooth tips distally. As the tooth moves distally, the resin is relieved to make space.

Mesio-Distal Movement of Posterior Teeth

The same appliance design used for the anterior teeth fulfills the needs of this operation. In general, a heavier wire will be used on a molar than on an incisor, since the root area is larger. For example, a 0.025 inch wire might be used for an incisor, whereas a molar probably would need a 0.028 or 0.030 inch wire for the lever.

Frequently it will be necessary to free the occlusion when tipping a posterior tooth, since cuspal interdigitation can counteract the force exerted by the appliance. To prevent full closure, the resin on the lingual of the incisors on a maxillary retainer is built up to act as a stop against the

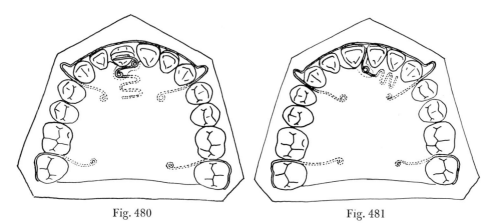

Fig. 480   Fig. 481

FIGURE 480. Diagram showing the use of a double cantilever spring to effect labial tipping of an incisor.

FIGURE 481. Distal tipping of a central incisor using a single cantilever spring.

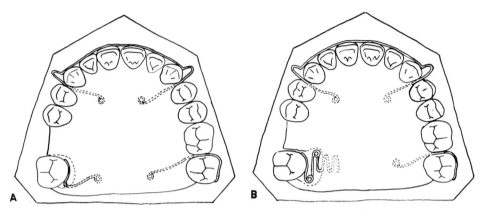

FIGURE 482. *A,* Single cantilever spring to tip a molar buccally. *B,* Double cantilever spring as used to tip a molar buccally.

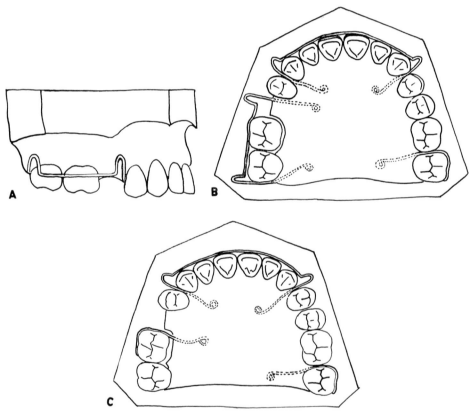

FIGURE 483. *A,* Buccal view of appliance used to effect lingual tipping of a molar. *B,* Occlusal view of appliance in *A.*

C, Diagram showing the use of a single cantilever spring to effect lingual movement of a molar.

mandibular incisors. A posterior opening of 1.0 to 2.0 mm. should be ample.

Bucco-Lingual Movement of Posterior Teeth

Molars and bicuspids may be tipped buccally or lingually with the working retainer. While this is being executed, it may be necessary to keep the posterior teeth out of occlusion. Buccal movement may be induced with a single-armed or double-armed cantilever spring (Fig. 482).

When using the double cantilever spring, both the primary and the secondary coils must be freed from the base to obtain a direct buccal thrust. The single lever spring can be used when rotating molars by having the free end of the lever resting on the surface that is to be moved the farthest. As in Figure 482A, the mesial of the second molar will be pushed farther buccally than the distal.

Lingual movement of the posterior abutment tooth may be brought about by a single lever or an inset in a buccal arch. This inset is placed in the wire in the same manner as in the labial arch wire used to tip incisors lingually. The force is generated in the vertical loops (Fig. 483).

Rotation of Incisor Teeth

Rotation of incisor teeth with the working retainer presents some difficulties. It is essential to apply two forces to the tooth, one from the labial and one from the lingual, with the distance between the two points of application as great as possible (Fig. 484).

There are two methods. The first consists of a labial arch wire acting on the labial surface, and selective relief of the acrylic resin on the lingual, to force the tooth to rotate instead of tipping lingually (Fig. 485). The second is to have a spring acting from the lingual instead of having a fulcrum point on the base (Fig. 486).

The tooth is braced on the mesial by an acrylic resin tooth, which fills the edentulous space. This double action will cause the tooth to rotate in situ rather than being tipped lingually to some degree, as in Figure 485. Therefore, the choice of design will depend on the type of correction desired.

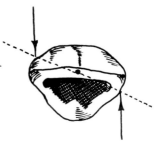

FIGURE 484.   Diagram showing necessary force application to effect rotation of an incisor.

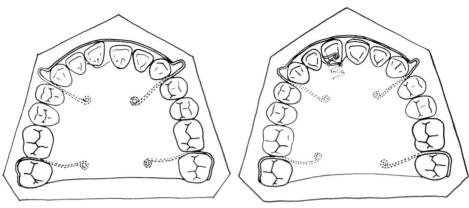

Fig. 485   Fig. 486

FIGURE 485. Design of appliance used to reposition the mesial of the incisor lingually.
FIGURE 486. Use of labial arch and double cantilever spring to rotate an incisor in situ.

Eruption of Posterior Teeth

The final type of tooth movement to be considered is that of eruption of posterior teeth. This can be brought about by using a bite plane to the lingual of the maxillary incisors, which serves as a stop to prevent the posterior teeth from occluding. There should be an opening in the posterior segments of approximately 1.0 mm. As these teeth erupt into occlusion, acrylic resin is added to the bite plane to keep the interocclusal space 1.0 mm. in height.

Detailed instructions for fabrication are purposely omitted from this chapter. Reference to the standard texts on this subject will supply such information.

REFERENCES

1. Orban, B. J.: Textbook of Histology. 4th ed. St. Louis, The C. V. Mosby Company, 1957.
2. Hemley, S.: Orthodontic Theory and Practice. New York, Grune & Stratton, 1953.
3. Oppenheim, A.: Human tissue response to orthodontic intervention of short and long duration. Am. J. Orthodont. & Oral Surg., 28:263, May 1942.
4. Reitan, K.: The initial tissue reactions incident to orthodontic tooth movement. Acta Odont. Scand., Suppl. 6, 1951.
5. Salzmann, J. A.: Principles of Orthodontics. 2nd ed. Philadelphia, J. B. Lippincott Company, 1943.
6. Adams, C. P.: The design and construction of removable orthodontic appliances. Bristol, John Wright & Sons, Ltd., 1955.

Jarabak, J. R.: Orthodontic treatment preparatory to fixed partial denture prosthesis. D. Clin. North America, March 1959, p. 31.

31

CROWN AND BRIDGE PROCEDURES FOR THE YOUNG-AGE GROUP

Until very recently construction of fixed partial prostheses for the preadolescent or adolescent patient was thought to be ill advised. Such restorative procedures were considered wholly acceptable only for a period starting with the early twenties and ending in the middle fifties. Reflecting on the difficulties formerly attending the preparations of abutment teeth, these limitations may have been warranted. However, with the advent of speedier procedures, indirect techniques, and the clinical research directed by Castaldi, Mink, Davis, Starkey, and other advanced pedodontists, the scope of the fixed prosthesis has been widened. To construct at least short-span bridges for young patients as soon as permanent teeth have erupted into occlusion, and even for very young patients when deciduous teeth are congenitally missing, is now recognized as safe and advantageous (Fig. 487).

The authors have been privileged to observe rather extensive fixed partial prostheses and crowns placed in the mouths of patients as young as 4 years, and have watched or have participated in the construction of many bridges for patients 16 years of age and younger. For the very young, because the deficiencies responsible for the spaces probably will have affected the contours of the teeth, it is usually necessary to use full gold or veneered gold crowns. Often, except at the cervical margin, little preparation will be needed (Fig. 488).

When using newly erupted permanent teeth as abutments, clinical experience has dictated that inlays are better retainers biologically than either partial veneer or full veneer gold crowns. Almost always the preparations for inlays will be two-surface and will follow in detail those described in Chapter 8, The Inlay Retainer. Proximal and occlusal depth of the

519

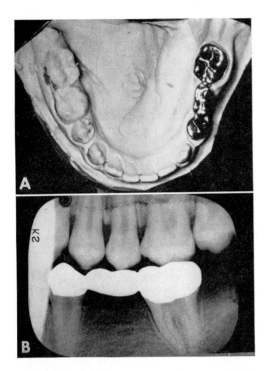

FIGURE 487. Bridge restoring continuity of mandibular arch for patient 14 years of age. Built in late 1960.

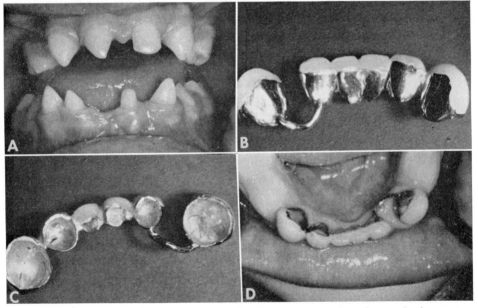

FIGURE 488. Bridge built for preadolescent to improve function, esthetic appearance, and attitude. Approximate age, 4 years; built in July, 1963.

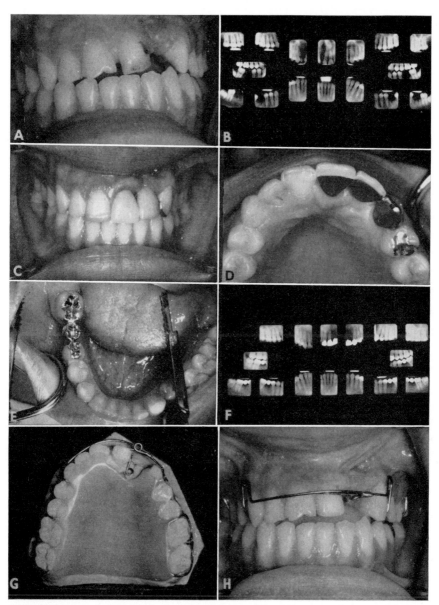

FIGURE 489. *A, B,* Patient, female, 17 years old, with operated cleft. Central incisor abutment realigned orthodontically. Pulp was large.

C, D, Anterior maxillary bridge. *C* shows right central incisor restored with a porcelain incisal edge bonded to a pinlay casting.

E, One mandibular bridge with inlay retainers.

F, Radiograph of completed mouth.

G, H, Appliance used to reposition abutments. Constructed in early 1962.

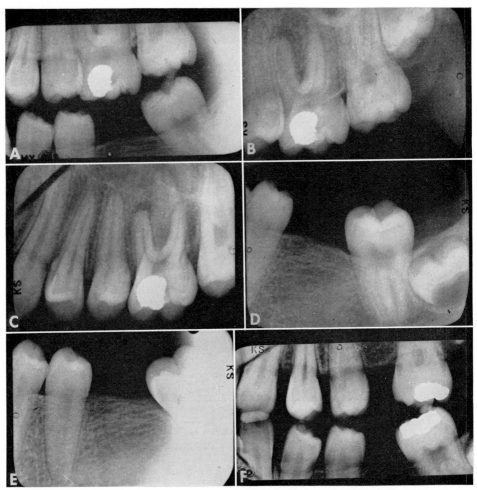

FIGURE 490. Radiographs of preadolescent patient with mandibular first molar already lost and condemned maxillary first molar, which was extracted. *F*, Situation thirteen months later. This patient is a dental cripple, needlessly.

cavities must be governed by information obtained from carefully-made radiographs. Pinholes must be judiciously positioned (see Fig. 489*E* and *F*).

Because of the potential mobility of teeth in the adolescent patient, bridges should be constructed with rigid joints. It is of the utmost importance that bridges built for young patients have adequate embrasure form and *minimal* ridge contact under the pontic. Before and after cementation, owing to the rapidly changing jaw relationships in the growing patient, these bridges must be critically equilibrated and should be examined at approximately three-month intervals so that the occlusion may be checked and corrected.

Anterior bridges are less easy to construct because of shorter clinical crowns and large pulps (Fig. 489), but if the abutment teeth are analyzed and meticulously prepared for pin-supported retainers, many extraordinary replacements may be accomplished.

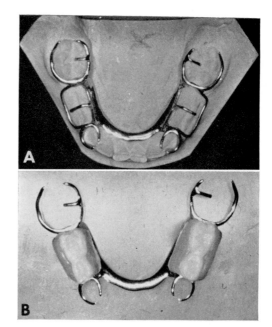

FIGURE 491. *A,* Frame for combination space maintainer and masticating prosthesis. Retentive arms for resin base are spaced so that areas may be cut out to permit eruption of bicuspids.

B, Completed temporary partial denture.

(Figs. 487, 488 and 491, courtesy of Dr. Bailey Davis.)

When a first molar is lost at a very early age, a decision must be made about maintaining the space and the opposing teeth in position (Fig. 490). If the second molar has already erupted, a space maintainer should be built and cemented; this will stabilize the prospective abutment teeth and also prevent extrusion of the opposing tooth or teeth. If the first permanent molar has erupted and the first and second deciduous molars are lost, unilaterally or bilaterally, a removable space maintainer should be built to provide occlusion for the opposing teeth. It should be constructed of a material that will permit an opening to be made later to accommodate the eruption of the underlying tooth or teeth (Fig. 491).

The span of life of such bridges is difficult to predict. Many have been in the mouth five years or more. Some of the early ones were built using full veneer gold crowns as retainers. Gingival acceptance of these retainers was often unsatisfactory, particularly at the linguo-cervical margins; as yet it has not been possible to determine the etiology. There also has been some, and similarly located, tissue disturbance from partial veneer crowns. Such reactions seemingly do not occur with much severity following puberty, and do not appear at all when inlays are used as the retainers.

This is the type of fixed partial prosthodontic service that should be practiced zealously.

REFERENCES

Mink, J. R.: Restorative dentistry for children. J.A.D.A., *66*:227, Feb. 1963.
Scures, C. C.: Porcelain baked to gold in pedodontics. J. Den. Children, *30*:9, 1st quar., 1963.

32

THE RESTORATION OF MUTILATED ANTERIOR TEETH

Mutilations of anterior teeth can be caused by fracture, by caries, or by excessive cutting away of tooth structure (sometimes unavoidable) for access in endodontic treatment.

The vitality of a fractured tooth often can be maintained if the pulp is not actually traumatized and if it is possible to treat the patient very soon after the injury. The exposed fractured surface immediately over the pulp should be coated with a palliative or neutral dressing and all of the surface covered with cement. This, in turn, is shielded by some device that has been made compatible with the occlusion. Steel crowns or plastic crown forms may be used, but orthodontic bands, extending 0.3 to 0.5 mm. to the incisal of the fracture, are beginning to be substituted for crowns of all types. The cemented band will retain the dressing on the fractured surface. Protection should be continued until it can be determined whether vitality has been preserved or whether, through no response to the accepted stimuli, it seems that the tooth is no longer vital.

When a tooth has gross carious lesions that undermine one or both incisal angles, it must be explored by removing the caries and be insulated against shock throughout a waiting period long enough to ascertain whether endodontic therapy will be needful.

There are three highly recommended means by which vital fractured teeth may be rebuilt:

1. If a portion of a proximal surface and an angle are involved, a wire-retained-and-supported resin restoration may suffice, making it unnecessary to resort to a less conservative repair, such as the jacket or veneered gold crown.

2. When all of the incisal edge is missing, but without extensive in-

524

volvement of the labial and proximal surfaces, the remaining tooth structure can be prepared for a partial veneer crown and the incisal portion of the casting filled with either silicate cement or resin. This is a well-established and meritorious method.

3. If a major portion of the incisal edge has been broken away, particularly if the fracture is a diagonal one across the labial surface, a casting to which porcelain has been bonded will restore contour, function, and usually esthetic appearance, in a most gratifying manner.

The objective of each of these three techniques is definitive and not solely an intermediate treatment preliminary to the construction of a jacket or veneered crown. Future developments in individual mouths may make the latter approach mandatory eventually.

CLASS IV RESIN RESTORATIONS

Resin restorations, retained and supported by wire, have been widely accepted for rebuilding proximal surfaces and incisal angles, and portions of incisal edges of incisors. Such restorations must be replaced periodically, but if the need for this is anticipated and if it is done when indicated, radical restorative measures can be postponed indefinitely.

Cavity Preparation. When restoring a tooth by this technique, a box-type preparation is made on the proximal surface. A typical Class IV step may be extended approximately three-fourths of the way across the incisal edge, or a retentive angle can be cut on the axial wall just inside the dentinoenamel junction. A pinhole capable of accepting an 0.020 inch stainless steel wire is placed in the cervical seat, somewhat to the lingual of the center of the tooth. The second pinhole is placed in the tooth structure supporting the remaining incisal angle, or on the proximal surface, parallel to the incisal edge, to the lingual of the center of the tooth, but inside the dentinoenamel junction. These holes should be 1.0 mm. deep (Fig. 492).

Threaded wire is cut and shaped so that it will extend into the holes for their full depth. With the holes filled with cement, the wire is placed first in the cervical hole and then flexed so that it may be pushed into the hole at the incisal. As a precaution against the possibility that a shadow will show through the labial surface of the restoration, the wire should be bent slightly toward the lingual half of the tooth. The excess hardened cement is chipped away and the restoration is built to form.

Building Restoration. Either the brush or the crown form technique may be used to build up the resin to contour. It is important that the occluding surface be equilibrated to accommodate mandibular movements. The restoration should be checked regularly and replaced if there is any

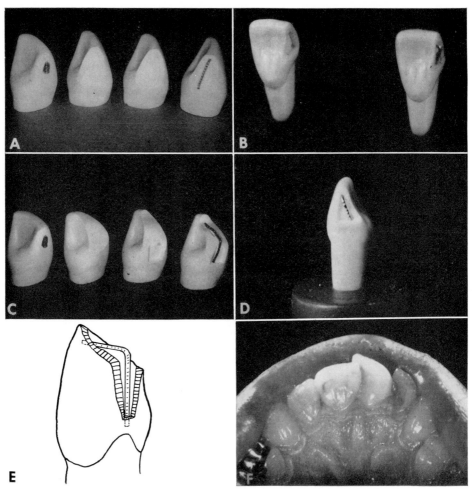

FIGURE 492.   *A, B,* Class IV preparation involving angle.
C, D, Class IV preparation involving angle and incisal edge.
E, Diagram of preparation in *C* and *D.*
F, Both centrals restored with wire-supported acrylic resin restorations.
(Courtesy of Department of Operative Dentistry, Indiana University School of Dentistry.)

evidence of marginal seepage. Opposing incisal edges and angles should be rounded to minimize any sheering incising movement.

VENEERED PARTIAL VENEER CROWN

When a partial veneer crown with a window is to be used, the proximal and lingual surfaces are reduced without extending the proximal margins labially beyond the line angles. The grooves may run parallel to the long axis of the tooth, they should be shallow, and their retentive properties should be supplemented by two or three shallow pinholes in the lingual surface, 0.7 mm. deep. Lingual clearance should be approximately 0.5 mm. and reduction of the proximal surfaces should be minimal. Labial extension for prevention can be disregarded. If caries should ever develop around the proximal margins, the tooth can then be restored with a jacket or veneered crown (Fig. 493).

An indirect technique is indicated. In order that the metal casting can be contoured to function without premature contact in any position, full arch occluding casts are needed. The area of the prepared tooth should be poured first. When this stone has set for 1 hour, it is removed and from it the die will be made. The full arch working cast is then poured. The casts may be mounted with a face-bow on an adjustable articulator, although the occluding unprepared anterior and posterior teeth should adequately guide the casts for carving the pattern even if freehand mounting has been used.

The wax pattern should be carved to cover the incisal edge. Lingual and incisal contours must be exact; otherwise, when equilibrating the casting, holes may appear in the metal through which the resin or silicate can be distorted or abraded. There must be a greater thickness of wax to ensure casting and bulk of metal for equilibration. The casting can be thinned at the labial margins for esthetic purposes. If the casting is to have minimal bulk, a hard crown and bridge or partial denture alloy is indispensable.

When the casting has been equilibrated and polished, it is cemented on the tooth, undercuts are made in both the tooth structure and the metal, and the resin or silicate veneer is built.

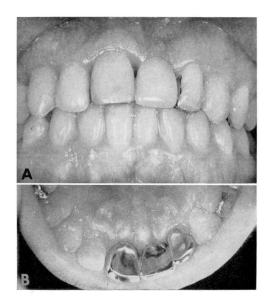

FIGURE 493. Bridge replacing maxillary left central incisor. Mesial angle of central abutment and inciso-lingual of lateral were fractured. Patient was immature; pulps were large. Shallow partial veneer preparations were made and exposed areas of castings were veneered with acrylic resin. Silicate cement could have been used and would have been equally effective.

PORCELAIN INCISAL BONDED TO A
METAL SUBSTRUCTURE

When the operator understands the fabrication of ceramic restorations, a casting with a bonded porcelain incisal edge probably is the most satisfactory restoration for the vital fractured anterior tooth. Assuming that he is capable of making castings that fit, the first requisite is a sound ceramic technique. Second, and even more consequential, is a discerning sense of shade and shade matching. Third, the clinician must have a concept of tooth form and the ability to mold the restoration into harmony with the surface contours remaining.

A workable and productive ceramic technique is not beyond the grasp of the average diligent and determined dentist or technician. Matching shades is a skill that even those who lack true color sense can acquire. In such cases as these, there is a great deal of remaining tooth surface which should guide the operator in contouring his restoration with comparative ease.

A bite-wing radiograph, or one that shows minimal coronal distortion, is essential (Fig. 494).

Preparation of Tooth. When preparing a fractured tooth for a bonded porcelain restoration, the incisal edge should be smoothed and any abrupt angles or curves eliminated. If the fracture line is close to or bisects one of the incisal angles, this portion of the tooth should be shortened to provide not less than 1.5 mm. of space.

The lingual surface of the tooth usually is prepared in the same way as for a pinledge retainer (0.5 mm. clearance is sufficient) except that the incisal pinholes are placed on the fractured incisal edge, mesially and distally to the pulp horns. However, when bulk of tooth structure permits, a ledge is cut cervically to the linguo-incisal edge of the tooth to increase the area of bonding. While the pinholes, 2.0 mm. in depth, can be made with a taper fissure bur, a spirec drill is preferable. When a long 0.023 inch drill is being used, a paralleling device may be helpful.

The Working and Firing Casts. Nylon bristles, 0.022 inch in diameter, are placed in the pinholes and a silicone rubber impression is taken in a custom-built tray. The path of removal should be parallel to the direction of insertion for the pins. A stone master cast is poured and allowed to set for 1 hour. The impression is very carefully removed and a second cast is made of porcelain investment.* This should not be separated sooner than 60 minutes or later than 2 hours after pouring (Fig. 495).

---

* Myken Porcelain Inlay Investment, Westwood Dental Mfg. Co., Inc., Los Angeles, Calif.
Loma Linda Porcelain Inlay Investment, Surgident, Ltd., Los Angeles, Calif.
Whip-Mix Porcelain Inlay Investment, Whip-Mix Corporation, Louisville, Ky.

Waxing and Investing the Pattern. The wax pattern is made on the original stone die after 0.020 inch nylon bristles have been cut, roughened, and placed in the pinholes. It should cover all of the lingual preparation except the extension over the incisal edge, where it should be approximately 0.35 mm. short of the proximal and labial peripheral margin.

A large sprue pin is attached to the center of the wax pattern, parallel

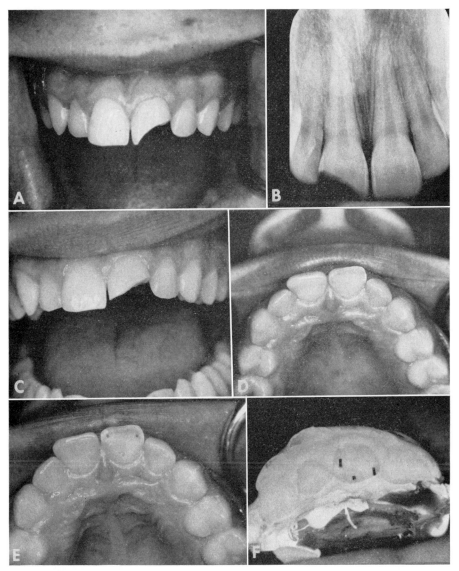

FIGURE 494.   *A*, Fractured maxillary left central incisor.

B, Fracture is in close proximity to pulp. Faint color was visible but there was only nominal sensitivity. Tooth did and does test normally.

C, D, Preliminary preparation.

E, F, Prepared tooth and elastic impression.

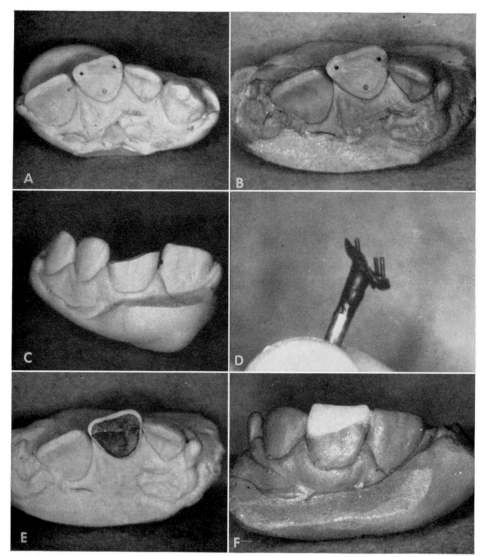

FIGURE 495.   *A, B, C,* Casts poured from single elastic impression.
D, Wax pattern.
E, Casting on stone cast.
F, Porcelain fired and bonded to casting.

to the path of withdrawal, and the pattern is removed from the die. No vents are needed. The investing and casting technique is the same as for crowns to be veneered with porcelain. The casting is made from a gold in balance with the porcelain to be used. The authors have always used Ceramco No. 1 Improved alloy and porcelain.

Building Technique with Ceramco Alloy and Porcelain.   The casting is seated on the stone master cast, and the surface that will be exposed is polished; that which is to receive the porcelain is ground with a coarse wheel stone. It is immersed in hydrofluoric acid for 8 hours, or this time may be reduced to 30 minutes if the acid container is placed in an ultrasonic cleaner.

The casting is placed on the porcelain investment cast and both are degassed in the porcelain furnace at 1900° F. (For degassing cycle, see Chapter 22, The Construction of Bonded Porcelain Veneer Crowns.) They are cooled, and opaque is applied to the metal only. It has not been found necessary to extend the opaque application beyond the edge of the metal casting.

Using the Ceramco porcelain firing cycle (described in Chapter 22), the opaque is fired to 1720° F. in vacuum. The vacuum is released and the temperature is increased to 1820° F. in air. The assembly is cooled and the body and incisal-colored porcelains are applied. The cast is wetted and the porcelain is condensed by capillary action. It is built about 1.0 mm. high but *not* to full contour *at this time,* as shrinkage will pull the porcelain from the labial margin.

The porcelain is dried and fired to 1700° F. in vacuum, then to 1800° F. in air. The second application of porcelain is built to an overcontour and the firing cycle is repeated.

After cooling, the restoration is deinvested and cleaned with hydrochloric acid in an ultrasonic cleaner, after which it is roughly ground to form on the stone master cast. Contour and occlusion are refined in the patient's mouth, using fine disks for contouring and small stones for adjusting occlusion (Fig. 496).

The restoration is reinvested in ceramic investment up to the porcelain margin and is allowed to set for 30 minutes. After drying, it is fired in air at 1780 to 1800° F. to bring the desired glaze to the surface. After deinvesting, the cavity surface is again cleaned in hydrochloric acid in the ultrasonic cleaner. It may be cemented with either zinc phosphate or silicophosphate cement.

Pulpless Teeth

Teeth in which much dentin has been lost, through caries and endodontic therapy, require other means of restoration than those that may be applied to the vital fractured incisor. Following preparation of the tooth structure that still remains, the tooth stump must be built to prepared form in order that the subsequent restoration will be amply supported, and also as insurance against the fracture of the remaining coronal tooth substance.

A pulpless tooth will best resist fracture if the restoration and tooth structure are supported by a post extending into the root canal for a distance equal to the coronal length of the restoration, and with a core rebuilding the tooth to prepared form. Even though a pulpless tooth has an intact labial surface and incisal angles, some endodontists and restorative

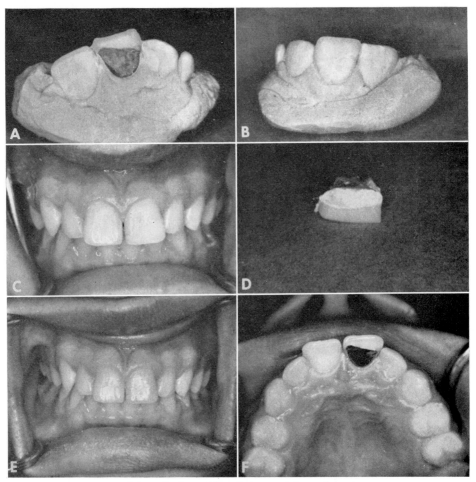

FIGURE 496. *A*, Lingual view of bonded porcelain and casting.
B, Porcelain contoured on stone cast.
C, Porcelain contoured and equilibrated in mouth.
D, Restoration reinvested for glaze firing.
E, *F*, Cemented restoration.

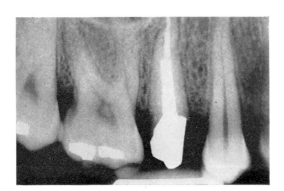

FIGURE 497. Relationship of post to crown-root ratio.

dentists feel that a post should be inserted in the root canal to extend approximately one-half the distance from the opening of the pulp chamber to the apex. Despite the fact that there is considerable insistence that pulpless teeth are *not* more brittle than vital teeth, it has been the clinical observation of the authors that they are more prone to fracture unless supported internally by a post (Fig 497). This is especially true when a tooth is serving as an abutment.

Direct Technique for Cast Post and Core.   The root canal is enlarged with a round bur (or with a reamer) to a depth equal to or greater than the inciso-cervical coronal measurement of the restoration. A post of high-fusing, nonoxidizing wire* is fitted and cut to extend from the extreme

* Ney PGP wire; Jelenko No. 6 wire.

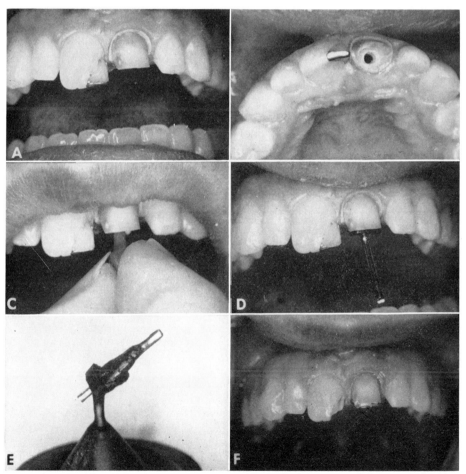

FIGURE 498.   *A, B,* Partially prepared tooth ready for wax and post for carving core.
C, Placing wax in enlarged canal.
D, Serrated wire post forced through wax into canal.
E, Wax pattern.
F, Post and core cemented.

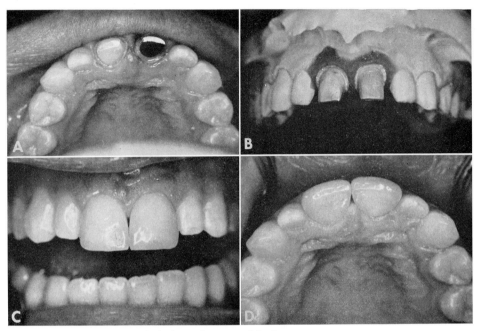

FIGURE 499.   *A,* Incisal view of prepared incisors.
B, Cast and dies of prepared incisors.
C, D, Teeth restored with porcelain jacket crowns.

depth of the hole to approximately 3.0 mm. beyond the incisal edge of the prepared tooth.

Casting wax is softened and forced into the posthole. The wire post, serrated in the coronal two-thirds, is heated and forced as far as possible through the wax into the root canal. The wax is built and carved to the form of the prepared tooth. The casting may be made with a regular crown and bridge gold if the pattern has bulk, or with a partial denture gold if the incisal half is thin (Figs. 498 and 499).

Indirect Technique for Cast Post and Core.   When using an indirect technique, the wire post may be serrated throughout its entire length. The apical portion is coated with wax and is repeatedly seated in the root canal until it can be removed with minimal resistance. The serrated coronal portion will be so firmly gripped by the rubber base impression material that an accurate relationship will be maintained when the cast is poured. Since the wire has been coated with wax, it can be warmed and readily removed from the cast.

The core is waxed, cast, polished, and cemented. Then the preparation is refined.

Rebuilding Vital Tooth to Prepared Form.   When there has been much loss of coronal dentin and enamel and the tooth is still vital, the favored restoration will be a jacket or veneered crown. The remaining tooth structure should be prepared for the type of crown selected. The core, which will rebuild the tooth to prepared form, can be retained by pins or a ferrule, or both. Pinholes, running in a long-axis direction, must extend into the dentin from 1.0 to 2.0 mm. While taper fissure burs can be used, drills are more effective, because the diameter of the holes will be smaller and there can be more and longer pins extending into the dentin.

The pattern can be made by direct waxing. If an indirect technique is elected, nylon pins must be placed in the nontapered pinholes before a silicone rubber impression is taken. Dies, working casts, patterns, and castings are made, as described previously.

Some operators complete the crown before cementation of the casting, but it is considered wiser to cement the casting and to check and make any needed refinements in the preparation before proceeding with the construction of the restoration.

REFERENCE

Baum, L., Hayden, J., Jr., and Bonlie, D.: Cast restorations with baked porcelain incisal edges for fractured young permanent incisors. J. Den. Children, *28*:177, 3rd quar., 1961.

33

OCCLUSION FACTORS
IN BRIDGE CONSTRUCTION

Occlusal disharmony, either before or after the construction of a bridge, or the added load on the abutments subsequent to the building of a prosthesis, can definitely alter the attachment apparatus. The manifestation of expanded function upon the periodontium may be divided into clinical symptoms and radiographic and histologic changes in supporting structures.

Clinically there may be a more pronounced mobility of the teeth, tenderness to masticating pressure, hyperemia of the soft tissues, and eventually, according to some authorities, a cleftlike formation of the gingiva. More acute sensitivity to heat, cold, and sweets can be experienced, also.

Radiographic differences may include a widening of the periodontal membrane space, a more discernible and compact lamina dura, an increased trabeculation of the alveolar bone, and a wedge-shaped radiolucent area, or funneling, of the alveolar crest at the coronal third.

Histologically the cementum may be thickened, even to the point where "spurs" will be formed, the periodontal membrane may become wider and heavier (Table 24), with more dense bundle fibers, and the alveolar bone may be recontoured.

Following the placement of a dental restoration, a patient may report discomfort ranging from a feeling of "lameness" to severe and constant pain. Sensitivity is due, in most cases, to pulp irritation from traumatic contact or greater leverages. When the occlusion has been adjusted, each type of discomfort may be relieved almost instantly and should disappear shortly.

The thought has been advanced that a tooth with hypercementosis and irregular projections, or spurs, will have an enlarged root surface and a strengthened root attachment and thus will be a better abutment. Within limits this may be true.

536

In the process of making the adjustment to supplemented or varied function, the alveolar bone often recontours. Resorption occurs first, then the periodontal membrane and cementum widen, the lamina dura of the alveolar bone becomes more dense, and trabeculae multiply. All of these are physiologic responses to additional stresses placed on the teeth.

With a fixed partial prosthesis, it is possible to stabilize a tooth, minimize or eliminate shock from occlusion, and improve the health of the supporting structure in every way, especially if the tooth in question can be made an intermediate abutment. However, unless everything has been done that will further a tranquil functional relationship between the abutments and occluding teeth, the opposite may ensue, with the clinical symptoms of tenderness becoming magnified.

The histologic picture of periodontal traumatism may include hyperemia, hemorrhage and thrombosis, tearing and hyalinization of fibers, both osteoclastic and osteoblastic activity, and necrosis of bone or periodontal fibers, or both. In short, injury of tissues and physiologic tissue response is seen. There is little inflammatory cell infiltration and therefore no inflammation in the true sense of the word.

The adaptability of the periodontium may result in satisfactory adjustment which takes care of the additional function, but later in life, because of changes in local or systemic conditions, a breakdown may occur.

In the construction of crowns and bridges and in the preparation of mouths for removable partial dentures, occlusal equilibration, reduction of occlusal areas, and accentuation of spillways are frequently mandatory to lessen occlusal forces.

Teeth subjected to intemperate stress may be more mobile than is normal. The simplest test for detecting mobility is to grasp the tooth with the index finger of each hand and apply force laterally. Sometimes such movement can be noted by retracting the lips and watching the chewing cycle. Also, the gingiva may blanch as pressure displaces the tooth. A check

*TABLE 24. Thickness of Periodontal Tissues in Varying Conditions of Function**

	ALVEOLAR CREST MM.	MIDROOT MM.	APEX MM.	AVERAGE MM.
Teeth in heavy function, 44 teeth from 8 jaws	0.20	0.14	0.19	0.18
Teeth not in function, 20 teeth from 12 jaws	0.14	0.11	0.15	0.13
Embedded teeth, 5 teeth from 4 jaws	0.09	0.07	0.08	0.08
Malposed and drifting teeth	0.22	0.16	0.18	0.19

* From Coolidge, E. D., and Hine, M. K.: Periodontology, 3rd ed. Philadelphia, Lea & Febiger, 1958, p. 359.

must be made not only for excessive lateral but also increased vertical movement.

The patient's history can reveal symptoms indicative of temporomandibular joint disturbance, habit neuroses, wandering teeth, and pain. These factors usually can be related to some form of intercuspal malrelationship.

To aid in the detection of occlusal disharmonies and in the study of wear patterns and facets, and to enable the operator to design restorations that will not create interferences, diagnostic casts of the patient's dental arches should be mounted on an instrument capable of simulating, if not really duplicating, the motions of the mandible.

The accuracy with which records must be obtained for this procedure probably is related to the patient's individual needs. Almost all persons have some occlusal discrepancies, and few people possess dentitions that allow centric occlusion and centric relation to coincide. Unless the patient has conditions such as periodontal disease, temporomandibular joint disturbance, extreme wear, mobile or tender teeth, or a large majority of the teeth carious or missing, it seems sensible to let the mandible continue to function in its acquired relationship and to make no gross change in the dentition other than to correct the clinically evident occlusal disharmonies, to restore mutilated teeth, and to replace any missing teeth.

In symptom-free cases, diagnostic casts often may be related on an articulator by an arbitrary face-bow mounting and a centric occlusion registration (such as the Kerr Bite Frame and impression paste registration). The condylar guidance mechanism may then be set by the use of wax eccentric registrations or even by merely observing the patient's mandibular movements and adjusting the articulator to conform while at the dental chair. Minor wear facets seen on the casts may also be used in setting the instrument. While restorations planned or executed on an instrument adjusted by such patently empirical means cannot relate to the opposing dentition in the mouth exactly as on the articulator, the discrepancies in the mouth should be within remediable limits.

For a patient who has one or more of the previously mentioned conditions, a more precise method of relating diagnostic casts and adjusting the articulator must be sought. The opening and closing center of rotation for each condyle should be found with a hinge axis locator and an arbitrary third reference point selected, such as the infra-orbital notch (Fig. 500). Casts then may be mounted in the right relationship to the hinge axis formed by the two centers of rotation and to the plane formed by this axis and the third reference point. If there must be more than one mounting of diagnostic apparatus or casts, the three reference points may be marked permanently on the patient's skin. This is done so that later mountings will not require the relocation of these points, taking new registrations, and readjustment of the instrument. As a matter of convenience, the infra-orbital point is placed on the side of the nose rather than at the rim of the orbit.

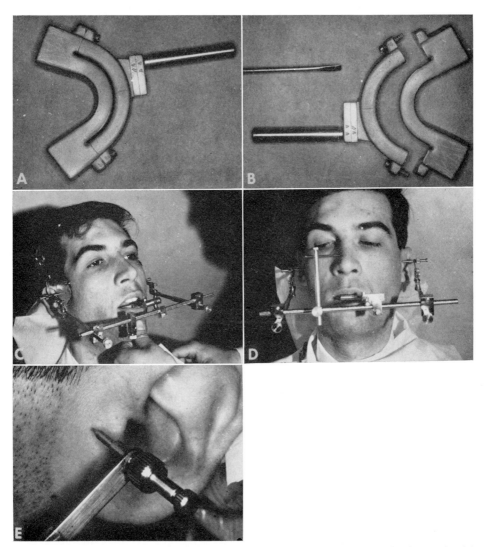

FIGURE 500. *A, B,* Two-piece clutch which is attached to the mandibular teeth with impression plaster in order to join the hinge axis locator to the mandible rigidly. The clutch is separable to allow easy removal from the mouth.

C, Locating the hinge axis by gently guiding the patient in pure rotary opening and closing movements of the mandible. When the points of the axis rods have been adjusted so that they rotate without arcing against the grids just anterior to the patient's ears, the axis of rotation has been located. The points then may be marked on the skin.

D, The face-bow related to the maxillary teeth by means of a bite fork covered with wax. The axis rods are adjusted to the hinge axis marks on the skin over the condyles and infra-orbital marker to the mark on the patient's nose.

E, Axis rod adjusted to axis mark on left side.

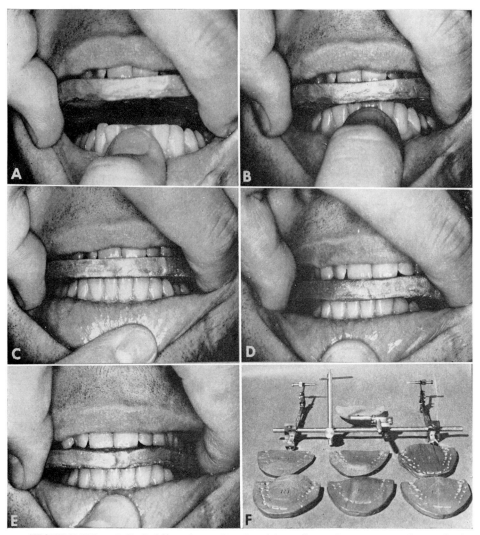

FIGURE 501. *A, B,* Guiding the patient in a hinge closure into a wax wafer to obtain a centric relation registration. Opposing teeth should not make contact. Three of these records are made. Note that upper and lower midlines do not coincide.

C, Obtaining a protrusive registration in wax. The anterior teeth are in an end-to-end relationship but do not touch through the wax.

D, Right lateral registration being made. The right posterior teeth are in a cusp-to-cusp relationship. They do not touch.

E, Left lateral registration.

F, The face-bow transfer, three centric relation registrations, and right lateral, left lateral, and protrusive registrations in wax.

A face-bow is adjusted to the three marked reference points and to the maxillary arch and used to mount the maxillary cast on the articulator. (See Fig. 500*D.*) In this way the maxillary cast is related to the opening and closing axis of the instrument in the same way as the maxillary teeth are related to the hinge axis of the patient. (See Fig. 502*A.*)

The mandibular cast is related to the maxillary cast by a wax centric relation registration (Figs. 501 and 502). This registration is procured by guiding the patient in a hinge movement, and while so doing having him close part way into softened strips of double-thickness hard baseplate wax or

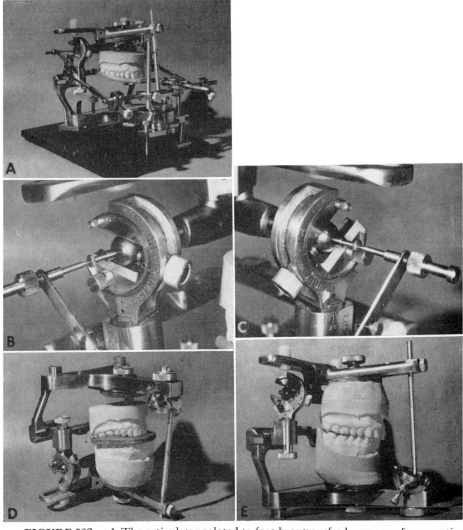

FIGURE 502. *A,* The articulator related to face-bow transfer by means of a mounting board. The articulator is adjusted so that the axis-orbital plane indicator aligns with the axis-orbital pointer on the face-bow and the extendible axis rods of the articulator with the axis rods on the face-bow. When this is accomplished, the upper cast is attached to the instrument with low expansion dental stone or plaster. (Hanau face-bow, Hanau 130–13 articulator, Hanau mounting jig.)

B, C, The axis rods on the articulator equally extended to meet the axis rods of the face-bow.

D, The upper cast has been mounted. The lower cast is related to the inverted assembly by means of one of the centric relation registrations and fastened with stone or plaster.

E, Both casts mounted on the instrument.

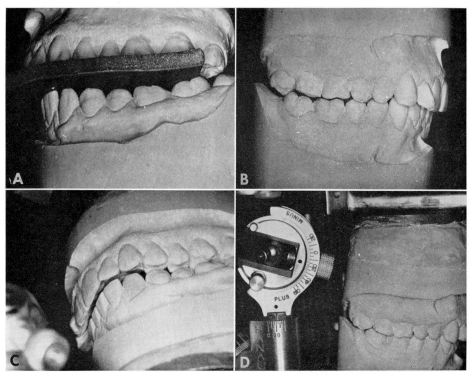

FIGURE 503.   *A,* A second centric relation registration inserted between the mounted casts with the condylar guides locked in centric relation. The perfect interdigitation of the teeth into the wax record indicates an accurate centric relation mounting.

B, The articulator closed to find the first contact during hinge closure. The only contact is made by the right mandibular second molar with the right maxillary third molar.

C, Amount of opening in anterior region caused by the centric prematurity.

D, Release of the right condylar ball allows the mandibular cast to move forward with the teeth interdigitating similarly to the patient's acquired centric occlusion.

into a wafer of Aluwax.* (See Fig. 501*A* and *B.*) The wax should not be perforated during the procedure, since contact between opposing teeth invariably results in a false centric relation registration. The best wax registrations are those indented only by the cusp tips. Three separate centric relation records are made, one of which is used in mounting the lower cast on the articulator, the other two being used to verify the first. If the mounted casts seat properly in all three registrations, the records are accurate (Fig. 503*A*). Since the wax records cannot be identical in thickness, **it is** only with a suitable relationship of both casts to the hinge that the instrument can accept all three centric relation registrations. Inaccuracy demonstrated at this point necessitates new centric registrations and remounting of the lower cast. Existing premature contacts in centric closure may now be demonstrated on the instrument (see Fig. 503*B* and *C*).

---

* Hickok Specialties Co., Grand Rapids, Mich.

When an articulator is used to study prematurities in eccentric movements, the instrument must be adjusted to the patient's individual condylar guidance. The recording device used will depend on the precision with which the dentist wishes to do this operation. The most uninvolved technique uses wax eccentric interocclusal records, which are acceptable with articulators having straight or simple paths of motion and with the condylar ball on the upper member of the instrument and the condylar guidance mechanism on the lower member.* Such instruments will not reproduce jaw movements without some latitude, and the errors introduced by wax records are likely no greater than those inherent to the articulators themselves.

The wax records generally consist of protrusive, right lateral, and left lateral registrations, with some clinicians recommending the use of three of each. (See Fig. 501C, D, E, and F.) However, it must be recognized that since the operator cannot control the patient to a degree that will ensure that the mandible is in the same position for each registration, these registrations may not be interchangeable.

The registrations are made in a hard baseplate wax or Aluwax, with the patient's teeth in an end-to-end or cusp-to-cusp relationship. To avoid rocking or shifting of the mandible, no teeth should make actual contact.

The condylar guidance is made to conform first to the protrusive record. The Bennett movement adjustment is opened about 15 degrees to allow for a possible deviation by the patient from a pure protrusive movement and the wax protrusive record is placed between the casts (see Fig. 504A). The condylar guidance is set and locked on each side so that the teeth on the casts make maximal interdigitation with the wax record (see Fig. 504B). Next, the left lateral record is placed between the casts, and the lateral adjustment is made for the Bennett movement on the right side of the instrument, or the side representing the gliding condyle (see Fig. 504C, D, and E). The condylar guidance adjustment is checked against that made with the protrusive record. The right lateral record is then used to adjust the left side of the instrument, and again it may be used as a check against the protrusive record (see Fig. 504F). There are some who obtain only a single protrusive record, which is used to adjust the condylar guides, with the Bennett setting being arbitrarily selected. The articulator settings should be recorded in order that the instrument may be realigned in case of inadvertent movements of parts, or because of the need to mount more than one patient's casts on the same articulator.

The patient's occlusion in both centric and eccentric relationships of the mandible may now be studied and occlusal prematurities located (Fig. 505).

---

* Instruments such as the Hanau #130-13 (Hanau Engineering Co., Inc., Buffalo, N. Y.) and the Dentatus (distributed by the Kerr Mfg. Company, Detroit, Mich.).

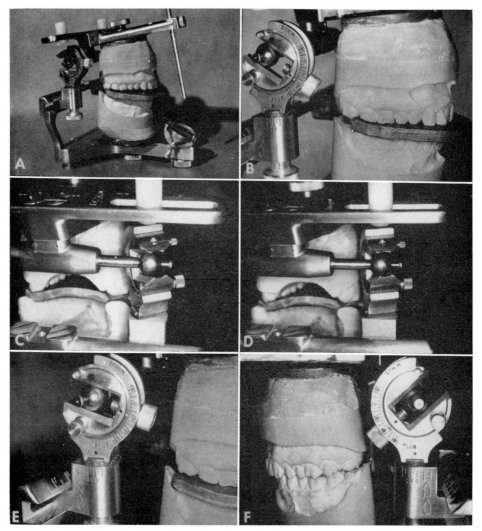

FIGURE 504. *A,* Protrusive registration placed between the casts on the articulator before adjustment. The anterior teeth cannot be placed into the indentations made in the mouth.

B, After increasing the condylar guidance, all teeth go to place in the registration. This adjustment must be made on both sides of the articulator.

C, Left lateral wax registration in the instrument with excessive rotation of the condylar posts to allow easy insertion of the record. Note that the condylar ball does not make contact with the shoulder on the instrument's axle.

D, Condylar ball brought into contact with the shoulder on the axle. This limits the sideward or Bennett shift to that which occurred during taking the wax registration.

E, Adjustments completed on right side: 18 degrees of condylar inclination, 21 degrees of rotation of condylar post to accommodate the lateral shift.

F, Left adjustments made in manner described for the right side of instrument: 42 degrees of inclination of condylar guide, 7 degrees for the lateral shift.

The purpose of equilibration should be relief of traumatic occlusion and establishment of improved function. These objectives can be attained by removing premature contacts, both centric and eccentric, and by eliminating the working of facets against facets.

Some operators prefer to remedy all discrepancies on the articulated casts before going to the mouth. If this is done, a written record is made of all changes on the casts. Centric prematurities should be removed first. Since all prematurities involve at least two opposing teeth, a decision must be made as to which offender is to be recontoured. If one of the surfaces is also in a traumatic relationship in an excursive movement, it is the one to be changed. For example, if the prematurity exists between a cusp of one tooth and a fossa of another, and the cusp is also making excessive contact in an eccentric position, the cusp should be shortened (Fig. 506). Conversely, if no eccentric prematurity exists, either the cusp can be reshaped or the sulcus deepened. In this circumstance, altering the sulcus may be indicated to maintain existing excursive relationships and chewing

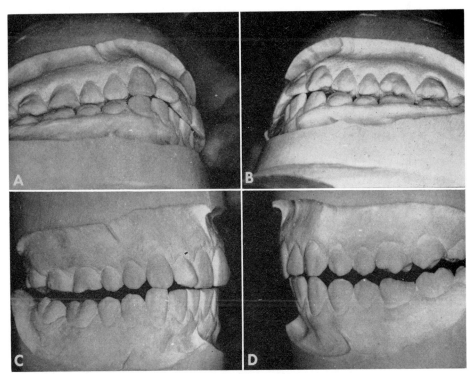

FIGURE 505. *A,* In right lateral movement the two first bicuspids are the only teeth that make contact. Note wear on tip of buccal cusp of the maxillary first bicuspid.

B, Casts on adjusted articulator moved into left lateral excursion. There is excessive contact between the maxillary and mandibular laterals and the two first bicuspids as well. There is no contacting of the two cuspids.

C, D, Right and left lateral protrusive movements. The articulated casts closely follow the facets of wear on the cuspids.

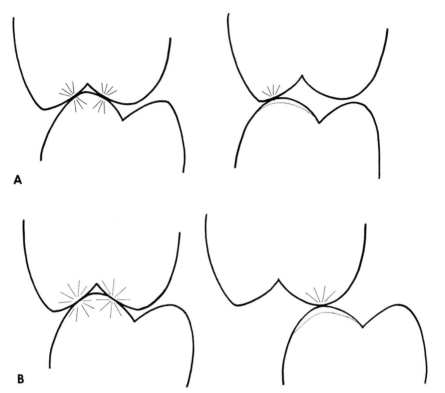

FIGURE 506. *A,* Traumatic relationship in centric occlusion relieved by reducing the lower buccal cusp, which is also striking excessively in the working or functional relationship.

B, Another traumatic relationship in centric occlusion relieved by reducing the lower buccal cusp, which is also in a traumatic relationship in the nonfunction movement.

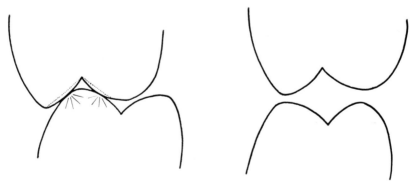

FIGURE 507. Sulcus is reduced as indicated to eliminate a centric prematurity, rather than reducing the lower buccal cusp, causing it to pass still farther away from its opponent in working excursion.

efficiency, which might be reduced if the cusp were shortened or blunted (Fig. 507).

A more obvious example is traumatic centric occlusion involving anterior teeth. If the teeth have a good incising relationship, the premature contact is removed by grinding the lingual aspect of the maxillary tooth, since shortening the mandibular tooth would take the teeth out of occlusion in protrusive movement (Fig. 508). If both centric and protrusive relationships are traumatic, the lower incisal edge is altered (Fig. 509). Should removal of the faulty centric contact fail to eradicate the protrusive interference, the incisal edge of the maxillary tooth is ground also.

Once centric occlusion has been corrected, along with removal of any directly related excursive prematurities, a check is made for other eccentric traumatic relationships. Since centric occlusion has been established, all subsequent improvements must be made on surfaces *not* making centric contact. To destroy centric contact while adjusting lateral and protrusive relationships would create an unstable occlusion, making eruption of teeth and recurrence of eccentric prematurities possible.

If, for example, during the masticating stroke, the buccal cusp of a mandibular bicuspid strikes the buccal cusp of its opposing tooth, the buccal cusp of the maxillary tooth is shortened (Fig. 510). To alter the buccal cusp of the lower tooth would take it out of centric occlusion, perhaps inviting the teeth to extrude and causing the lateral prematurity to recur.

It has been claimed that premature contact on the nonworking side (often called balancing side) is the most destructive of all occlusal defects.

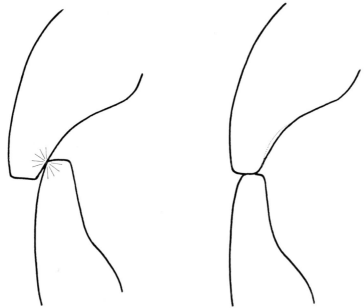

FIGURE 508.   An anterior centric prematurity between teeth with a satisfactory protrusive relationship is corrected by altering the upper lingual surface.

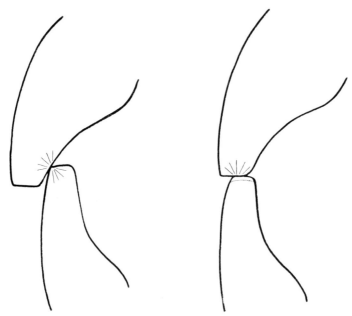

FIGURE 509.   An anterior traumatic relationship which occurs in both centric and protrusive relationships is corrected by reducing the lower incisal edge.

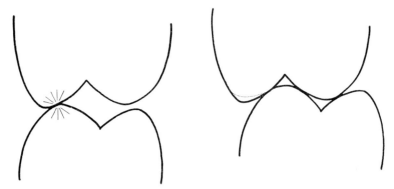

FIGURE 510.   Excessive contact between buccal cusps in lateral excursion is eliminated by shortening the upper buccal cusp while maintaining the original centric occlusion.

This contention is reasonable, since the posterior tooth relationships that occur during this phase of chewing do not direct forces along the long axes of the participating teeth. Whether such contacts should be eliminated completely, or just reduced enough to make them no more forceful than those on the working side, is open to argument. However, it seems logical to err on the side of no contact rather than to gamble on forces that may exceed the physiologic limits of the supporting structures.

Nonworking contacts involve the lingual cusps of maxillary posterior teeth and the buccal cusps of mandibular teeth. Both areas form centric contacts. Fortunately, centric contact generally occurs on cusp planes rather

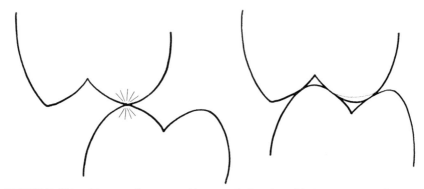

FIGURE 511.   Traumatic nonworking or "balancing side" contacts at times may be eliminated by reducing the cusp tips without interfering with centric stops.

FIGURE 512.   If a cusp loses its centric stop following removal of cuspal interference, the opposing sulcus or marginal ridge will have to be built up by means of a restoration.

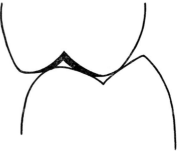

than on the tips of the cusps. Consequently, shortening the cusp to rid it of a nonworking contact will not necessarily cause loss of centric occlusion (Fig. 511). If this should occur, there is no recourse other than to place a restoration that builds up the sulcus or the marginal ridge area of the opposing surface, or both (Fig. 512).

The type of occlusion that is best for most patients is a subject of much controversy. In the past, completely balanced occlusion has been widely advocated. Recently there is growing support for a tooth arrangement having an anterior guidance that permits little contact of posterior teeth away from centric occlusion. Most natural dentitions appear to be some modification of the latter type.

The principles briefly outlined here can be applied to both the equilibration and the restoration of natural dentitions. There is only scant evidence to support the use of either procedure as a prophylactic measure in the absence of a pathologic condition.

REFERENCES

D'Amico, A.: The canine teeth. J. South. California D. A., *26:*64, 1958.
Granger, E. R.: Practical Procedures in Oral Rehabilitation. Philadelphia, J. B. Lippincott Company, 1962.

Lucia, V. O.: Modern Gnathological Concepts. St. Louis, The C. V. Mosby Company, 1961.

Moulton, G. H.: Importance of centric occlusion in diagnosis and treatment planning. J. Pros. Den., *10*:921, Sept.–Oct. 1960.

Schuyler, C. H.: Considerations of occlusion in fixed partial dentures. D. Clin. North America, March 1959, p. 175.

Schweitzer, J. M.: Masticatory function in man. J. Pros. Den., *12*:262, March–April 1962.

Stallard, H.: Functions of the occlusal surfaces of the teeth. J.A.D.A., *13*:401, 1930.

Stallard, H., and Stuart, C. E.: Eliminating tooth guidance in natural dentitions. J. Pros. Den., *11*:474, May–June 1961.

Wilson, W. H., and Lang, R. L.: Practical Crown and Bridge Prosthodontics. New York, McGraw-Hill Book Company, Inc., 1962.

34

BRIDGE FAILURES: INDICATIONS AND CORRECTIVE MEASURES

The prosthodontist who constructs bridges must be well aware of both gross and subtle indications of failure and have some knowledge of corrective procedures. The failure of a bridge can be manifested in various ways. There may be discomfort, the bridge may become loose, caries may recur, the supporting structure may atrophy or a pulp degenerate, the framework or a facing may fracture, a veneer may be lost, the prosthesis may have ceased to function, or there may be a complete loss of tissue tone or tissue form.

Changes in environment may necessitate the removal and remaking of a bridge. Also, a bridge may simply wear out. After all, no bridge, nor the teeth approximating or opposing it, can carry a lifetime guarantee. Replacement for these two reasons cannot be classified under failures.

DISCOMFORT

It is only natural that discomfort will claim the attention of the patient more readily than any other type of failure, with the possible exception of fracture. Discomfort may be caused by

(1) malocclusion or premature contact;

(2) an oversize or poorly positioned masticating area, with retention of food by pontics or retainers;

(3) torque produced from the seating of the bridge or from occlusion;

(4) an excess of pressure on the tissue;

(5) plus or minus contact areas;

(6) overprotected or underprotected gingival and ridge tissue;

(7) sensitive cervical areas;

(8) thermal shock; and

(9) certain intangible sources, usually relatively unimportant and easily remedied if diagnosed.

Discomfort from *malocclusion* can be traced to a high marginal ridge, central fossa, cusp tip, or an inclined surface on one of the cusps in lateral excursion, and also to mobility and extrusion from loss of supporting bone. *Areas of premature contact* will be indicated by burnished metal. All or any of these can be corrected by equilibration, using either a small knife-edge stone or a round bur. Mobility from lack of support may have occurred because of faulty diagnosis and planning; that is, too much having been expected of too few abutment teeth. There is no cure except to rebuild the bridge, including a greater number of abutment teeth, or to construct a removable prosthesis with bilateral bracing.

An *oversize or poorly positioned masticating area* is difficult to correct if the operation requires grinding porcelain, which cannot be reglazed. When the food table is too wide, an attempt may be made to narrow the distance between the cusp tips by reducing the bucco-lingual measurement, often at the expense of the lingual cusp; by opening the embrasures, again at the expense of the lingual cusp or cusps; and by cutting auxiliary escape grooves through the marginal ridges to both the lingual and the buccal of the connectors.

Tenderness during chewing and a reluctance to utilize the bridge will be evidence that food is being retained on the occlusal surface of a crown or a pontic. The height and form of the marginal ridges and the contour of the inclined surfaces of the cusps must be examined. It is often necessary to widen the embrasures, diminish the lingual cusp, and increase the number and size of the grooves crossing the marginal ridges and emptying into the embrasures. Occasionally auxiliary grooves to the buccal of the solder joint will aid the escape of food from the occlusal surface of a pontic or retainer.

Torque, generated when the bridge was seated, may be eliminated in time by resorption and rebuilding of the alveolar process. It must be remembered that no bridge should be cemented if seating changes the natural long-axis relationship of the abutments. Torque from occlusion stems from a cusp extended too far buccally or lingually, or a premature contact at the extremity of a lateral excursion. This can be corrected by reduction of the bucco-lingual dimension or by equilibration.

Pressure on tissue may have been present at the time the bridge was seated, or it may be caused by a foreign body, such as food or cement particles lodging under the pontic ridgelap.[1] For the first of these two conditions there is no cure other than removal and reconstruction of the bridge. If the pressure results from a removable irritant, the area should be cleansed by passing dental floss mesio-distally between the pontic and mucous membrane, and treated by flushing with a mild antiseptic and painting the surrounding tissue with a mild counterirritant.

The *strength of contact areas* may be increased or diminished by malocclusion, which would tend to force the bridge either toward or away from an approximating tooth. Equilibration, either on the occluding surfaces of the bridge or the opposing teeth, is the remedy. No bridge should be seated if contact with an approximating tooth is faulty. However, to correct such a situation, it may not be necessary to remove the bridge. Sometimes it is possible to prepare a small proximo-occlusal cavity in the retainer and to make and cement an inlay that will bring the strength and location of the contact to the desired point.

Overprotected gingival tissue probably will show some swelling and hemorrhage. The overcontoured areas of a crown or pontic may be reduced, reshaped, and repolished. For *underprotection of gingival tissue* there is no treatment except reconstruction of the prosthesis.

Exposed sensitive cervical areas are caused by overdisplacement of gingival tissue before taking impressions, by overextended temporary crowns worn for too long a period during construction of the prosthesis, and by recession due to exposed margins of preparations or ill-fitting, underextended, overpolished, or overextended castings. Zinc chloride and stannous fluoride seem to be effective medicaments. Frequently a cavity preparation can be made at the margin of the restoration and a restoration placed that will protect the patient from further inconvenience. While this is a makeshift operation, it is better than removing an otherwise satisfactory bridge.[2, 3]

Thermal shock, if it persists for many days following the seating of the crown or fixed partial denture, may point to a serious pulpal involvement, premature contact, or an exposed margin or cementoenamel junction. Malocclusion is indicated not only by tenderness of the supporting structure but also by sensitivity to sweets and cold. A reaction to heat is more significant, since it seldom occurs without pulpal abnormality. Correction of malocclusion and exposed margins has been discussed. Sensitivity to heat is sometimes corrected by natural reparative action; therefore, usually the sensible procedure is to wait for more definite developments before deciding on a course of treatment that might necessitate endodontics or extraction.

LOOSENESS OF BRIDGES

When a bridge becomes loose at one end, it may be possible to remove and recement it, provided that the cause of failure is correctable. More often, however, it will be necessary to reprepare the abutments and rebuild the prosthesis.

A bridge becomes loose because of

(1) deformation of the metal casting on the abutment;

(2) torque;

(3) technique of cementation;

(4) solubility of cement;

(5) caries;

(6) mobility of one or more abutments;

(7) lack of full occlusal coverage;

(8) insufficient retention in the abutment preparation; or

(9) poor initial fit of the casting.

Deformation of a retainer may result when the yield point of the alloy is low, or when the casting is too thin because of insufficient reduction of the abutment in the areas that will receive forces from opposing teeth. Deformation may also be caused by wear or equilibration brought about or necessitated by reduction of vertical dimension in other quadrants; by a sharp cusp on an opposing tooth, which should have been rounded or reshaped prior to the construction of the bridge; or by an opposing restoration, made of a harder metal or of unglazed porcelain, which will bring about undue wear. Deformed cast retainers must be corrected by reconstruction of the restoration.[4]

Torque, which will break the cement bond and allow a retainer to become loose, generally is caused by a premature contact in lateral excursion, or by different types of occlusion; that is, a natural tooth opposing one end of the bridge with a tissue-supported removable partial denture opposing the other, or an absence of any occlusion on a terminal abutment. Torque may be eliminated by equilibration, by recontouring or reducing occluding areas, or by the construction and insertion of an occluding prosthesis.

If a bridge becomes loose because of the *technique of cementation,* it can be assumed that either the abutment tooth (or teeth) or the inside surface of the retainer was not dry or clean, or that the cement was poorly mixed. If the bridge can be removed and recemented, with the field, the abutment teeth, and the retainers dry, and if it is *held in position without movement* until cement has hardened, success may be expected.

Cement dissolves for one of three reasons: the margins were open originally; the retainer has been deformed, creating an open margin; or a hole has been worn through an occluding surface of the retainer. There are no means of improving this situation except by remaking the bridge.

When a bridge becomes unseated, partially or totally, because of *recurrent caries,* it must be removed, the abutment teeth must be reprepared, if possible, and the bridge must be reconstructed. Caries will develop because of a leaking margin, gingival recession, or an exposed cervical margin. Also, there are many cases on record in which illness seemingly has predisposed the patient to caries, and exposed enamel areas, healthy at the time the bridge was seated, have become susceptible to caries.

Mobility of an abutment may cause a bridge to loosen. Lack of judgment by the prosthodontist, an increased load on the abutment teeth due to malfunction in another segment of the arch, or periodontal disease from an undetermined origin might be responsible. The bridge and the area should be evaluated carefully to ascertain whether more abutment teeth and splinting will correct the fault, or whether the offending abutment must be lost.

Sometimes *when the buccal cusp of a bicuspid has not been covered* in the construction of a retainer, because of esthetic demands, a force applied directly to the occluding enamel surface will tend to drive the tooth out of the retainer. Unless the bridge is very short, with inlay retainers and one broken-stress joint to allow greater individual tooth movement, all occluding surfaces of all abutment teeth should be covered by metal that will absorb and dissipate forces from the occluding teeth.

If a bridge comes off because of *too little retention* in the prepared abutments, a new bridge is mandatory. Even though teeth are short or conical, auxiliary grooves and pins may be used to increase parallelism and frictional retention.[1]

A bridge that becomes loose because a *retainer casting did not fit* should not have been seated in the first place.[5] Often only one retainer will develop movement on the abutment, and the patient will not be cognizant of the condition or the possible sequelae. It is the duty of the dentist to recall the patient periodically for prophylaxis and examination, at which time any fixed prosthesis should be thoroughly inspected for signs or evidence of loosening, or of developments which might terminate in such a situation. Precautionary equilibration, polishing, or a small restoration may forestall failure of this type.

RECURRENCE OF CARIES

Caries may recur because of
(1) overextension of margins;
(2) short castings;
(3) open margins;
(4) wear;
(5) a retainer coming loose;
(6) pontic form which fills the embrasures;
(7) poor oral hygiene;
(8) use of the wrong type of retainer, which will promote caries susceptibility; or
(9) because temporary protection of the abutment uncovered the neck of the tooth by a prolonged or permanent displacement of the gingiva.

Overextended margins cannot be adapted to the converging convexity of the enamel at the cervix of the tooth. While the space between the margin of the casting and the tooth may be filled with cement at the time the bridge is seated, cement is soluble, and later a crevice may appear that will be filled with saliva or food debris. This can stimulate recession of the gingival tissue and induce disintegration of enamel and cementum, and caries. Occasionally it is possible to polish off the excess casting, prepare a cavity, and place a restoration. Usually, however, the affected area will go so far occlusally beyond the margin of the retainer that it becomes necessary to remove the bridge, explore the tooth, and be guided in reconstruction by what remains.

A *short casting* leaves the cervical margin of the prepared tooth surface exposed. This rough enamel or dentin collects debris, and caries results. Sometimes it may be removed and the area can be restored with a casting or a resin restoration.

Open margins, regardless of the cause, allow the entry of saliva and cariogenic organisms, and require the remaking of the prosthesis.

Wear, producing an opening through the occluding surface, will expose cement or tooth structure, and caries may occur. If detected in time, a plastic restoration or an inlay may be sufficient to return the tooth to normalcy.

Saliva and food particles that infiltrate into the space between a *loose retainer* and the tooth have no means of escape. Through the pumping action or movement of the casting, especially if there are pinholes in the preparation, the destruction is accelerated, and within only a very short time the entire coronal dentin may be affected.

When cleaning embrasures is impossible, owing to overcrowding from *poor pontic form,* and this results in caries, the only remedy is to remove the bridge and build one of correct design.

Oral hygiene should be stressed and preventive therapy should be employed when retainers are used that do not cover all surfaces of the crown.

Many times *small carious areas* on the labial or buccal surface of a tooth carrying a partial veneer crown, or on a proximal surface supporting an inlay retainer, may be restored without disturbing or unseating the casting. Judgment must be exercised in this respect. If there is any doubt at all about the stability of the retainer or the depth of the caries, the bridge should be removed and the tooth reprepared. In mouths showing a relatively high caries index, partial veneer crowns, pinledges, MacBoyle-type restorations, and inlays should not be used unless the dentist is reasonably sure that the tendency toward caries has been arrested, or is being controlled by frequent prophylaxis, stannous fluoride treatments, and correct diet. Otherwise, retainers with long marginal lines are susceptible to recurrent caries in a period of time shorter than the normal life of the restoration or prosthesis.

When the *temporary protection* for the prepared abutment has uncovered the neck of the tooth because of overextension, or because it was used for too long a period of time, this area may be attacked by caries. In such a situation, repreparing the abutment tooth and extending the cervical margin of the preparation to a less susceptible point should be seriously considered.

RECESSION OF SUPPORTING STRUCTURE

Loss of the supporting alveolar process[6] may result from overloading due to

(1) length of the span;

(2) size of the occlusion table;

(3) embrasure form;

(4) contour of the retainers; or

(5) too few abutment teeth;

or it may develop because of

(6) an overextension of the cervical margins of the preparation, which interferes with or traumatizes the peripheral attachment of the periodontal membrane.

(7) Indiscreet band impression technique can also stimulate recession of the alveolar process. Too much pressure might have been exerted in taking the impression, forcing the band up beyond the attachment of the periodontal membrane and either cutting or tearing it loose. These same things will happen if the band is not contoured to the proximal curvatures of the gingival line.

Overloading can be avoided by correct diagnosis and planning of the restoration. If the *span is too long,* or if there are not enough teeth suitable for abutments, a fixed partial denture should not be constructed. Often the *size of the occlusion table* can be reduced, *embrasure form* can be changed, or *contour of the retainers* can be altered to decrease the load during mastication. If *too few abutment teeth* have been used, the bridge must be removed and remade with multiple terminal abutments. If these are not available, the prepared abutment teeth should be recontoured for the support and retention of a removable prosthesis. An *overextended margin* must be ground and polished to contour. If this cannot be done, the restoration should be removed and rebuilt. *Loss of the alveolar process* often can be retarded or eliminated by periodontal treatment, reestablishing a correct occlusal plane, or equilibrating the existing occlusion.

DEGENERATION OF PULP

Supporting structure, or root length, may be lost owing to periapical involvement brought about by the method of preparation, lack of protection of the prepared abutment teeth during construction, hidden caries, and malocclusion. It seems that a latent, low-grade pulp infection can be activated by the preparation of the abutment tooth and the building of the bridge, irritation from temporary coverage, lack of temporary coverage, or malocclusion. There is no method by which such a pulp condition may be discovered, and discomfort or pulp degeneration, occurring several months after the insertion of a fixed prosthesis, may be the result of such infection.[7]

A *pulp might degenerate* because of too-rapid preparation of the tooth or because of improper lubrication during preparation. Teeth unprotected during the construction of a bridge are exposed to saliva and the resulting irritation. Caries under a retainer sometimes cannot be discovered by radiographs. Marginal examination with a mirror and explorer should supplement radiographic examination.

Endodontic therapy may be possible without removing the bridge. However, if apical resection, rather than apical curettage, is deemed necessary, the change in crown-root ratio can create the need for splinting. If such treatment is not in order, the prosthesis must be cut, the pontics and the affected retainer removed, and the abutment extracted. The casting should be left on the remaining abutment until a new plan of treatment has been established.

FRACTURES OF BRIDGE COMPONENTS

A *bridge framework will fracture*[8, 9, 10] because of (1) a faulty solder joint, (2) incorrect casting technique, and (3) overwork of the metal due to the length of the span or to struts or parts that are too small. *Imperfections in solder joints* or from *casting technique* have been discussed in the appropriate chapters. *Overwork* or *strain hardening* caused by *a span being too long,* with springing in the center of the bar, may result in brittleness, loss of strength and ductility, and subsequent fracture. When *parts are too small,* there is a similar situation and result. Redesigning and remaking the prosthesis will be necessary.

A *facing may fracture* because, in its final form, a shelf of porcelain was left exposed to opposing surfaces or cusps and was subjected to either *leverage* or *spot contact.* Checks in a facing, or susceptibility to fracture, may be caused by *over-rapid heating* or *cooling* during glazing. A satisfactory replacement can be made in most instances, provided that it is given correct form. It should not be necessary to disturb the bridge.

When a pontic has been constructed so that the metal protecting the porcelain facing is insufficient to resist deformation from occluding teeth, fracture or loosening will ensue. Under such conditions equilibration is indicated before another facing, or perhaps a different type of facing or veneer, can be substituted. The force that caused the deformation must be directed to another area, or the tooth supplying the force must be reshaped to eliminate the force, malocclusion, or premature contact.

LOSS OF VENEERS

Veneers are lost from the labial and buccal surfaces of crowns or pontics because of
  (1) too little retention;
  (2) badly designed metal protection;
  (3) deformation of the protecting metal;
  (4) malocclusion; and
  (5) improper curing or fusing technique.

If a resin veneer is lost because of *insufficient retention,* a resin substitute must be constructed. Usually it will be retained by incorporated metal pins and projections from the veneer fitting into holes in the metal structure. If a porcelain veneer fractures or comes off, a resin substitute frequently will be necessary.

Lack of metal protection or *deformation of metal protection* requires equilibration, reduction of the force from occlusion, some change in the form of the occluding areas, and an increase in the number of pinholes supplying the retention.

If *malocclusion* has been responsible for the loss of a veneer, a change in occlusal form is in order.

A veneer which becomes unsatisfactory because of *curing or fusing technique* may be replaced with some expectation of success.

Broken facings and lost veneers do not always suggest the removal of the prosthesis. However, if the situation recurs consistently, rebuilding the bridge is the only solution.

LOSS OF FUNCTION

Bridges are failures at times because
  (1) they do not function in occlusion;
  (2) they have no contact with opposing teeth; or
  (3) they have premature contact.
  (4) Overcarved or undercarved occlusal surfaces may impair efficiency, as may
  (5) loss of opposing or approximating teeth.

The esthetic effect that the patient expected may have required that the bridge be built in such a way that *function is at a minimum or lacking completely.*

"No contact with the opposing teeth" does not necessarily indicate failure of the bridge. Loss of a tooth in the opposing arch without subsequent replacement may permit drifting, rotation, and tilting of teeth occluding with the bridge. Such movement, of necessity, reduces the efficiency of the occlusion, and the opposing arch must be reconstructed.

When function is reduced because of *premature contact* with an opposing tooth, either the occlusal plane of the bridge or the offending cusp of the opposing tooth should be recontoured.

When a bridge performs with subpar efficiency because of an *overcarved occlusal surface,* it must be rebuilt. If the *occlusal surface is undercarved,* usefulness will be increased by cutting grooves and spillways and by sharpening cusps, so long as this recontouring does not destroy contact with the opposing teeth in centric occlusion and in lateral movements.

If function is lost because of the *extraction of the opposing teeth,* replacement of those teeth is mandatory.

LOSS OF TISSUE TONE OR FORM

Loss of tissue tone or form may be due to
(1) pontic design;
(2) position and size of the joints;
(3) embrasure form;
(4) overcontouring or undercontouring of retainers; or
(5) the oral hygiene practiced by the patient.

The health of the tissue can be affected by too much pressure from the *pontic,* by improper clearance between the pontic and the ridge tissue, or because the cervical half of the pontic is oversize. In such cases the bridge must be removed, the tissue allowed to reorganize, and the bridge reconstructed.

If tissue is overprotected by the *position and size of the solder joints,* these joints probably can be reduced in contour, which in turn will increase the size of the embrasures and allow more adequate massage of the tissue by the food bolus during mastication.

If *embrasure form* is too small, lingual portions of the pontic[11] and bulky retainers may be recontoured. However, when a bridge was so *badly designed* that considerable change is required in the form of the pontic or of the retainer to make it biologically acceptable, everyone concerned would be better off if the bridge were removed and rebuilt.

Oral hygiene is largely up to the patient, provided that the bridge is built in such a way that oral hygiene is possible. He should be instructed in methods of using dental floss, Stim-U-Dents,* and toothbrushes. If, at a subsequent visit, there is evidence that the patient is not following advice concerning mouth cleanliness, instructions should be repeated and their importance emphasized in no uncertain terms.

---

* Stim-U-Dents, Inc., Detroit, Mich.

FAILURE TO SEAT

Why is it that occasionally a bridge will fail to seat, even though constructed with some care over abutment preparations that contained no undercuts and had been checked to verify the seating and fit of the retainer castings? (1) The abutment preparations may not be parallel, or (2) the soldering assembly may have been incorrect, or the relationship of the retainers may have been altered during soldering.

If the abutment preparations are *not parallel,* one or more teeth must be reprepared and the associated retainers reconstructed. It is relatively easy to check parallelism of the abutment teeth by taking an alginate impression and pouring a cast in impression plaster, which sets quite rapidly. After transferring the cast to a surveyor, the acceptability of all prepared surface planes on the abutments may be substantiated with the analyzing rod of the surveying instrument.

When castings do not fit, *undercuts* may be detected on one or more surfaces of the preparations by using the surveyor. The tooth or teeth must be reprepared and new retainers constructed.

If the individual parts of a bridge have been incorrectly related in the *soldering assembly,* or if alignment has been changed during soldering, one or more joints must be broken and the bridge must be reassembled and resoldered.

Such discernible factors as poor preparations, bad waxing and casting techniques, incorrect assembly and application of heat during the soldering operation, and a general lack of attention to pertinent details may be to blame when a bridge does not fit. It is true that intangible or unknown factors occasionally crop up; for instance, it is not always possible to control the shelf life of materials being used, or to prevent contamination. Likewise, there are inherent variables in the casting procedure and other manipulative steps in the bridge fabrication that cannot be controlled perfectly. For the most part, however, failures in bridge construction are due to attempted short cuts or positive indifference and inexcusable ignorance on the part of those concerned with building the prosthesis.

REFERENCES

1. Willey, R. E.: Why do bridges fail? J. Florida D. Soc., *31*:110, Fall 1960.
2. Agnew, R. G.: Impregnation of tooth surfaces with zinc chloride and potassium ferrocyanide. California D. J., *26*:228, Sept. 1950.
3. Pelton, W. J.: The effect of zinc chloride and potassium ferrocyanide as a caries prophylaxis. J. D. Res., *29*:756, Dec. 1950.
4. Rieser, J.: Periodontal aspects of fixed bridge failure. J. Pros. Den., *5*:677, Sept.–Oct. 1955.
5. Teteruck, W. R.: A study of the fit of certain dental casting alloys using different investing materials and technics. Master's thesis, Indiana Univ. School Den., 1963.

6. Dykema, R. W.: Fixed partial prosthodontics. J. Tennessee D. A., *42*:309, Oct. 1962.
7. Brecker, S. C.: How to prevent failures in crowns and bridges. D. Practitioner & D Record, *14*:261, March 1964.
8. Dykema, R. W.: A study of the effects of certain variables on the comparative strengths of soldered and cast bridge joints. Master's thesis, Indiana Univ. School Den., 1961.
9. Simpson, R. L.: Failures in crown and bridge prosthodontics. J.A.D.A., *47*:154, Aug. 1953.
10. Pokorny, D. K.: Fixed bridge failures. J. Michigan D. A., *43*:203, July–Aug. 1961.
11. Henry, P. J.: An investigation into the changes occurring in the oral mucosa beneath fixed bridge pontics. Master's thesis, Indiana Univ. School Den., 1963.

Thin, Vu thi: A study of the Brinell hardness of metals used in conjunction with the porcelain fused to metal technic. Master's thesis, Indiana Univ. School Den., 1962.

35

COMPLETE ORAL REHABILITATION

To rehabilitate means "to restore to a former capacity." Oral rehabilitation is the restoration of the form, function, and esthetic qualities of the masticatory mechanism. The rehabilitation of a mouth therefore can be the *satisfactory* placement of a single restoration, or it can encompass the rebuilding of the remaining teeth and replacing of any number of missing teeth. It follows then that not all oral rehabilitation procedures entail complete restoration and not all full mouth reconstructions can correctly be called oral rehabilitation.

Unfortunately, the terms oral rehabilitation, oral reconstruction, full mouth rehabilitation, full mouth reconstruction, occlusal reconstruction, and occlusal rehabilitation are used interchangeably by members of the dental profession. Even the word *gnathology* is used by some in place of these terms. However, the definition of gnathology is the *science* of the masticatory system, including physiology, functional disturbances, and treatment. While gnathological principles may form a basis for complete oral rehabilitation, all full mouth reconstruction operations cannot be considered to be the practice of gnathology.

Perhaps the best term to designate extensive restorative treatment that involves most or all of the teeth and that is accomplished according to sound anatomic and physiologic concepts might be "complete oral rehabilitation."

The indications for complete oral rehabilitation are:

1. Loss of large amounts of tooth structure necessitating the replacement or restoration of most or all of the dentition.

2. Temporomandibular joint disturbances that can be attributed to the patient's faulty occlusion.

3. The treatment of periodontally diseased mouths in which defective occlusion seems to play a major role as a contributing factor.

Many techniques have been advocated and used in endeavors to achieve complete oral rehabilitation. In the early 1920's McCollum and his group of investigators attempted to demonstrate the existence of rotational centers about which the mandible moved. They designed apparatus for the purpose of locating and recording these centers of rotation with extraoral tracing devices, transferring this information to a dental articulator, which was then adjusted to follow the recorded motions of the mandible. In an effort to minimize the amount of force on any one tooth during mastication, Mc-Collum taught the usage of balanced occlusion; that is, synchronous contact of all teeth in centric occlusion and during all movements of the mandible.[1]

Relatively recently Granger[2] and Stuart[3, 4] each produced tracing equipment and articulators intended to be improvements over those of McCollum.* Granger[5] is an advocate of balanced occlusion; Stuart[6] teaches the use of tooth arrangement in which the posterior teeth have simultaneous contact in centric occlusion but no contact in any eccentric position of the mandible.

These techniques and devices are complicated and time-consuming and not particularly well understood by the dental profession as a whole. This has led many to continue the use of the more simple, albeit less accurate, procedures that came before, and to the development of other, some-times simplified, methods that are expected to afford more exactness and control than altogether arbitrary approaches.

Pankey and Mann[7]† make use of the Bonwill triangle and the Monson sphere to rebuild the lower arch, the upper arch being coordinated with the rebuilt lower by means of a functionally generated path obtained in the mouth. After the occlusion has been effected, it is altered to have some degree of "long centric" and barely to eliminate contact between cusps on the "balancing side." The proponents of this technique believe functional centric occlusion to be an area, *not* a point.

De Pietro[8]‡ has designed a partially adjustable instrument which is set by using extraoral checkbites. The manufacturer of this instrument plans its conversion to one that can be set by means of an extraoral tracing apparatus.

Several simplified articulators are on the market. Included among these are the Hanau and Dentatus instruments. These are characterized by having straight paths of motion, with the guiding elements on the lower member and the condylar ball on the upper, which is just the opposite of the human mechanism.

One of these, the Hanau #130, may be converted so that the condylar

* Granger Gnatholator, Gnatholator Co., Inc., Pelham Manor, N. Y. Stuart Articulator, Charles E. Stuart, Ventura, Calif.

† P-M Instrument, J. F. Jelenko & Co., Inc., New Rochelle, N. Y.

‡ Ney Articulator, The J. M. Ney Company, Hartford, Conn.

ball is on the lower member and most of the guiding mechanism on the upper, but with the paths of motion remaining straight lines. An instrument recently introduced by the Whip-Mix Corporation has the condylar elements on the lower and the guiding elements on the upper member.

Intraoral checkbites are used to set all three of these instruments, and casts may be mounted on them either by an arbitrary face-bow or a hinge axis transfer-bow.

A patient who suffers from any of the conditions requiring the rebuilding of his dental arches deserves the best his dentist has to offer. Since the successful handling of such cases may depend on the degree of accuracy with which the operator can capture and utilize the highly individual functional characteristics of the patient's masticatory mechanism, the dentist should use the most faultless methods and machines within his capabilities.

In most complete oral rehabilitation cases, it is necessary to prepare and restore *at the same time* many, if not all, of the teeth in order to have total control over the occlusal relationships that are to be established. Once this is done, the patient's original occlusal relationship, be it good or bad, is destroyed forever. Under these circumstances, it seems wise, if not imperative, that the patient's diagnostic and working casts be related exactly to the hinge axis through a hinge axis transfer and centric relation registrations.

The care with which eccentric records are made and transferred to the instrument is probably related equally to the patient's needs and the dentist's skills. One such method is discussed in Chapter 33 (Occlusion Factors). It is logical to assume that since the precision required for individual cases cannot be wholly comprehensible, it would be better to err on the side of too much, rather than too little, effort in this direction; conversely, that the operator is well advised not to employ techniques over which he does not have unqualified control, owing to lack of proficiency or understanding.

As in the case of occlusal equilibration or adjustment, there appears to be no excuse for the use of complete oral rehabilitation as a prophylactic measure.

REFERENCES

1. McCollum, B. B.: Fundamentals involved in prescribing restorative dental remedies. D. Items Interest, *61*:522, 641, 724, 852, 942, 1939.
2. Granger, E. R.: Practical Procedures in Oral Rehabilitation. Philadelphia, J. B. Lippincott Company, 1962.
3. McCollum, B. B., and Stuart, C. E.: Gnathology, A Research Report. South Pasadena, Scientific Press, 1955.
4. Stallard, H., and Stuart, C. E.: Eliminating tooth guidance in natural dentitions. J. Pros. Den., *11*:474, May–June 1961.

5. Granger, E. R.: The establishment of occlusion. The articulator and the patient. D. Clin. North America, Nov. 1960, p. 536.
6. Stuart, C. E., and Stallard, H.: Diagnosis and treatment of occlusal relations of the teeth. Texas D. J., *75:*435, Aug. 1957.
7. Mann, A. W., and Pankey, L. D.: Oral rehabilitation. Part I. The use of the P-M instrument in treatment planning and in restoring the lower posterior teeth. Part II. Reconstruction of the upper teeth using a functionally generated path technique. J. Pros. Den., *10:*135, 151, Jan.–Feb. 1960.
8. De Pietro, A. J.: Concepts of occlusion. D. Clin. North America, Nov. 1963, p. 607.

Courtade, G. L., ed.: Symposium on occlusal rehabilitation. D. Clin. North America, Nov. 1963.
D'Amico, A.: The canine teeth. J. South. California D. A., *26:*6, 1958.
Kazis, H., and Kazis, A. J.: Complete Mouth Rehabilitation through Crown and Bridge Prosthodontics. Philadelphia, Lea & Febiger, 1956.
Lucia, V. O.: Modern Gnathological Concepts. St. Louis, The C. V. Mosby Company, 1961.
Schweitzer, J. M.: Masticatory function in man. J. Pros. Den., *12:*262, 1962.
Schweitzer, J. M.: Oral Rehabilitation Problem Cases. St. Louis, The C. V. Mosby Company, 1964.

36

CASE HISTORIES

This chapter includes two case histories depicted through illustrations and brief captions.

The first case, for an adolescent, required orthodontic treatment of the opposing arch and some recontouring of the repositioned teeth. The abutments were surveyed for the best path of insertion, construction was indirect on a cast, and dies were made from an elastic impression. One post-seating adjustment was made.

The second case was complicated by the skepticism of the patient and the intricacies of the abutment preparations. Extent of the cutting was determined after the facings were shaped, aligned, and approved. After this was accomplished, construction proceeded by the indirect technique. Three post-seating checks were made, only the first showing a minimal prematurity.

Each bridge was seated without interference.

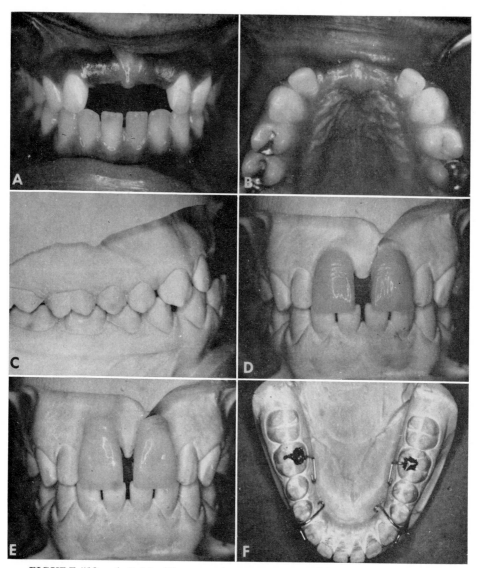

FIGURE 513. *A, B,* Maxillary anterior space, young adolescent.

C, Lateral view. Poor relationship between mandibular incisors and maxillary ridge.

D, Largest facings. Diastema much too large.

E, Large denture teeth. Diastema still overwide. Decision made to move mandibular incisors lingually and to shorten them to improve situation for building bridge.

F, Wires bent for a working retainer; those on molars to support appliance. The anterior loops were to hold an elastic which would force incisors lingually.

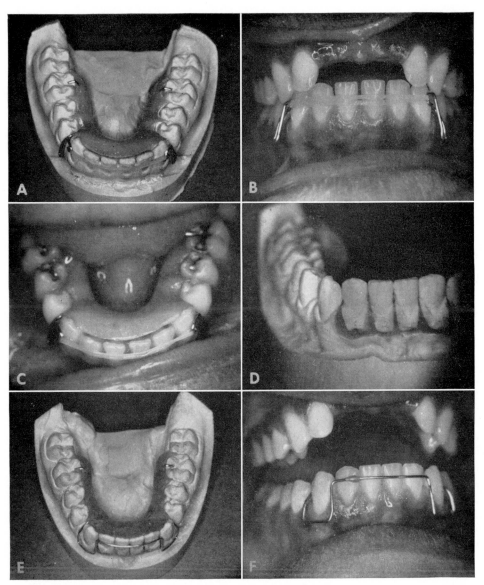

FIGURE 514. *A, B, C,* Appliance showing wire support on molars and elastic against incisors. Lingual movement by this method was 50 per cent of that desired.

D, Teeth sectioned and aligned for Hawley retainer.

E, F, Hawley retainer on cast and in mouth. Patient was uncomfortable for a few hours. This was worn for several weeks.

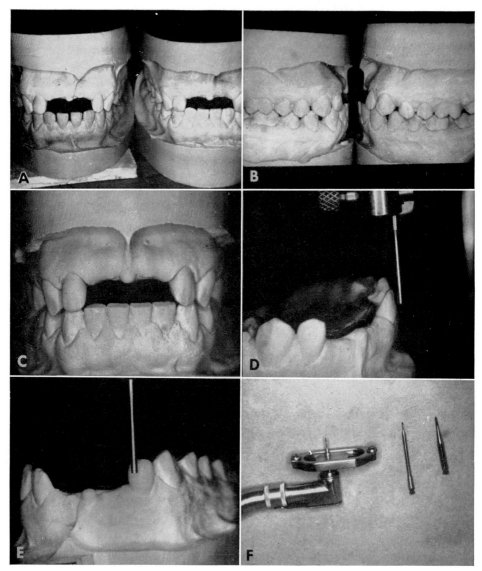

FIGURE 515. *A, B,* Casts before and after orthodontic treatment. While mandibular incisors were tipped, instead of being moved bodily, realignment produced a situation readily treatable. Vertical overlap of bridge should maintain new positions.

C, Mandibular incisors shortened on cast. Radiographs showed this to be feasible.

D, E, Determining best path of insertion.

F, Loma Linda Parallelometer and drills for pinholes.

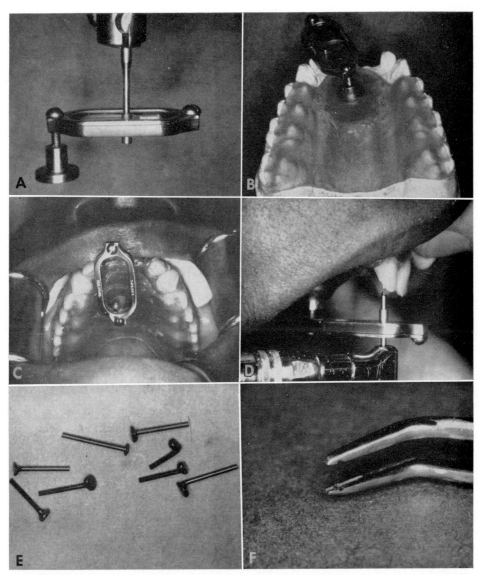

FIGURE 516. *A,* Parallelometer on analyzing rod of surveyor, ready to be attached to baseplate. Holes will be drilled in line with pre-established path of insertion.

B, C, Device attached; on cast and in mouth. Plate covers parts of occlusals of posterior teeth and is well adapted to lingual surfaces and embrasures. It is quite stable when seated in mouth.

D, Disk with bur sleeve moves forward and back and rotates so that drill can reach any of the four anterior teeth.

E, Nylon bristles cut and headed.

F, Cross-grooved pliers for handling either headed or straight bristles.

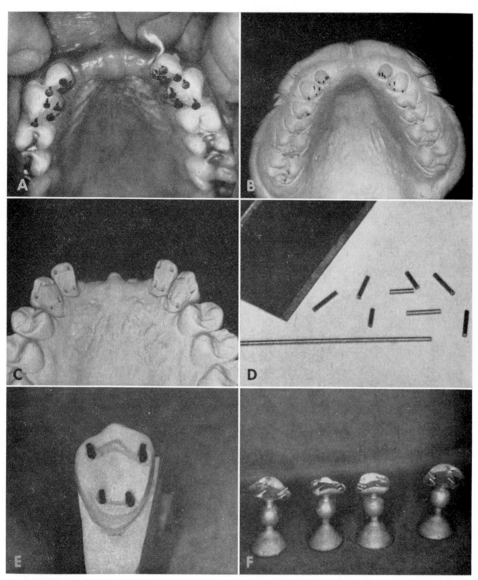

FIGURE 517. *A, B,* Abutments packed to displace gingival tissue. Nylon bristles placed in pinholes. When cotton fibers were removed (*B*), impression was taken with silicone.

C, Cast of prepared arch. Another was poured prior to this one, to be sectioned for dies.

D, Cut nylon bristles. Drills were 0.023 inch in diameter. Bristles for impression were 0.022 inch. These are 0.020 inch.

E, Die, lubricated and with bristles in place, ready for waxing retainer patterns.

F, The retainer castings. Pinholes in teeth must be very slightly countersunk with round bur so that castings will seat. Investment breaks down minutely where pin and lingual plate join. This cannot be machined safely.

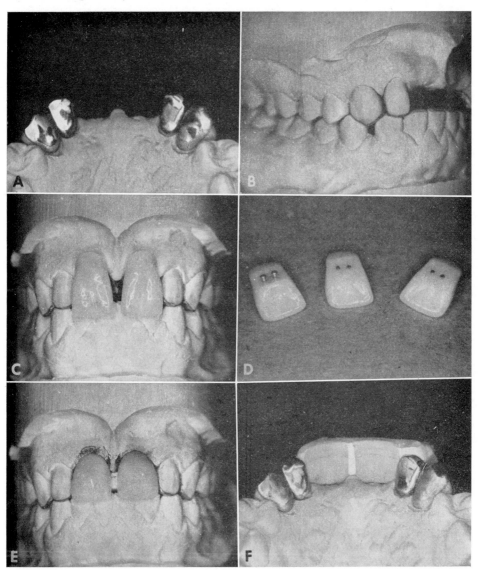

FIGURE 518. *A, B,* Castings on working cast, ready for equilibration.

C. D, Denture teeth from which facings will be made. Pins are cut off, are partly drilled out, and then are finally removed with aqua regia.

E, F, Facings ground to form and alignment. Pencil line shows extent of hollow-ground incisal bevel.

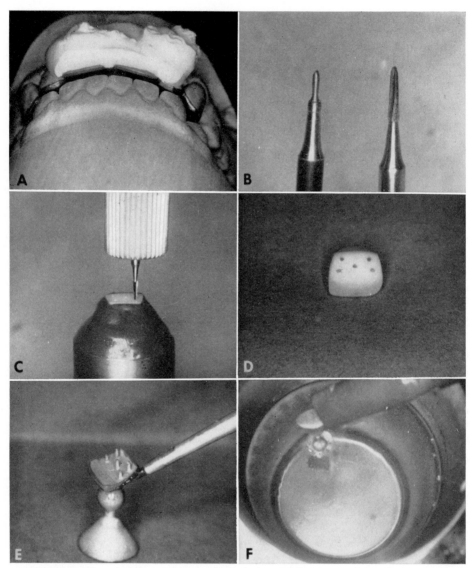

FIGURE 519. *A,* Aligned facings, incisal view. Hollow-ground bevel gives room for bulk of metal to protect facing at incisal edge.

B, Drills made from carbide burs.

C, Facing mounted on table with modeling compound for drilling holes.

D, Completed facing.

E, Cast pontic being coated with lacquer before "stripping." This is necessary to reduce size of cast pins so that facing will seat without causing stress in porcelain. Also, holes must be countersunk very slightly with round-end diamond stone.

F, Casting in stripping machine. Stripper is Model 300 Stripper/Plater (Westwood Dental Mfg. Co., Los Angeles, Calif.).

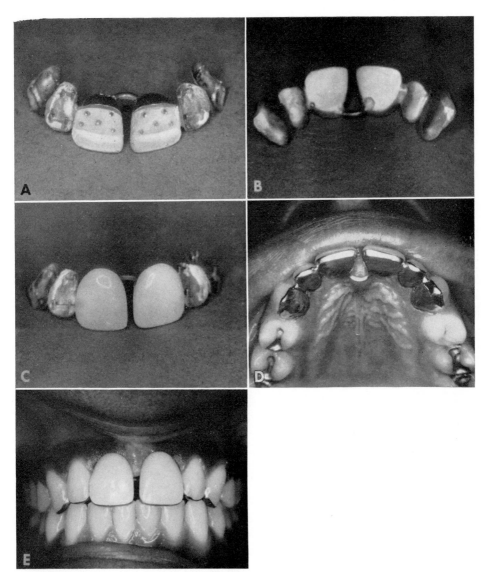

FIGURE 520. *A, B,* Assembled framework. Each pair of retainers was soldered. Pontics were then soldered to retainers. Loop was soldered to one pontic in third assembly. One pontic was cast to loop, but this joint was reinforced with solder to give better contour to joint.

C, Facings glazed and cemented.

D, Bridge from incisal. Loop is contoured from 17-gauge, high-fusing clasp wire and is set in a rugae depression. It contacts tissue without pressure.

E, Bridge in occlusion. Overlap is sufficient to maintain mandibular incisors in new alignment.

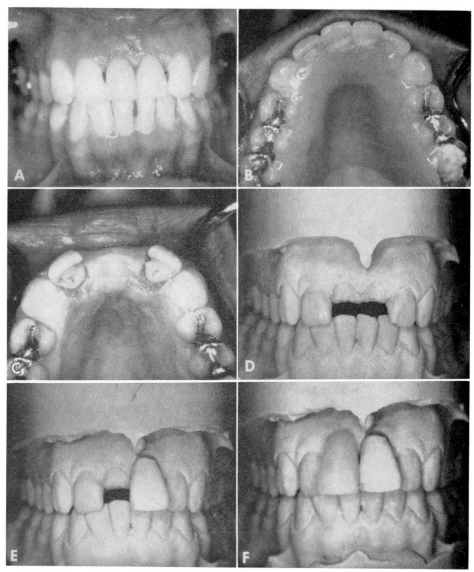

FIGURE 521. *A, B,* Maxillary arch showing patient wearing temporary partial denture replacing central incisors. Space is narrow. Centrals are in alignment but are narrower than laterals.

C, D, Upper arch and cast with denture removed.

E, Occluded casts with a stone replica of patient's extracted central incisor. Instead of recommending orthodontic treatment, patient had been advised to have overlapping centrals extracted.

F, A wax incisor has been added, closely duplicating alignment of maxillary teeth before extraction.

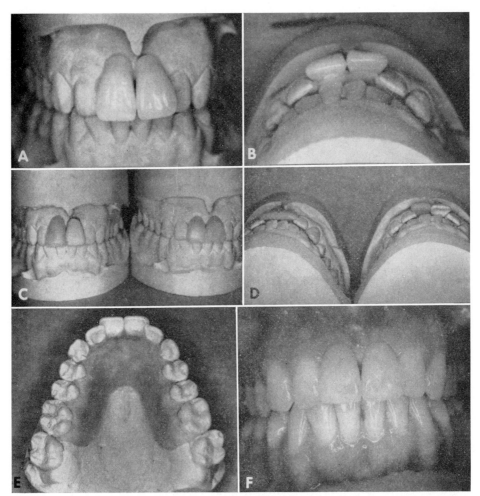

FIGURE 522. *A, B,* Denture teeth selected for facings. In a situation in which there must be irregular alignment or overlapping, the reverse-pin facing is very adaptable.

C, D, Two wax teeth have been carved and aligned to simulate expected esthetic result.

E, F, Denture teeth ground to contour and alignment and attached to resin base and seated in mouth (*F*). This was done to help persuade patient that end result would be desirable and to help plan preparations on lateral incisors.

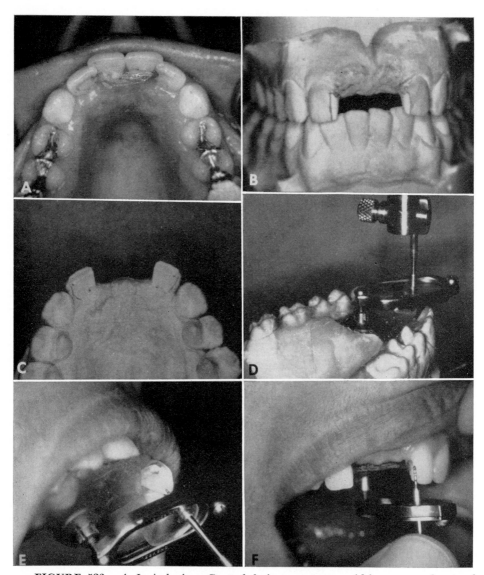

FIGURE 523. *A,* Incisal view. Central facings are same width as natural central incisors and have been adapted and aligned in a manner pleasing to patient.

B, C, Simulated preparations on diagnostic cast. Extensions on labial determined by contacting surfaces of the facings.

D, Loma Linda Parallelometer attached to baseplate parallel to calculated path of insertion so that preparations may be duplicated in mouth.

E, Drill used to cut lingual pinholes.

F, Drill used to check alignment of labio-proximal grooves.

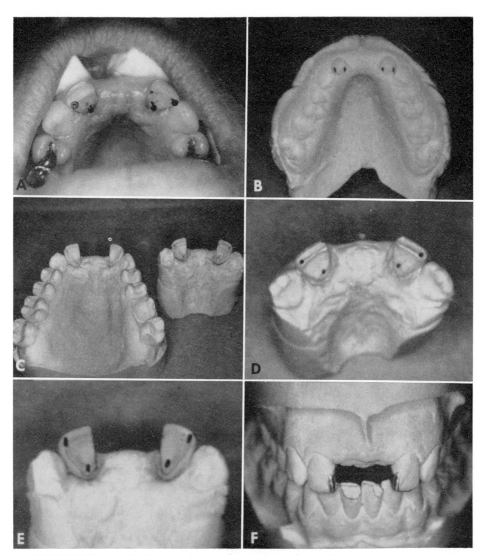

FIGURE 524. *A,* Nylon bristles in place prior to impression.

B, Silicone impression.

C, D, Working cast and cast to be used for carving patterns.

E, Nylon bristles on lubricated die cast.

F, Castings on working cast with reduced areas on occluding teeth outlined in pencil. This grinding was done when finished bridge was fitted.

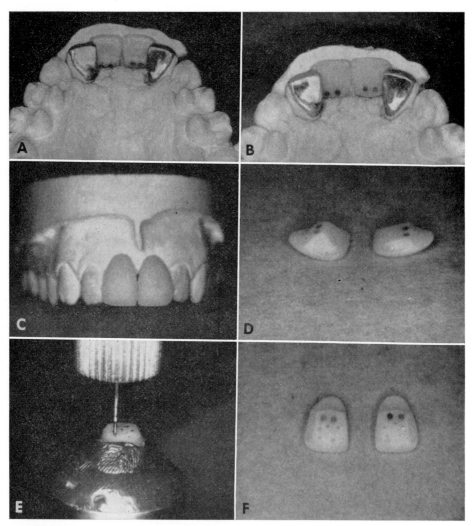

FIGURE 525. *A, B,* Facings before and after preparing lingual surfaces and beveling and hollow-grinding incisal edges.

C, Final alignment of facings.

D, Showing concave grinding to effect overlapping.

E, F, Holes for reverse-pins.

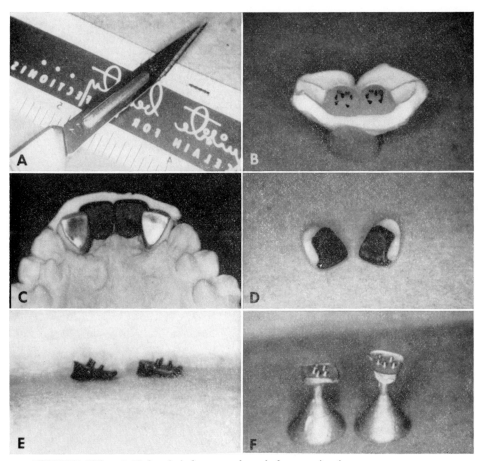

FIGURE 526. *A,* Nylon bristle cut to length for pontic pin.
B, Facings seated in labial index ready for waxing of pontic patterns.
C, D, E, Pontic patterns carved.
F, Pontic castings.

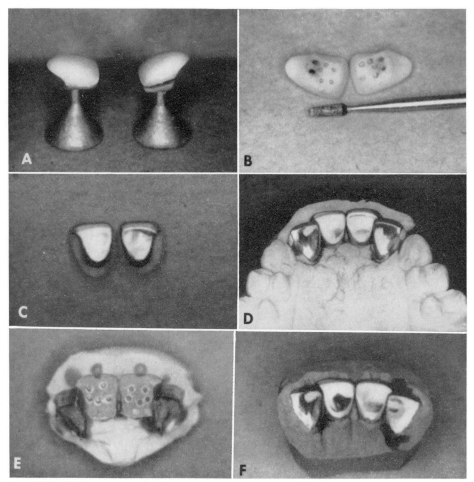

FIGURE 527. *A, B,* Facings will not seat on castings until castings have been "stripped" and (*B*) pinholes have been countersunk slightly with a round-tip stone.

C, Polished pontics.

D, Bridge aligned using labial plaster index.

E, Bridge assembled in lingual splint ready to pour soldering assembly after painting index with separating medium and soaking for 5 minutes.

F, Soldering assembly trimmed and washed.

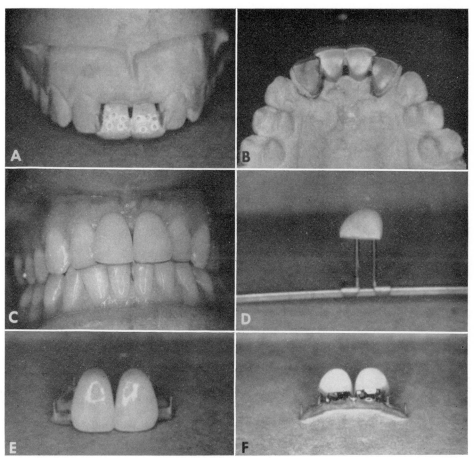

FIGURE 528. *A, B,* Soldered bridge on working cast. Size and location of solder joints and size and contour of embrasures correct.

C, Bridge, with unglazed facings, checked for occlusion.

D, Facing, on holder, ready for glazing.

E, Bridge with glazed and cervically stained facings.

F, Tissue-contacting surfaces highly polished and glazed.

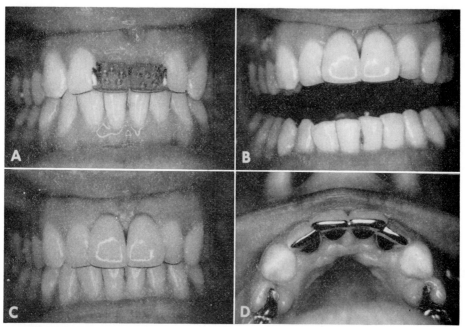

FIGURE 529. *A*, Bridge frame cemented. Margins polished. Bridge could not be seated with facings in place.

B, Facings cemented. Extra care needed to remove all particles of cement from labial embrasures and under pontics.

C, *D*, Bridge, labial and incisal views.

"Thus we may see," quoth he, "how the world wags.
'Tis but an hour ago since it was nine;
And after one hour more 'twill be eleven;
And so, from hour to hour, we ripe and ripe."

Shakespeare, *As You Like It.*

APPENDIX

Manufacturers of the materials mentioned in the text are listed below. Special thanks are due those marked with asterisks for their help in the assembly of illustrations and reference material.

Julius Aderer, Inc.
Long Island City, N. Y.

*Claudius Ash, Sons & Co., Inc.
Niagara Falls, N. Y.

Aurora Dental Specialties Co.
Hillside, Ill.

Austenal Company
Chicago, Ill.

Barkmeyer Electrical Mfg. Co.
Redlands, Calif.

Beuhler, Ltd.
Evanston, Ill.

Blue Island Specialty Co., Inc.
Blue Island, Ill.

Harry J. Bosworth Co.
Chicago, Ill.

*Buffalo Dental Mfg. Co., Inc.
Brooklyn, N. Y.

The Carborundum Company
Niagara Falls, N. Y.

The L. D. Caulk Company
Milford, Del.

Ceramco, Inc.
Woodside, N. Y.

Chayes Dental Instrument Corp.
Danbury, Conn.

*The Cleveland Dental Mfg. Co.
Cleveland, Ohio

*The Columbus Dental Mfg. Co.
Columbus, Ohio

*Densco, Inc.
Denver, Colo.

Dental Development & Mfg. Corp.
Brooklyn, N. Y.

*The Dentists' Supply Company
York, Penna.

William Dixon, Inc.
Newark, N. J.

*Hanau Engineering Co., Inc.
Buffalo, N. Y.

*Harmony Dental Products Corp.
Pasadena, Calif.

Hickok Specialties Co.
Grand Rapids, Mich.

*K. H. Huppert Co.
Chicago, Ill.

The Hygienic Dental Mfg. Co.
Akron, Ohio

587

*J. W. Ivory, Inc.
Philadelphia, Penna.

*J. F. Jelenko & Co., Inc.
New Rochelle, N. Y.

Johnson & Johnson
New Brunswick, N. J.

H. D. Justi & Son, Inc.
Philadelphia, Penna.

*Kerr Manufacturing Company
Detroit, Mich.

K and R Dental Products Co.
Blue Island, Ill.

Lever Bros.
New York, N. Y.

Linde Co. Div. of Union Carbide Corp.
Speedway, Ind.

*L&R Manufacturing Company
Kearny, N. J.

Mizzy, Inc.
Clifton Forge, Va.

E. C. Moore Company
Dearborn, Mich.

The J. Bird Moyer Co., Inc.
Philadelphia, Penna.

National Keystone Products Co.
Philadelphia, Penna.

*The J. M. Ney Company
Hartford, Conn.

The Niranium Corp.
Long Island, N. Y.

Pfingst & Company, Inc.
New York, N. Y.

Premier Dental Products Company
Philadelphia, Penna.

*The Ransom & Randolph Co.
Toledo, Ohio

Slaycris Laboratories
Portland, Ore.

The Snow Dental Company
Tonawanda, N. Y.

*Star Dental Mfg. Co., Inc.
Philadelphia, Penna.

Stim-U-Dents, Inc.
Detroit, Mich.

Stuart, Charles E.
Ventura, Calif.

Surgident, Ltd.
Los Angeles, Calif.

Tempil Corp.
New York, N. Y.

Tooth Corporation
Cambridge, Mass.

Torit Manufacturing Co.
St. Paul, Minn.

Dr. Wagner's Dental Specialties
Janesville, Wis.

Western Gold and Platinum Co.
Belmont, Calif.

Westwood Dental Mfg. Co., Inc.
Los Angeles, Calif.

*Whip-Mix Corporation
Louisville, Ky.

*The S. S. White Dental Manufacturing Co.
Philadelphia, Penna.

The Wilkinson Company
Santa Monica, Calif.

*Williams Gold Refining Co., Inc.
Buffalo, N. Y.

INDEX

Page numbers in *italics* refer to illustrations.

Abutments. See also *Foundations.*
abnormal position of, 47–48
caries in, 41
crown for, 41
definition of, 5
exploration of, 37
multiple, definition of, 45
orthodontic positioning of, 40–41, 505–518
appliance design in, 513–518
diagnosis in, 512
physiologic considerations in, 508–511
treatment planning in, 512
preparation of, for hydrocolloid bridge, 180
tooth form and, 72
pulpless teeth as, 43
relationship of, 41
root of, 14
rotation of, 48
tipping of, 48
tooth form and, 72
Accelerated speeds, for MacBoyle retainer, 154
for veneered gold crown, 343
in tooth reduction for porcelain jacket crown, 402
Acrylic resin, physical properties of, 430
precautions with, 431
Acrylic resin veneer, retention form for, *435*
Adolescent, mouth of. See *Mouth, in adolescent.*
Alginate, in diagnostic cast, 27, *30*
Alginate impression, 189–190
Alloys, casting, 247
gold, melting range of, 240

Alum, in tissue displacement, 160, *160*
Aluminum shell, as temporary protection, 89
Amalgam, condensing of, 85
Amalgam core, pin-retained, for carious teeth, 79–86
Amalgam die, 204, *205*
Anterior teeth, distal tipping of, 515, *515*
fractured, restoration of, 524–535
with class IV resin restoration, 525
with porcelain incisal and metal substructure, 528–535
instrumentation system for (tables of), 107–108
mesial tipping of, 515
patterns of, for partial veneer crown, 109
pontic form of, 292
reduction of, for veneered gold crown, 344
splinting of, 485
Ante's law, 11
Antiflux, 304
Appointments, scheduling of, 41
Articulator, *33*
relation of diagnostic cast on, 538
transfer of face-bow registration to, *171*
Asbestos liner, for investment, 224
Axial angles, reduction for veneered gold crown, 341
Axial preparation, for porcelain jacket crown, 401

"Back pressure" porosity, 222
Backing, of pontic facing, 267
Balanced occlusion, 564

589

Band, copper, for porcelain jacket crown, 401
  preparation of, for working cast, 157, 197–199, *198*
Bennett setting, 543
Beveling, of maxillary bicuspid, 113
Bicuspids, instrumentation system for (tables of), 116–117
  mandibular, form in pontic, 293
    partial veneer crown for, 122–124
    patterns of, 477–478
  maxillary, partial veneer crown for, 112–116
    contraindications to, 111
    form in pontic, 291
    patterns of, 467–473
  reduction, for veneered gold crown, 344
Bite frame, Kerr. See *Kerr Bite Frame*.
Bonded porcelain veneer crown. See *Crown, bonded porcelain veneer*.
Boxes, cutting of, in maxillary bicuspid, 113
Bridges. See also *Pontics*.
  alignment of, 323
  assembly of, 272
  benefits of, 9
  case histories, 567–584
  cementation of, 320–335, *329*
    failure due to, 554
    postoperative treatment, 333–335
    checking of, 322–325
  construction of, *6, 15*
    occlusion factors and, 536–550
    prior to baking veneers, 387–394
    requirements in, 5–9
    with bonded porcelain veneers, 385–397, *386*
    with resin veneers, 89–91, *90, 91,* 430–443, *439, 440*
  contraindications to, 13–18
    in abnormal occlusion, 17
    in adolescent mouth, 16
    in elderly, 16
  crowns and, in preparation for removable partial dentures, 487–504
  definition, 3
  equilibration of, 323
  failures of, 551–562
    discomfort in, 551–553
    fracture of components in, 558
    looseness in, 553–555
  malocclusion in, 552
    pulp degeneration in, 557
    recession of supporting structure in, 557
  recurrent caries in, 555–556
    seating failures in, 561
  for adolescent mouth. See *Mouth, in adolescent*.

Bridges (*Continued*)
  hydrocolloid, abutment preparations for 180
  indications for, 10–13
  initial seating of, 322–325
  inlay-retained, *148*
  patterns for, 459–479
    mandibular, 473–479
    maxillary, 460–473
  pickling of, 310
  polishing of, 272
  removable. See *Removable partial denture*.
  resin, temporary, 89–91, *90, 91*
  ridge adaptation of, 323
Brightness, definition, 359
Brush technique, in class IV resin restoration, 525
Buccal surface, convex, preparation of, 62–64
  reduction of, 77
    for veneered gold crown, 341
Burnishing of matrix, instrumentation in, *447*
Burnout, 235–236, *236*
Broken-stress joint, 272–276
Burs, carbide, 52, *56, 58*
  steel, *57*

Cantilever spring, for tipping abutments, 513, *513,* 515, *515,* 517
Carbide burs, 52, *56, 58*
Caries, in abutment, 41
  recurrent, in bridge failure, 554–556
Case histories, 567–584
Cast, diagnostic. See *Diagnostic cast*.
  pouring of, for reversible hydrocolloid impression, 185
  study. See *Diagnostic cast*.
  working. See *Working cast*.
Cast post, core and, direct technique, 533
    indirect technique, 534
Cast transfer, 193–195, *194*
Castings, 237–243
  against backing, 268
  alloys for, 247
  cleaning, 242
  cleaning metal for, 237
  contamination of, 246
  failure of, 246
  fluxing for, 239
  for bonded porcelain veneer crown, 367–372
  full veneer gold crown, 320–322

Castings (*Continued*)
   hardening, 242
   in bridge failure, 555–556
   melting gold for, 239–242
   of pontic, 268–272, *269*
   of resin veneer crown, 435
   polishing, 243–246, *244, 245*
   splinted, *495*
   stability of, 226
   veneered, 367–372
      finishing, 371
      investing, 369
      spruing, 369
      wax pattern for, 368
Casting core, 79
Casting machine, centrifugal, *238*
Casting pressure, "back pressure" porosity
      and, 223
Cavity, preparation of, for class IV resin
      restoration, 525
   for inlay retainer, 145–148, *146, 147*
   varnishes for, 325
Cement, dissolution of, in bridge failure, 554
   solubility of, *328*
   zinc phosphate, 327–332
Cementation, of bridge. See *Bridge, cemen-
      tation of.*
   of crown, 320–335
      bonded porcelain veneer, 382
      porcelain jacket, 428
      resin jacket, 457
   with resin cement, 333
   with zinc oxide-eugenol cement, 332
   with zinc phosphate cement, 327–332
Centrifugal casting machine, *238*
Ceramic restoration. See *Crown, porcelain
   jacket.*
Cervical contact technique, 416–420, *417*
Cervical ditching technique, 420–428
Cervical margin, 64, *64*
   checking of, 216
   locating, for noncarious teeth, 77
Cingulum reduction, for MacBoyle retainer,
      153
   in preparation of maxillary central in-
      cisor, 97
Clasps, for porcelain veneer crown, 382
   for splinting, 485
   Roach-Akers, *8*
Clasp-retained prostheses. See *Removable
   partial denture.*
Cocoa butter, as coolant, 51
Color, selection of, for porcelain jacket
      crown. See *Crown, porcelain jacket,
      shade selection for.*
   for resin jacket preparation, 444
Condensing of amalgam, 85

Connector, definition, 5
   nonrigid, 272–276
Consultation with patient, 36
Contour heights, 359
Contouring, 418, *419*
Contrast enhancement, 360
Control powder, for investment, 227, 229
Coolants, 51–52
Copper band, for porcelain jacket crown,
   402
Copper-plated die, from polysulfide rubber
   impression, 202–204, *202*
Core, cast post and, direct technique, 533
   indirect technique, 534
Cristobalite investment, 227
Crowns. See also *Bridges.*
   bonded porcelain veneer, castings for,
      367–372
   construction, 365–384
   porcelain shoulder in, 377–380
   preparation of frame, 372–377
   bridges and, in preparation for removable
      partial dentures, 487–504
   cementation of, 326–333
   checking of, 320–335
   definition, 3
   for abutment, 41
   for adolescent mouth, 519–523
   for clasp-retained removable prosthesis for
      partially edentulous mouth. See *Re-
      movable partial denture.*
   full veneer gold, 74–93
      checking casting 320–322
      contraindications to, 75
      indications for, 74
      preparation of carious teeth for, 79–86
      preparation of noncarious teeth for, 75–
         79
      seating casting, 320–322
      wax occlusion registration in, 91–92
      wax pattern for, 211
   partial veneer, 94–129, *101*
      contraindications to, 94–95
      for first maxillary, 117–118
      for mandibular bicuspid, 122–124
      for mandibular cuspid, 119–122
      for mandibular incisor, 118–119
      for mandibular molar, 124–129
      for maxillary bicuspid, 112–116
      for maxillary central incisor, 95–100, *98,
         99*
         modified preparation, 100–103
      for maxillary cuspid, 103–105
      indications for, 94–95
      instrumentation system for (tables of),
         107–108
      spruing for, 109–110, *111*

Crowns (*Continued*)
    partial veneer, for fractured anterior teeth, 526–527
        wax pattern for, 213
    porcelain jacket, 398–429
        breakage of, 428
        building of, 415
        cementation of, 428
        cervical contact technique in, 416–420
        cervical ditching technique for, 420–428
        die for, 408–411
        firing of, 415
        for fractured anterior teeth, 528–535
        for pulpless teeth, 531–535
        matrix for, 412–415
        Nuttall preparation for, 403–405
        preparation of, 399–408
        shade selection for, 358–363
            additive primary colors in, 361
            color distribution chart for, 362
            light reflection in, 359
            pigments in, 352
            psychological primary colors in, 360
            subtractive primary colors in, 361
        temporary crown in, 411
        working cast for, 408–411
    resin, temporary, 89–91, *90, 91*
    resin jacket, 444–458
        cementation of, 457
        construction, for pulpless tooth, *455, 456*
        laboratory procedures in, 449–457
        matrix for, 445–448
        preparation for, 444
        wax pattern for, 448
    resin veneer, 430–443
        casting for, 435
        finishing of, 439–441
        mold for, 436
        processing of, 439–441
        selection of resin for, 436–439
        wax pattern for, 432–434
    veneered gold, 336–350, *337*
        accelerated speeds for, 343
        contraindications to, 337
        controlled depth in tooth preparation, 347–350
        conventional speeds for, 341–343
        for anterior teeth, 344
        indications for, 337
        instrumentation system for (tables of), 345
        preparation of tooth for, 338–346, *340*
        reduction of bicuspid for, 344
        reduction of molars for, 344
Crown length, 78
Crown-root ratio, 11

Crucible, high-heat, 371
Cuspid, bridge patterns for, 463–474
    height of contour, 288
    mandibular, preparation for partial veneer crown, 119–122, *121, 122*
    maxillary, form in pontic, 287
        preparation, for partial veneer crown, 103–106
    Vedder's preparation on, *104–105*
Crown form technique, in class IV resin restoration, 525
Curve of Spee, excessive, correction of, 512
Cutting depth, for veneered gold crown, 347–350
Cutting instruments, 51–58, *76*
    for carious teeth, 86
    for maxillary central incisor, *98, 99*

Decalcified areas, staining of, 318
Deflasking, of resin jacket crown, 454
Denstply facing, 250
Denture, partial, 3, *8*
    fixed. See *Bridges.*
    removable. See *Removable partial denture.*
Diagnostic cast, construction of, 27–29
    examination of, 12
    registration in, 29–34
    relation of, on articulator, 538
    value of, 34–35
Dies, for porcelain crowns, 366, 408–11
    for resin bridge and crown, 431, 444
    from tube impressions, 166–168, 197–206
        amalgam, 204, *205*
        copper-plated, 202–204
        fitting band, 197–199, *198*
        stone, 204
    separate from working cast, 170–173
Direct technique, for cast post and core, 533
    for wax pattern, 207
Direct waxing, for MacBoyle retainer, 154
    for pinledge retainer, 139–143, *142*
    for resin jacket crown, 448
Disks, diamond, *55*
    Moore's, *53*
    paper, 52
    separating, *58*
Distal surface reduction, for MacBoyle retainer, 153
    in maxillary bicuspid, 112
    in maxillary central incisor, 96
    in noncarious teeth, 75
    with conventional speeds, 341
Distortion of wax pattern, 208

Dovetailed occlusal rest, 273, *275*, 276
Drilling, in pinhole preparation. See *Pinholes, drilling of.*
Drills, for grinding reverse-pin facings, 262

Edentulous space, temporary bridge for, 90
Equilibration of bridge, 323
Eruption of posterior teeth, 518
Examinations, oral, 12
   radiographic, 11, 22–27
Expansion of investment, 225, 226, 234

Face-bow registration, 169–170, *169*
   transfer to articulator, *171*
Facial surface reduction, for noncarious teeth, 76
Facings for pontics. See *Pontics, facings for.*
Feldspar, in porcelain restoration, 351
Finishing line(s), *64*
   for pinledge retainer, 139
   of maxillary bicuspid, 113
   of maxillary central incisor, 100
Firing, of porcelain jacket crown, 415
      cervical contact technique, 416–419, *417, 418*
      cervical ditching technique, 423–428
      reaction to, 352
Firing cast, for ceramic restoration, 528
Flasking pattern, for resin jacket crown, 449–454, *450, 452, 454*
Flatback facing, 253
Fluxes, 303, 351
Fluxing, 239, *390*
Foundations, 41–45. See also *Abutments.*
Fractured anterior teeth, ceramic restoration for, 528–535
Frame, preparation, opaque mixing in, 372
Full veneer gold crown. See *Crown, full veneer gold.*
Furnace, glazing, *316*
   porcelain, 351–356, *354, 355*
Fusing temperature, of porcelain, 352

Gelation of hydrocolloid, 177
Gingival crevice, examination of, 157, *158*
Gingival recession, tooth preparation in, 79
Gingival resin, 437
Gingival tissue, bridge discomfort and, 553
Glazing, of bonded porcelain veneer crown, 376
   of porcelain, facings, 312–319
      applying glaze, 313–315, *313, 314*
      firing glaze, 315–316, *316, 317*

Gnathology, definition, 563
Gold alloys, melting range of, 240
Gold crown, full veneer. See *Crown, full veneer gold.*
Gold melting, for casting, 239–242
   oxidation during, 239
Gold plating, 431
Gold solders, 301
Grinding, of facings, 256–263, *261, 262*
   pulpal reaction to, 51
Grooves, making of, 66
      in preparation of maxillary central incisor, 97
Guide lines for band fitting, 198

Hairline check of stains, 317
Hand investing, 230
Handpiece, with water spray attachment, *61*
Harmony facing, 250, *252*, 253, 259, *261*
Hemodent, 160
Hue, defined, 359
Hydrocolloids, conditioning of, 177–180, *178, 179*
   time-temperature combinations, 180
Hygroscopic expansion of investment, 225, 234

Imbibition, definition, 185
Impression, alginate, 189–190
   for clasp-retained prosthesis, 493
   irreversible hydrocolloid, 189–190
   plaster of Paris, 190–195
   polysulfide rubber, 155–169
      die for, 166–168
      examination of gingival crevice for, 157
      for tube technique, 199
      mouth preparation for, 158
      precautions with, 165
      preparation of band for, 157
      preparation of tray for, 157
      syringe in, 163–165
      tissue displacement for, 159–162
   reversible hydrocolloid, 176–189
      construction of die for, 187
      preimpression steps in, 182
      pouring cast for, 185
      selection of tray for, 181
      taking impression in, 183
      tray filling for, *182*
      treatment of, 184
      use of syringe in, 183
   rubber, of pinledge preparation, 173–176

Impression (*Continued*)
  tube, individual dies from. See *Dies, from tube impressions.*
Incisal, porcelain, for bonded porcelain veneer crown, 374
  for fractured anterior teeth, 528–535
Incisal edges, reduction of, 62, *62,* 341
Incisal veneer, 438
Incisors, central, bridge patterns for, 461–466
    maxillary, form in pontic, 281–285
      partial veneer crown for. See *Crown, partial veneer, for maxillary central incisor.*
      preparation for pinledge retainer, *134–135, 136*
  lateral, maxillary, form in pontic, 285–287
  mandibular, partial veneer crown for, 118–119
    patterns for, 474–479
    preparation for MacBoyle retainer, 152
  maxillary, patterns for, 460–473
  rotation of, 517
  tipping of, 514, *514*
    with double cantilever spring, 515, *515*
    with single cantilever spring, *515*
Indentations for pinledge retainer, 133
Indirect technique, for cast post and core, 534
  for casting pattern, 170–173
  for veneered partial veneer crown, 527
  for wax patterns, 207
  with tapered pinholes, 174–176
Indirect-direct technique, for wax pattern, 207
Indirect-direct wax pattern, 215
Indirect wax pattern, 209–211
Inlay, two-surface, for adolescent mouth, 519
Inlay retainer, 144–150
  cavity preparation for, 145–148, *146, 147*
  contraindications to, 145
  indications for, 144
  wax pattern for, 148–149, 214
Insertion, path of. See *Path of insertion.*
Intracoronal attachment of veneers, 381
Investing, for veneered casting, 369–371
  hand, 230
  vacuum, 231
    equipment used in, 232–233, *233*
Investments, 224–235
  asbestos liner for, 224
  burnout following, 235
  expansion of, 225, 226, 234
  for ceramic restoration, 528
  proportioning of, 227–230
  soldering, 301, 388, 396

Investments (*Continued*)
  water-added technique for, 235
  weighing of, 227–230
Irreversible hydrocolloid impression, 189–190

Joint, broken-stress, 272–276
  definition, 5
  proximal, matrix with, 412–415

Kaolin, in porcelain restoration, 351
Kerr Balance, *228,* 229
Kerr Bite Frame, *32,* 168
  registration with, 169

Labial "line angle," 96
Labial surface, preparation of, 62–64
Lateral incisor, patterns for, 460, 462, 465, 467
Ledges, making of, 67
  for pinledge retainer, 133
Light reflection, in porcelain restoration, 359
"Line angle," labial, 96
Lingual joint, matrix with, 446–448
Lingual rest, 276, *276*
Lingual surface, preparation of, 62–64
  reduction of, 77
    for MacBoyle retainer, 153
    for pinledge retainer, 133
    for veneered gold crown, 341
    in maxillary bicuspid, 113
    in maxillary central incisor, 96
    in noncarious teeth, 76
Long-pin facing, 250, *251*

MacBoyle retainer, 151–154, *152*
  schematic explanation of, *153*
  wax pattern for, 213
Malocclusion, bridge discomfort from, 552
Mandibular arch, pinledge retainer for, 132
Mandibular cast, relation to maxillary cast, 541
Mandibular patterns, 473–479
Mandibular Sanitarypontic, 263–266
Mandrel, Moore's, *53*
Margin, cervical. See *Cervical margin.*
  open, in recurrent caries, 556
  overextended, in recurrent caries, 556

Masking, of resin veneer, 437
Matrix, burnishing of, instrumentation in, 447
    for carious teeth, 84
    for porcelain jacket crown, 412–415, *413, 414*
    for resin jacket crown, 445–448, *446*
    with proximal joint, 412–415
Maxillary arch, pinledge retainer for, 131
Maxillary cast, relation to mandibular cast, 541
Maxillary patterns, 460–473
Mesial surface, reduction of, for MacBoyle retainer, 153
    for veneered gold crown, 341
    in maxillary bicuspid, 112
    in maxillary central incisor, 96
    in noncarious teeth, 75
Metal, cleaning of, 237
Metal substructure, porcelain incisal and, for fractured anterior teeth, 528–535
Metalizing, of copper-plated die, 203
Mixing slab, for zinc phosphate cement, 330
Mobility of abutment, in bridge failure, 554
Mobility of teeth, test for, 537
Modeling compound technique, for tube impression, 199–200, *200*
Molar, mandibular, partial veneer crown for, 124–128
    patterns for, 477
    preparation of, *123*
    maxillary, partial veneer crown for, 117–118
    patterns for, 469–473
    pontic form of, 292
    preparation of, for inlay retainer, 146
        for removable partial denture, *497*
    reduction of, for veneered gold crown, 344
Mold for resin veneered crown, 436
Moore's disk and mandrel, *53*
Moskey technique, in construction of resin jacket crown, 449–453
Mouth. See also *Oral.*
    checking wax pattern in, 216
    examination of, 35–37, *23*
    in adolescent, bridges for, 519–523, *520, 521*
        case history, *568–575*
        contraindications to, 16
        pattern for, 464
        crowns for, 519–523
    in aged, contraindications to bridge in, 16
    partially edentulous, construction of crown for clasp-retained removable prostheses. See *Removable partial denture.*

Mouth (*Continued*)
    preparation of, for polysulfide rubber impression, 158
    restoration of, *501*
Mouth hygiene, choice of prosthesis and, 15
Muffle, in porcelain furnace, 355

Nuttall preparation for jacket crown, 403–405

"Occluded gas" porosity, 239, *240*
Occlusal surface, reduction of, 61
    for veneered gold crown, 341
    in maxillary bicuspid, 113
    in noncarious teeth, 76
Occlusion, abnormal, contraindications to bridge in, 17
    balanced, 564
    registration of, for full veneer gold crown, 91–92
Occlusion factors in bridge construction, 536–550
Opaque, application of, in cervical ditching technique, 421
    mixing of, in frame preparation, 372
Open margin, in recurrent caries, 556
Opposing arch, preparation of, 48–49
Oral. See also *Mouth.*
Oral examination, purpose of, 12
Oral hygiene, in maintenance of tissue tone, 560
    in recurrent caries, 556
Oral rehabilitation, complete, 563–566
Orostat, in tissue displacement, 160
Orthodontic positioning of abutments. See *Abutments, orthodontic positioning of.*
Overextended margins, in recurrent caries, 555
Overextension, in full veneer gold crown casting, 321
Oxidation, during melting of gold, 239
    of solder, 309

Paper disk, 52
Paralleling device, *68,* 135–139, *136, 137, 138*
Partial denture. See *Denture, partial.*
Partial veneer crown. See *Crown, partial veneer.*
Path of insertion, 45–47, *46*
    for pinledge retainer, 137

Periodontal factors in treatment planning, 38–40
Periodontal membrane, characteristics of, 508–511
Periodontal traumatism, 537
Peripheral form, in porcelain restoration, 357
Pickling, 242, 310
Pier, definition, 10
Pin facings, for pontics. See *pontics, facings for.*
Pinholes, drilling of, 67
  in carious teeth, 81–82
  in maxillary central incisor, 100
  for pinledge retainer, 133–139
  in class IV resin restoration, 525
  tapered, indirect technique with, 174–176
Pinledge pattern, spruing of, *222*
Pinledge preparation, rubber impression of, 173–176
Pinledge retainer, 130–143, *139*
  advantages of, 130
  direct waxing for, 140–143
  indications for, 131–135
  preparation of, 132–140
  wax pattern for, 213
Pins, direct waxing with, 142
  preparation of, 83–84
Pinwaxer, 140
Plaster of Paris impression, 190–195
Plastic beads for crown retention, 434
Plating, of copper-plated die, 203
  quadrant, 205
Platinum, for porcelain jacket matrix, 412
  for resin jacket matrix, 445, *446*
Polishing, of bridge, 272
  of casting, 243–246, *244, 245*
  of resin jacket crown, 454
Polysulfide rubber impression. See *Impression, polysulfide rubber.*
Pontics, 249–277. See also *Bridges.*
  broken-stress joint for, 272–276
  casting of, 268–272, *269*
  contact with ridge, 297–299
  definition, 5
  facing for, backing of, 267
    Dentsply, 250
    flatback, 253
    glazing of, 312–319, *313*
    grinding of, 256–263
    Harmony, 250, *252*, 253, 259, *260, 261*
    long-pin, 250, *251*
    mandibular porcelain-incisal, 266
    modification of, 253
    protection of, 262, *263*
    reverse-pin, 254, 260–262, 270

Pontics (*Continued*)
  facing for, Sanitarypontic, 253, 263–266, *264, 266*
    seating of, 319
    selection of shade, 249–250
    stabilization of, 267, *267*
    staining of, 312–319, *318*
    Trupontic, 253
      grinding of, 259
    types, 250–255
    waxing with, 270
  fitting of, *269*
  form of, 278–299
    factors in anterior construction, 288–290
    in recurrent caries, 556
    mandibular anterior, 292
    mandibular bicuspid, 293
    maxillary bicuspid, 291
    maxillary cuspid, 287
    maxillary central incisor, 281–285
    maxillary lateral incisor, 285–287
    maxillary molar, 292
    posterior, 294–297, *295*
  nonrigid connector for, 272–276
  waxing of, 268–272, *268*
  with bonded porcelain veneers, 385–387
Porcelain, composition of, 351
  firing of, 351–356, *354, 355*
  glazing of, 312–319, 376
  high-fusing, 352
  low-fusing, 352
  maturity of, 352
  medium-fusing, 352
  mixing powder, 415, *416*
  shade selection for. See *Crown, porcelain jacket, shade selection for.*
Porcelain incisal, metal substructure and, for fractured anterior teeth, 528–535
Porcelain jacket crown. See *Crown, porcelain jacket.*
Porosity, "back pressure," 222
  "occluded gas," 239, *240*
  shrinkage, *219*, 220, *220*
Posterior teeth, eruption of, 518
  instrumentation system for (tables of), 86–88
  splinting of, 485
  tipping of, 515–517
Premature contact, bridge discomfort from, 552
Preoperative study, 3–18
Prepared form, definition, 42
  for rebuilding vital tooth, 534
Proportioning of investment, 227–230
Prosthesis, choice of, mouth hygiene and, 15
  clasp-retained. See *Removable partial denture.*

Proximal joint, matrix with, 412–415
Proximal slice, 60, *60*
Proximal surface, reduction of, for pinledge retainer, 132
    in modified preparation of maxillary cuspid, 106
Pulp, degeneration of, in bridge failure, 557
Pulpal reaction to grinding, 51
Pulpless teeth, porcelain jacket crown for, 531–535
Pyrometer, 353
    precautions with, 235

Quadrant plating, 205
Quartz, in porcelain restoration, 351

Radiographic examination, 11, 22–27
Reduction. See *Teeth, reduction of.*
Registration, 29–34
    centric relation, wax, 541
    face-bow, 169–170, *169*
        transfer to articulator, *171*
    occlusion, wax, for full veneer gold crown, 91–92
Rehabilitation, oral, complete, 563–566
Removable partial denture, 487–504
    definition, 3
    impression for, 493
    indications for, 492
    preliminary design in, 492
    rationale for, 488–492
    splinted castings for, *495*
    surveying of wax pattern for, 495–500
    tooth preparation for, 493
    treatment planning for, 492
Resin, acrylic. See *Acrylic resin.*
    gingival, 437
    self-curing, for temporary crown, 411
        for tray construction, 156
    veneering, 436
Resin bridge, temporary, 89–91, *90, 91*
Resin cavity varnish, 325
Resin cement, 333
Resin crown, temporary, 89–91, *90, 91*
Resin jacket crown. See *Crown, resin jacket.*
Resin restoration, class IV, 525, *526*
Rest, subocclusal, 273–275, *274*
Rest seat, for removable partial denture, 493
Retainer, definition, 5
    deformation of, in bridge failure, 554, 556
    inlay. See *Inlay retainer.*
    MacBoyle. See *MacBoyle retainer.*
    pinledge. See *Pinledge retainer.*
    working, 505, *507*

Retention, extended, lever arm and, *14*
    fundamentals of, 72
    lack of, in bridge failure, 555
Retention form, for acrylic resin veneer, *435*
Retention wire, for resin veneer crown, 433
Reverse-pin facings, 254, 260–262, 270
Reversible hydrocolloid impression. See *Impression, reversible hydrocolloid.*
Ridge, contact of pontic with, 297–299
Ridge adaptation, of anterior facings, *284*
Roach-Akers clasps, 8
Root length, of abutment, 14, *20, 24,* 41
Rosin cavity varnish, 325
Rotation of incisors, 517

Sanitarypontic, mandibular, 263–266, *264, 266*
Saturation, definition, 359
Seating, failures in, 561
    initial, of bridge, 322–325
    of facing, 319
    of full veneer gold crown casting, 320–322
Setting expansion of investment, 225
Self-curing resin, for temporary crown, 411
Shade selection, for porcelain jacket crown. See *Crown, porcelain jacket, shade selection for.*
Shoulders, forming of, 65
        in tooth reduction for porcelain jacket crown, 402–405
    in bonded porcelain veneer crown, 377–380
    in veneered gold crown, 341–343
Shrinkage porosity, *219,* 220, *220*
Silica, in thermal expansion, 226
Silicone rubber impression, for working cast, 176
Silver-plated die, from polysulfide rubber impression, 201
Slice, proximal, 60, *60*
Soldering, 300–311
    antifluxes for, 304
    fluxes for, 303
    heating assembly, 307
    investment for, 296, 301, 388
    preparation of assembly, 301–303, *304, 305, 306*
        for bonded porcelain veneer bridge, 387–396, *390*
    technique of, 308–310
Solders, gold, composition of, 301
    selection of, 300
Space lengths, in treatment planning, 47
Spee, curve of, excessive, correction of, 512
Splinting, 43–45, *44,* 480–486, *481, 482, 483, 484, 485, 486*

Spring, cantilever, for tipping abutments, 513, *513*, 515, *515*, 517
Sprue, 220, 221
Sprue pin, placement of, 220
  precautions with, 219
  removal of, 235
Spruing, 219–224
  for inlay retainer, 149
  for MacBoyle retainer, 154
  for partial veneer crown, 109–110, *111*
    Starr method, 110
  for veneered casting, 369
Stability of casting, 226
Staining, of porcelain facings, 312–319
  of porcelain restoration, 364
Stains, hairline check of, 317
Starr method, in spruing, 110
Steel burs, *57*
Stone, carborundum, 52, *57*
  diamond, 52, *54, 56*
  for concave surfaces, 63
  for convex surfaces, 62
  for die construction, 188
  for occlusal surfaces, 61
  in diagnostic cast, 27
  in forming of cervical margin, 64
  in forming of shoulders, 65
Stopping, as temporary protection, 89
Storage of hydrocolloid impression, 185, *188*
Storage factors, in distortion of wax pattern, 208
Stress, in wax pattern, 208
Study cast. See *Diagnostic cast.*
Subocclusal rest, 273–275, *274*
Surveyor, *499*
Syneresis, definition, 184
Syringe technique for reversible hydrocolloid impression, 183
  for rubber base impression material, 163–165

Teeth, abutment. See *Abutments.*
  anterior. See *Anterior teeth.*
  incisor. See *Incisors.*
  mobility of, test for, 537
  posterior. See *Posterior teeth.*
  preparation of. See also specific procedures.
    crown length in, 78
    in gingival recession, 79
    precautions in, 52
  pulpless, as abutment, 43
    porcelain jacket crown for, 406–408, 531–535
    resin jacket crown for, *455, 456*

Teeth (*Continued*)
  reduction of, 59–73
    accelerated techniques in, 69–73
    for porcelain jacket crown, 401–405
    for veneered partial veneer crown, 526–527
    standard techniques in, 59–68
  splinting of, 43–45, *44*, 480–486, *481, 482, 483, 484, 485, 486*
  temporary protection of, 88–91, *88*
Tempering of hydrocolloid, 179, *179*
Temporary bridges and crowns, 89–91, *90*
Thermal expansion of investment, 225–226
Thermal shock, bridge discomfort from, 553
Thermocouple, in porcelain furnace, 355
Thermotrol, 242, *242*
Three-piece flask, 449–453, *452, 453*
Three-quarter crown. See *Crown, partial veneer.*
Tipping, bucco-lingual, 517
  distal, 515, *515*
  labial, 515, *515*
  lingual, 514, *514*
  mesial, 515
  mesio-distal. 515
  of abutments, 48
Tissue, displacement of, for polysulfide rubber impression, 159–162, *161*
  gingival, bridge discomfort and, 553
  loss of tone of, in bridge failure, 560
  pressure on, bridge discomfort from, 552
Torque, in bridge failure, 552, 554
Transfer, construction, 193–195, *194*
Trays, for alginate impression, 190
  for irreversible hydrocolloid impression, 190
  for plaster of Paris impression, 190
  for polysulfide rubber impression, 156, 157, 163–165
  for reversible hydrocolloid impression, 181, *182*
Treatment planning, 19–50
  diagnostic casts in, 27–35
  for removable partial denture, 492
  in orthodontic positioning of abutment teeth, 512
  methods in, 20–41
  periodontal factors in, 38–40
  radiographic examination in, 22–34
Trupontic facing. See *Pontics, facing of, Trupontic.*
Two-section flask, 453–454, *454*
Two-surface inlay, for adolescent mouth, 519

Underextension, in full veneer gold crown casting, 321

Vacuum-fired porcelain, 353, 380
Vacuum investing, 232–233, *233*
Varnish, cavity, 325
Vedder preparation on cuspid, *104–105*
Veneer, gingival, 437
    incisal, 438
    intracoronal attachment of, 381
    loss of, in bridge failure, 559
Veneered gold crown. See *Crown, veneered gold.*
Veneering resins, 436

Water, as coolant, 51
Water-powder ratio of investment, 230, 234, 235
Water spray attachment, *61*
Wax occlusion registration, for full veneer gold crown, 91–92
Wax centric relation registration, 541
Wax patterns, 207–217, *211, 212, 213*
    checking of, 216
    distortion in, 208
    for ceramic restoration, 529
    for full veneer gold crown, 211
    for inlay retainer, 148–149, 214
    for MacBoyle retainer, 154, 213
    for partial veneer crown, 213, 527
    for pinledge retainer, 143, 213
    for resin jacket crown, 448–450, *450*
    for resin veneer crown, 432–434
    for veneered casting, 368
    hand investing, 230
    indirect, 209–211
    indirect-direct, 215
    location in ring, 222

Wax patterns (*Continued*)
    stress in, 208
    surveying for removable partial denture, 495–500
Waxing, direct, for pinledge retainer, 140–143
    of pontic facings, 268–272, *268*
Wear, in recurrent caries, 556
Weighing of investment, 227–230
Wire, retention, for resin veneer crown, 433
Working cast, 155–196
    alginate, 189–190
    construction of, *173*
    for bonded porcelain veneer crown, 366
    for porcelain jacket crown, 408–411, 528
    for resin jacket preparation, 444
    indirect technique, 170–173
    irreversible hydrocolloid, 189–190
    mounting of, 169–173
    opposing, impression for, 168
    plaster of Paris impressions, 190–195
    polysulfide rubber impressions, 155–169
    relation of die to, 170–173
    reversible hydrocolloid impression for, 176–189
    rubber base impression materials, 155
    rubber impressions of pinledge preparations, 173–176
    silicone rubber impression, 176
Working retainer, 505, *507*

Zinc chloride, in tissue displacement, 162
Zinc oxide eugenol cement, 332
Zinc phosphate cement, 327–332